Best · Medical Record Practice · Medical Record Practice

이해하기 쉽게 풀이한

최신 의무기록실무

MEDICAL RECORD PRACTICE

필수 약어 및 의학용어 정리 수록

이성란 조혜영 최원창 신연순 조은희 이경미 김광애

현문사

서 론

최신 의무기록실무는 차트를 통하여 의료기관에서 실제 발생한 각종 정보를 수집·분석함으로써 진료 정보 생성의 간접적인 경험을 하도록 하는 과목이다. 본서는 의학, 의무기록, 보건학, 간호학 계열 및 병원계통의 종사자뿐만 아니라 일반인들에게 체계적이고 효과적인 학습에 초점을 맞추어 의무기록의 용어 사용 및 해독능력을 함양하는 데 있다.

본서는 우리나라 종합병원에서 현재 사용하고 있는 의무기록 중에서 학습에 필요한 내용만 선별하여 발췌하였다. 반면 환자의 개인적인 비밀보장에 손상이 가지 않도록 편집하고 학습효과를 높일 수 있는 내용으로 구성하였다.

그동안 실무 및 강의 경험을 토대로 기존의 내용과 최근의 학문적 동향을 체계적인 분석을 통해 쉽게 풀이하였다. 의무기록의 범위가 광범위하므로 기본적이며 개괄적으로 알아야 할 내용들을 수록하였다. 좀 더 자세한 부분은 그에 따른 전문서적으로 보완하길 바라며 향후 변화하는 사항은 독자들의 의견을 수렴하여 계속 수정·보완하고자 한다.

독자들은 거의 '반(半)무의식적으로 사용할 수 있는 수준에 이를 수 있도록 의식적인 노력'을 계속해야 할 것이다. 이를 위해 본서는 다음 몇 가지 사항에 중점을 두었다.

❑ 국가시험 최다 합격자 배출한 기적의 교재 ❑

- 최신 국가시험에 맞추어 전체 및 요약 차트로 구분하여 쉽게 풀이
- 의무기록을 해독할 수 있는 필수적인 실무용어 및 해석
- 실제 임상에서 사용되는 해부, 생리 및 병리적 상태를 쉽게 정리
- 필요한 해부학적 구조 및 기능을 설명하는 그림 삽입
- 질환의 이해를 돕고자 증상, 검사, 진단 및 처치 설명
- 임상에서 사용되는 약어를 원어와 해설 병행
- 질병분류상(KCD-7) 주의점 및 예제를 통한 학습효과
- 각 장마다 국가고시 실전문제를 수록하여 체계적인 정리 및 실전대비

본서가 발간되기까지 자료 수집에 많은 협조를 해주신 각 병원 관계자 여러분과 현문사 임직원분들께 깊은 감사를 드린다.

겨자씨가 자라 울창한 나무로 성장시키는 놀라운 하나님의 계획과 인도하심에 깊은 감사와 영광을 돌린다.

2018년 3월

저자

목 차

A • 의무기록 쉽게 찾는 방법

의무기록	내 용
차트의 내용 및 순서	· 경과기록(입원일~퇴원일 상세한 기록): 병력기록, 퇴원요약에도 기재됨 ‣ 순서: C.C(주소) → P.I(현재질병) → P.H(개인력), FH(가족력) → ROS(신체각계 조사), P/E(신체검진기록) → S(주관적), O(객관적), A(평가), P(계획) ‣ 상기순서 경과기록 1-2페이지 기록: 출제 필수 · 퇴원요약: 중요내용만 기록/진단, 검사, 치료, 약, 퇴원상태 등 ‣ 최종진단, 임상검사(CT, MRI, Endoscopy 등) 찾을 때 필수
입·퇴원일자	· 입퇴원기록, 경과기록, 의사지시기록, 퇴원요약(재원일 계산 시 사용)
입원과	· 입퇴원기록[경과기록, 병력 및 신체검진기록 → PI: present illness(현재질병)], 응급실기록 ‣ 병력 및 신체검진기록: 인턴(24시간 이내 작성)
입원경로	· 경과기록, 병력기록, 퇴원요약, 응급실기록 → PI ‣ ER: 응급실, OPD: 외래
퇴원과	· 입퇴원기록, 경과기록, 의사지시기록
전과	· 경과기록, 의사지시기록, 간호기록(재원일 계산 시 사용) 전과(타과): transfer out(전출), transfer in(전입) 예) transfer to GS(일반외과로 전과) · 동일과: 인수인계(duty on 또는 duty off): 전과 재원일수 계산 시 해당되지 않음
치료결과	·완쾌, 경쾌, 호전안됨, 진단뿐, 가망없는 퇴원, 48시간 이내 사망, 48시간 이후 사망 ·입퇴원기록, 경과기록, 퇴원요약 확인
퇴원형태	· 퇴원지시 후, 자의퇴원(discharge against medical advice; DAMA), 탈원(escape), 전원 · 입퇴원기록, 경과기록, 퇴원요약, 자퇴서약서 확인
중환자실(ICU)	· ICU(Intensive Care Unit) ‣ MICU(Medical Intensive Care Unit): 내과계 중환자실 - CCU(Cardiac Care Unit): 심혈관내과 중환자실 - RCU(Respiratory Care Unit): 호흡기내과 중환자실 ‣ SCU(Surgical Care Unit): 외과계 중환자실 - NCU(Neurological Care Unit): 신경외과 중환자실 ‣ NICU(Neonatal Intensive Care Unit): 신생아 중환자실
신생아	· 본원에서 출생한 출생아 ‣ 정상 출산력: 임신기간 37주~42주 미만, 체중 2,500g~4,500g 미만
산모구분	· 분만, 유산(임신 20주 이하, 500g 이하), 미분만, 산욕기(분만 직후~6주)
병원감염 (Infection in hosp.)	· 입원 시 깨끗한 상태 → 환자가 재원하고 있는 동안 병원내에서 감염 · 퇴원요약, 경과기록, 임상병리기록 등의 내용에서 감염사실 확인

* 상기 의무기록지 기재 순서는 차트찾는 우선순위임

A-1 • 의무기록 쉽게 찾는 방법

의무기록	내 용
감염종류	·수술 후, 기타처치 후, 비뇨기계, 호흡기계, 소화기계, 기타
감염부위	· urinary tract(비뇨기계)/UTI(요로감염), wound(상처), blood(혈액), repiratory(호흡기계)/URI(상기도 감염), G.I. tract(위장계), drainage site(배액부위), others(기타)
병원 합병증	· 병원 감염, 수술 및 처치 후 출혈, 수술부위 파열 등 · T80-T88에 해당 예) POD #1 UTI(수술 후 1일째 요로감염) → T81.4 + Y62.0
협의진단	· 협의진단 의뢰과와 시행과 ‣ 임상과, 진료지원부서가 다른 경우 각각 횟수 계산 ‣ 협의진단기록, 경과기록, 의사지시기록
수술	· 수술 건수: 수술기록, 경과기록 확인 · 수술 내용: 수술기록, 경과기록의 brief op. note(수술 요약기록) 확인
마취 종류	· 수술기록지(procedure의 첫번째 줄), 경과기록지의 brief op. 확인 ‣ 전신마취(General anesthesia): Endotracheal(기관내), Endobronchial(기관지내) IV(정맥내), IM(근육내), Rectal(직장), Open drop(개방점적식) ‣ 부분마취(Regional): Spinal(척추), Epidural(경막외), Nerve block(신경차단) ‣ 국소마취(Local): 회복실기록지 불필요
생검(Biospy)	· 생검의 분류(bx.) ‣ 진단: endoscopic, needle bx., aspirational bx. ‣ 치료/수술: surgical bx., frozen bx., incisional or excisional bx.
주진단	· 주진단 ‣ 가장 주가 된 진단명 ‣ 입원에서 퇴원까지 모든 검사결과 확진된 것 ‣ 환자의 치료나 검사를 가장 필요로 했던 상태 ‣ 의료자원의 소모가 가장 컸던 진단명
기타진단	· 기타진단 ‣ 입원 시 가지고 있는 질환(concurrent disease, 동반질환) 입원 후 발생한 상태(complication, 합병증) ‣ 치료나 재원기간에 영향을 주는 상태 ‣ 협의진단 등을 통해 나타난 진단
진단분류	·진단분류 번호 찾는 방법 ‣ 퇴원요약지, 조직병리보고서, 입퇴원기록지의 진단명 ‣ 수술기록지의 수술 후 진단명(postop. dx.) ‣ 경과기록지의 O(객관적), A(평가)의 진단명 ‣ 협의진단 imp.(의증), O(객관적)의 진단명 → 신체검진, 병력기록, 경과기록 등 타기록의 imp.는 제외 ‣ 임상병리 기록지(감염, 빈혈, 매독, 간염 등) 예) Hb 9.6: 빈혈 VDRL: reactive 매독 HBsAg(+), Anti HBs(-): 간염
원사인	· 사망환자: 선행사인 분류 · 경과기록, 퇴원요약의 최종기록(expire, 사망)

* 상기 의무기록지 기재 순서는 차트찾는 우선순위임

01. 내과계
Internal Medicine

I. 전체 차트 (Full Chart)

II. 요약 차트 (Summary Chart)

MEDICAL RECORD PRACTICE

01 신장암
Renal cell carcinoma

1.1 신장암(Renal cell carcinoma) = 신세포암

- 신장암(renal cell carcinoma): 성인 콩팥에서 발생하는 악성종양/성인 암의 2%
  - 윌름종양(Wilm's tumor): 아동기 신장의 악성종양
- 일차적 증상은 혈뇨(hematuria)
- 뼈와 폐로 전이 빈번
- 생존율(survival rate)은 종양의 진전 정도로 결정
- 치료는 신장절제(nephrectomy)

1.2 신장과 관련된 주요 질환

요붕증(Diabetes insipidus)

- 항이뇨호르몬(antidiuretic hormone; ADH)의 불충분한 분비/뇌하수체후엽(과소분비)
  - 내분비장기 9가지
    - 뇌하수체, 송과체(송방울샘), 갑상선, 부갑상선, 흉선(가슴샘), 부신, 췌장(이자)
    - 고환, 난소

신증후군(Nephrotic syndrome)

- 소변으로 과잉의 단백이 상실되어 생기는 증상군

신부전(콩팥기능상실, Renal failure)

- 신장(콩팥)의 요배설 부전

당뇨병(Diabetes mellitus): 내과계 요약차트 상세 설명 참조

- 인슐린의 결핍
- 내분비계 → 췌장: 과소분비

- Type I 당뇨병(Insuline-dependent diabetes mellitus; IDDM): 소아 E10.__
- Type II 당뇨병(Non-insulin-dependent diabetes mellitus; NIDDM): 성인 E11.__
  - 1차 합병증: 케톤산증(ketoacidosis), 혼수(coma), 저혈당증(hypoglycemia)
  - 2차 합병증: 당뇨병성 망막병증(diabetic retinopathy)
    - ▶ 당뇨성 신병증(diabetic nephropathy)
    - ▶ 당뇨병성 신경병증(diabetic neuropathy)

당부하 내성검사(Glucose tolerance test; GTT)

▶ GTT: 75g의 포도당(glucose)을 이용한 경구 당부하검사/혈당검사

▶ **당뇨병(DM) 진단**

- 공복 시 혈당(fasting blood sugar; FBS) 측정: 8시간 이상 비열량 섭취
  - 정상치: 126mg/dl 이하
- 식후 2시간째
  - 정상치: 200mg/dl 이하
- 당뇨병의 징후: 혈당이 정상치로 돌아오는 시간이 지연됨

2.1 처치(Procedures)

투석(Dialysis)

- 신장(콩팥)의 기능을 못할 경우, 혈류로부터 요소(urea) 등의 물질을 제거

▶ **혈액투석(Hemodialysis)**

- 인공신장기를 이용하여 노폐물이 가득찬 혈류를 여과

▶ **복막투석(Peritoneal dialysis)**

- 복강카테터(peritoneal catheter)를 이용
- 수액을 복강 속으로 삽입
- 이 액(fluid)은 복강의 모세혈관에 있는 노폐물질이 혈류에서 액으로 빠져나오도록 함
- 노폐물을 담은 수액은 복강카테터로 다시 나옴

복막의 종류

▶ **간헐적 복막투석(Intermittently peritoneal dialysis; IPD)**

- 기계장치의 도움으로 간헐적으로 수행

▶ **지속적 활동성 복막투석(Continuous ambulatory peritoneal dialysis; CAPD)**

- 기계 없이 환자에 의해 계속 수행

신장이식(Renal transplantation)

- 신부전(콩팥기능상실)이 있는 환자에게 이식

카테터 삽입법(Urinary catheterization)

- 유연한 관으로 된 기구를 요도를 통하여 방광으로 삽입
- 카테터는 소변을 빼내거나(drainage, 배액법), 방광으로 세척액(irrigation solution)을 넣을 때, 방광을 불릴 때 이용

체외충격파 쇄석술(Extracorporeal shock wave lithotripsy)

- 충격파가 요로석을 부수어 작은 조각으로 만듦
- 소변과 함께 빠져나갈 수 있게 함

2.2 종양의 분류

양성종양

- ~Oma [예: adenoma(선종)]
  - 단, Hepatoma(간암), melanoma(흑색종), seminoma(정상피종) → 악성

악성종양

- ~Sarcoma(육종) → Connective tissue(결체조직) [예: fibrosarcoma(섬유육종)]
  - 뼈, 근육, 지방, 섬유
- ~Carcinoma(암종) → Epithelial tissue(상피조직) [예: adenocarcinoma(선암종)]
  - 피부 [예: carcinoma(암종), adenoma(선종), papilloma(유피종)]

3.1 진료통계

- Off service note: 담당 의사(주치의)가 교대 근무자에게 인계하는 기록
- On service note: 인계받은 기록
- Transfer note: 임상과의 전입 또는 전출

(전과 재원일 계산 시 사용: 경과기록, 의사 기록, 간호기록 확인)

▶ Length of stay(LOS, 재원일수): 단입법(퇴원일-입원일)

예) 입원일: '17. 2. 18

퇴원일: '17. 3. 20

[풀이: 28-18+20=30 → 답: 재원일수 30일] * 2월은 28일

임상검사

- 정상 혈압(Blood pressure): 120/80 mmHg
- 고혈압(Hypertension): 140/90 mmHg 이상(성인)

표 1 • 상피 종양(Epithelial tumors)

양성(Benign Neoplasms)	악성(Malignant Neoplasms)	원발장기(primary tumor)
· Squamous cell papilloma (편평세포유두종)	· Epidermoid carcinoma(표피양암종) · Squamous cell carcinoma(편평세포암종) · Oat cell carcinoma · Basal cell carcinoma(기저세포암종) · Hepatocellular carcinoma(간세포암종)	· Skin(피부) · Lung(폐), esophagus(식도) · Skin(피부) · Liver(간)
· Cystadenoma(낭선종)	· Cystadenocarcinoma(낭선종암종) · Serous cystadenoma,borderline malignancy (악성경계형 장액성 암종)	· Ovary(난소) · Ovary(난소)
· Renal tubular adenoma (신관선종) · Transitional cell papilloma (이행성 세포 유두종)	· Endometrioid carcinoma(자궁내막암종) · Renal cell carcinoma(신세포암종)	· Ovary(난소) · Kidney [신장(콩팥)] · Bladder(방광)
· Hydatidiform mole(포상기태)	· Choriocarcinoma(융모막암종) · Seminoma(정상피종)	· Placenta(태반) · Teste(고환)
· Nevus(모반)	· Melanoma(흑색종)	· Skin(피부)

표 2 • 결체 종양 및 혼합 종양(Connective & Mixed tumors)

양성(Benign Neoplasms)	악성(Malignant Neoplasms)	원발장기(primary tumor)
Chondroma(연골종)	Chondrosarcoma(연골육종)	Cartilage(연골)
Lipoma(지방종)	Liposarcoma(지방육종)	Fat(지방)
Fibroma(섬유종)	Fibrosarcoma(섬유육종)	Fibrous tissue(섬유조직)
Leiomyoma(평활근종)	Leiomyosarcoma(평활근육종)	Smooth(visceral) muscle(평활근/내장근)
Rhabdomyoma(횡문근종)	Rhabdomyosarcoma(횡문근육종)	Striated(skeletal) muscle(횡문근/골격근)
Osteoma(골종)	Osteosarcoma(골육종)	Bones(뼈)
	Ewing's tumor(유잉종양)	Bones(뼈)
	Leukemia(백혈병	Bone marrow(골수)
	Multiple myeloma(다발성 골수종 = Plasma cell tumor(형질세포종양)	Bone marrow(골수)
	Hodgkin's disease(호지킨스 질환) Non-Hodgkin's lymphoma (비호지킨스 질환)	Lymph node(림프절), thymus(가슴샘), Spleen(지라), tonsil(편도), stomach(위) intestine[장(소·대장)], breast(유방)
Hemangioma(혈관종)	Hemangiosarcoma(혈관육종)	Blood vessel(혈관)
	Glioma(신경교종) Astrocytoma(성상세포종) Ependymoma(상의세포종) Glioblastoma multiforme(GM, 다형성 교모세포종)	Brain(뇌)
	Oligodendroglioma(핍지교종)	Cerebellum(소뇌)
	Medulloblastoma(수아종)	Meninges(수막)
	Meningeal sarcoma(수막 육종)	Embryonic nerve tissue(배아신경조직)
	Neuroblastoma(신경아세포종)	
Neurofibroma(신경섬유종)	Neurofibrosarcoma(신경섬유육종)	Nerve(신경)
	Nephroblastoma(신아세포종) = Wilm's tumor	Kidney[신장(콩팥)]

차트 용어

· Adhesion	유착	· Atherosclerosis	죽상경화증	· Calculus	결석
· Fibula	비골	· Foley catheter	소변줄	· Homovac(H/V)	배액관 = 피주머니
· Invasion	침입	· Suspect	의심하다	· Thick	두꺼운
· Tibia	경골	· Thoracoabdominal	흉복부의	· Upper pole	위쪽

약 어	원 어	
ADH	Antidiuretic hormone = vasopressin	항이뇨호르몬
ARF	Acute renal failure	급성 신부전(콩팥기능상실)
BUN	Blood urea nitrogen	혈액뇨질소
CRF	Chronic renal failure	만성 신부전(콩팥기능상실)
e′	Electrolyte	전해질
	예) e′ 133-4.1-102: 전해질 검사결과	sodium(Na)이 133mEq/L
ESRD	End stage renal disease	말기신장질환(콩팥병)
ESWL	Extracorporeal shock wave lithotripsy	체외충격파 쇄석술
FBS	Fasting blood sugar	공복 시 혈당/의사지시기록
HD	Hemodialysis	혈액투석
IDDM	Insuline-dependent diabetes mellitus	인슐린의존성 당뇨병
IMV	Inferior mesenteric vein	하부 장간막 정맥
I/O	Intake and output	섭취량 및 배설량
IVP	Intravenous pyelogram	정맥내 콩팥깔대기 조영술
K+	Potassium	전해질(electrolyte): 칼륨
KUB	Kidneys ureter, and bladder	신장, 요관 및 방광의 x-ray 검사
LLSB	Left lower sternal border	흉골(복장뼈) 하부 좌연
LN	Lymph node	림프절
Na+	Sodium	전해질: 나트륨
NIDDM	Non-insulin-dependent diabetes mellitus	비인슐린의존성 당뇨병
RGP	Retrograde pyelography	역행성 신우조영술
TNM	Tumor, nodes, metastasis	종양, 림프절, 전이
UA	Urinalysis	요분석, 소변검사
UTI	Urinary tract infection	요로감염
VCUG	Voiding cystourethrogram	배뇨성 요도방광조영술
WBBS	Whole body bone scan	전신골주사

등록번호	108 20 30	성별	M
성명	복 덩 이		
주민등록	781025－1234567		

입 퇴 원 기 록
Admission and Discharge Record

<table>
<tr><td colspan="3">본 적: 광주 광역시 서구 농성 2동</td></tr>
<tr><td colspan="3">주 소: 서울시 영등포구 당상 1동 210 직 업: 전 화 :</td></tr>
<tr><td colspan="3">연고자성명: 관 계: 주 소: 전 화:</td></tr>
<tr><td>입원: 2016년 2월 18 일 UR 과 병동 호</td><td rowspan="3">전과</td><td>20 년 월 일 과 병동 호</td></tr>
<tr><td>퇴원: 2016년 3월 20 일 과 병동 호</td><td>20 년 월 일 과 병동 호</td></tr>
<tr><td>재원일수:</td><td>20 년 월 일 과 병동 호</td></tr>
</table>

최종진단명	분 류 번 호
주진단명 : Renal cell ca. clear cell type, Rt	
DM nephropathy, intermediate stage	
기타진단명: DM	
Hypertension	
R/O Diabetic retinopathy	
GB, Tubular adenoma	
수술 및 처치명	
수술명 : Radical nephrectomy, Rt	
기타수술 및 주요검사: Cholecystectomy	
IVP, abd U/S,	
Abd－pelvic CT scan	

<table>
<tr><td colspan="2">치료결과: 1. 완쾌 2. 경쾌 3. 호전안됨 4. 진단뿐 5. 가망없는 퇴원 6. 48시간내 사망 7. 48시간이후 사망</td></tr>
<tr><td colspan="2">퇴원형태: 1. 퇴원지시후 2. 자의퇴원 3. 탈원 4. 전원</td></tr>
<tr><td colspan="2">병원감염: 1. 수술후 2. 기타처치후 3. 비뇨기계 4. 호흡기계 5. 소화기계 6. 기타</td></tr>
<tr><td colspan="2">원사인 : 부검: 예, 아니오</td></tr>
<tr><td colspan="2">계속적 진료 계획</td></tr>
<tr><td colspan="2">없음·있음 (약속일 20 년 월 일 시)</td></tr>
<tr><td>담당 전공의 서명: 윤동민</td><td>담당 전문의 서명: 정교식</td></tr>
<tr><td>의무기록 완성 : 2016 년 3 월 27 일</td><td>의무기록사 서명: 박동진</td></tr>
</table>

등록번호	108 20 30	성별 M
성명	복 덩 이	
주민등록	781025－1234567	

퇴 원 요 약
Discharge Summary

Final Dx. : 1. Renal cell ca. clear cell type (T_2 No Mo)
2. Diabetic nephropathy, intermediate stage
3. Hypertension
4. GB polyp
5. R/O Diabetic retinopathy

C.C: Rt flank pain
D: Remote 16. 2. 12
Recent 16. 2. 16

PHx: DM → 10년 전 Dx. → Diamicron 1Ⓣ/d 복용중
Diabetic retinopathy Dx.

ROS: Rt. flank pain: Diffuse, dull
Gross hematuria: painless, total
intermittent $\bar{c}$ clot

Lab: U/A (16. 2. 18) 1,020/5.0/protein 3t/gluc. 3t
RBC many
AC 256 (2.19)
PC 267 (2.19)

양일수 / 윤동민

퇴 원 요 약

IVP (16. 2. 18)

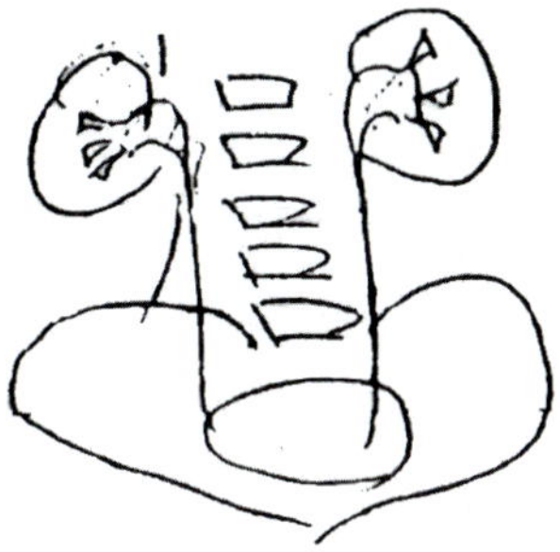

Lt. upper tr: WNL
Rt upper pole calyceopelvic
system이 mass effect에 의해
compression된 양상 보임

CT scan (16. 2. 22)

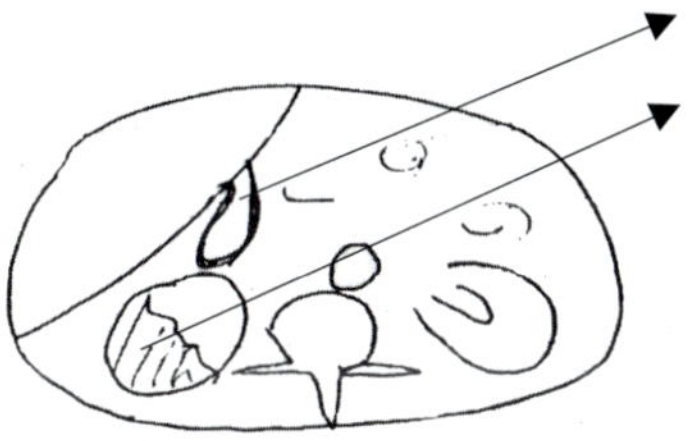

Diffuse GB wall thickening
6x5cm sized low density lesion on Rt posterolateral aspect of kidney possible confined to the renal capsule

16. 2. 24 BP 170/100mmHg

monopril, BASA, novasc — started

T,P/ AIb 5.3 / 3.0

OT/PT 17 / 31

Tx. (16. 2. 28) Radical Nephrectomy. Rt.
Cholecystectomy
Finding: ① Tumor mass located in upper pole of kidney and didn't invade to renal capsule
② one artery & one renal vein
③ no abnomal LN enlargement
④ Diffuse GB wall thickening

양일수 / 윤동민

퇴 원 요 약

POD #3 (3.3)	gas passing → S.O.W 시작, ventrol tube removal
POD #4 (3.4)	BP 170/80 mmHg BT 38.3°C Chilling, palpitation 호소 B−sugar 103 Hb/Hct 9.3/27.7 Hemovac 800cc (8시간 등) drainage H/V fluid Hb/Hct 1.0/3.0 → Transamine, Albumin replacement Cardio ⓒ → Almarl 10mg #2로 투여 시작
POD #6 (3.6)	Total I & O 2600/2500 H/V 23cc → Intraperitoneal H/V removal SMA T, P/ AIb 4.9/2.6 → Albumine 200ml replacement
POD #7 (3.7)	BP 180/100 mmHg → Almarl 10mg, HOVASC 5mg 투여 시작 T,P/Alb 4.5/2.7 (Albumng 200ml replace 후) retroperitoneal H/V removal
POD #8 (3.8)	Full stitch out 시행

양일수 / 윤동민

퇴 원 요 약

POD #10 24hr urin
(3.10) Ccr 50.8 (80~146)
Alb 7161 (3.9~24.4)

Plan) 1. periodic radiologic f/u (CT, WBBS)
2. evaluation of DM nephropathy
3. BP control
4. evaluation of diabetic retinopathy

Discharge Med)
① Diamicron 1 Ⓣ # Siq p.o (자가용)
② Novasc 5mg #1 Siq p.o × 6 ⓓ
Renitec 10mg #2 Siq p.o bid × 6 d
③ Tarivid 3 Ⓣ
Vonidase 3 Ⓣ ― # 3 Siq p.o bid × 6 d
Bithree 3 Ⓣ

OPD F/U
① URO 16. 3. 21 AM
② Eye Dept 16. 3. 21 PM
③ Nephro Dept.
④ Cardio Dept

양일수/윤동민

등록번호	108 20 30	성별	M
성명	복 덩 이		
주민등록	781025 - 1234567		

문 제 목 록
Problem List

Ward 23 Room 2012 Dept. URO

Problem No.	Date Entered	Problem List	Problem Resolved	Date Resolved
1	2/18	Ureter stone		
		→ Renal mass, Rt		
2		DM		
3	2/28	Radical nephrectomy, Rt		
		Cholecystectomy		
4				
		〈pathology〉		
5		kidney: renal cell ca, clear cell type		
		confined to renal capsule		
6		LN(0/4): free		
		pT_2 pNo iMo		
7		GB polyp: tubular adenoma		
8	3/4	Albumin, pro. replacement		
	3/6	Hemovac Removal		
9	3/7	Half stitch out		
	3/8	Full stitch out		
10				

Problem Letter	Temporary Problem List (Acute – Limited)		Date of Occurrences

등록번호	108 20 30	성별 M
성명	복 덩 이	
주민등록	781025 - 1234567	

경 과 기 록
Progress Notes

S: Subjective O: Objective A: Assessment P: Plan

〈 Admission Note 〉

2.18 본 38세 남자환자는
CC: Rt. flank pain
D: Remote 16. 2. 12
16. 2. 16
을 주소로 ER을 경유하여 UR에 내원하였다. 환자는 10년 전부터 당뇨로 oral medication 받던 것 이외엔 특별히 치료받는 일이 없었으나 16년 2월 11일 혈전을 동반한 육안적 혈뇨와 '16. 2. 12. 우측 측복부 동통으로 local 병원에 내원 치료받았다. 그후 동일한 증상이 2월 16일부터 다시 병발하여, 2개의 다른 인천병원을 경유 IVP 시행 후 further evaluation 및 proper Tx 위해 UR에 입원하였다.

PHx : No Tbc, HiBP, hepatitis
No Urethritis
No Previous stone
No dehydration
Diabetic retinopathy … Dx 초기
'13: Rt. tibia fx … 인천병원에 입원 Hx

FHx : 여동생 … Renal calculus
작은 아버지 … Atherosclerosis

윤수동

경 과 기 록

일 자	내 용	서 명

2.18 ROS: General weakness ⊖

Easy fatique ⊖

Fever / chill ⊖ / ⊖

N/V ⊕ / ⊕ → ⊖ / ⊖

D/C ⊖ / ⊖

Abd. pain ⊖

Rt. flank pain (±) diffuse, chill

Voiding: Nocturia 2/N

Frequency $\bar{q}$ 2, 3 hrs

Urgency ⊖

Hematuria ⊕

Painless intermittent $\bar{c}$ clot, total

Residual sense ⊖ → ⊕

1. P/Ex. BP 12O/80

Afebrile

2.18 (KUB) 16. 2. 18 at ER

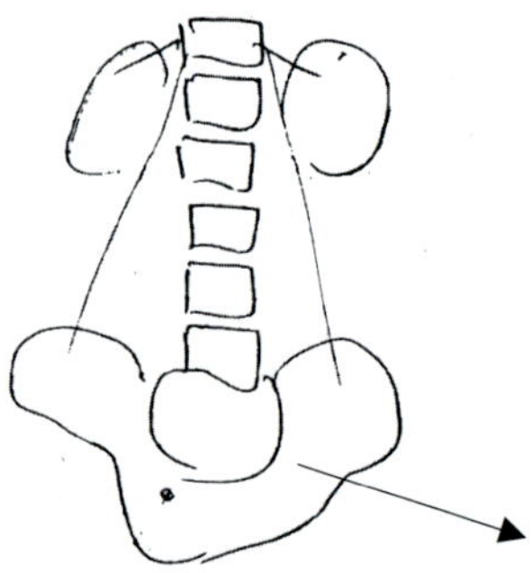

equivocal radiopaque density

8.8cm × 0.6cm sized

Rt pelvic cavity

U/A $\bar{c}$ ⓜ

CBC 11.0/35.6 8700 (65%)

254K

U/A $\bar{c}$ ⓜ 1.020 P115.0 pro/gli ♯ / ♯

cell: RBC many

bloody: Many

윤수동

경 과 기 록

일 자	내 용	서 명

2.22 (CT scan)

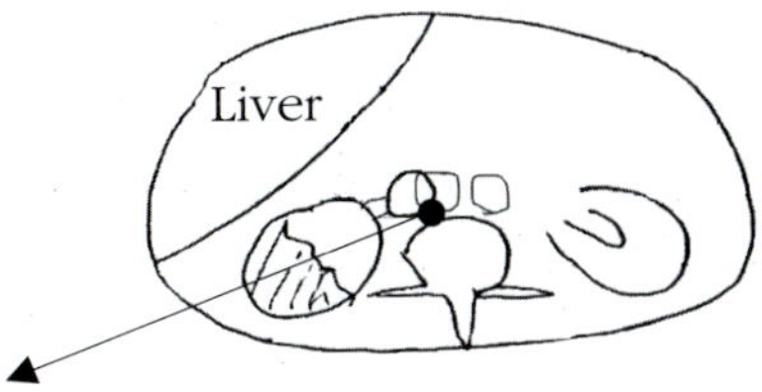

6×5cm sized
low density lesion , Rt
Post, lateral kidney
equivocal
low density lesion, 0.8cm sized
→ No LN

2.24 DM: well controlled, oral medication
HiBP: probably essential hypertension
Monopril, BASA, Nuvasc — started

Pro/AIb	5.3	3.0
OT/PT	17	31

2.26 〈 Off Service Note 〉

본 38세 남자 환자는 renal parenchymal origin tumor. Rt. 및 GB polyp, DM. hypertension으로 입원 9일째입니다. Rt. flank pain을 동반한 gross hematuria: clot이 16년 2월 12일과 16일에 시행한 IVP 및 U/S(타병원 시행)에서 renal tumor 의심되어 본원에 내원하여 시행한 Abd U/S 및 CT에서 비교적 parenchyme내에 국한되는 5x6cm sized heterogeneous soft tissue mass가 Rt. upper LUQ, lateral aspect에 관찰되며 LN enlargement와 perinephric fat involvement는 없는 것으로 추정됩니다. 동반된 문제로는 GB polyp c̄ wall thickening이 있어 윤호진 선생님께 협의진료 상태이며, 당뇨는 oral medication으로 조절되고 있습니다. proteinuria, invasive와 hypoalbuminemia는 renal origin으로 추정되며 surgical resection까지는 할 예정입니다. Gross hematuria는 없으나 Hb 9.0까지 저하되어 수술 전후로 transfusion 가능성에 대해 설명하였습니다. BP는 monopril, novasc로 조절되기 시작하며, renal origin의 hypertension에 대한 가능성을 배제할 수 없습니다. 가급적 2.28일 op.를 진행(외과, 비뇨기과)하시고, radiology confirm 후 치료 결정을 하십시오.

R1 윤수동

경 과 기 록

일 자	내 용	서 명
2.26	〈 On Service Note 〉 본 38세된 남환은 Renal parenchymal tumor, Rt. GB polyp, DM, Hypertension으로 현재 입원 9일째입니다. 16년 2월 11일 clot을 동반한 Gross hematuria 16년 2월 12일 Rt flank pain으로 local병원에서 시행한 IVP U/S상 renal tumor로 의심되어 본원 내원하여 시행한 Abd U/S 및 CT에서 비교적 parenchyme 내에 국한되는 5X6cm sized heterogenous soft tissure mass가 Rt upper pole, lat. aspect에 관찰되며 LN enlargement Lt perinephric fat tissue envolvement는 없는 것으로 생각됩니다. 동반된 문제로 초음파상 GB polyp c̄ wall thickening 있어 외과 양상수 선생님께 협의진료 상태이며 당뇨는 oral medication으로 잘 조절되는 상태입니다. proteinuria와 hypoalbuminemia는 renal origin으로 추정되며 surgical resection까지는 replace할 예정입니다. Gross hematuria는 없으나 Hb 9.0까지 down있어 수술 시 전후로 수혈 가능성에 대하여 설명한 상태이며 혈압은 novasc로 조절되기 시작하며 renal origin의 Hypertension 가능성을 배제할 수 없는 상태며 2.28일 외과, 심장내과, 마취과 해결 후 op. 진행 예정이며, pathology confirm 후 추가치료 예정입니다.	강일도
2.28	〈 Brief Op Note 〉 Preop Dx. : Renal tumor, Rt GB polyp Post op Dx. : same Op name : Radical nephrectomy, Rt Cholecystectomy Operator : Prof. P. K. Kim Assistant : 1st H. L. Jung 2nd O. K. Park 3rd E. R. Lee Findings ① Rt kidney: 10 x 7 x 5cm in size ② Tumor mass located on upper pole of kidney & invasion to renal capsule was not suspected. ③ Adrenal gland was normal. ④ There was no adhesion around ureter & kidney. ⑤ There was one renal artery & one renal vein. ⑥ There was no abnormal LN enlargement. ⑦ There was diffuse GB wall thickening.	강일도

경 과 기 록

일 자	내 용	서 명
2.28	〈 Procedure 〉 ① Under the endotracheal anesthesia op field was prep & draped in the usual manner. ② Shavrrong incision was done 20cm in length. ③ SG internal & ext oblique muscle was dissected & electrical cutting. ④ Transversal muscle was incised. ⑤ After confirming IMV. Rt renal vein, renal a. the renal vein & artery were dissected. ⑥ Renal a & vein were clamped $\bar{c}$ Rt−angle clamp & cutted and the ligated 5 silk. ⑦ The kidney was mobilized and gonadal vein was ligated & cutted, adrenal vein was ligated & cutted. ⑧ Rt. ureter was dissected and ligated as distancy as possible. ⑨ Rt. kidney, two third of adrenal gland ureter were extracted from op fieled. ⑩ There was no LN enlargement. ⑪ LN dissection was performed from renal hilum to mesenteric artery $\bar{c}$ sharp dissection. ⑫ All bleeding was controlled. Hemovac was placed on renal fossa & introperitoneal dependent position. ⑬ Transverse abdominal, int & ext oblique abdominal muscle was sutured by 1−0 Dexon continously. ⑭ The skin was closed $\bar{c}$ stapler. ⑮ Dressing was applied.	
3.3	POD #3 BT: 37.4℃ CBC: 11300/9.1/27.0/177K BP: 170/90 (Isocket 139tt/min으로 titrotron＋Adalat 30mg 투여 중) B. supar 166 (5AM) 109 (3PM) → 1040 D/W 1L ＋RI 20$\bar{u}$로 control 중 Total I & O 3050/2229 (H/V 165) 아직 gas passing 못하고 있으며, low abd distention 호소함 plan) rectal stimulation recommend Ambulation	강일도

경 과 기 록

일 자	내 용	서 명

3.4 POD #4

BP 170/80 mmHg

BT 38.3˚C

palpitation 호소

(PR → 136회)

→ B－sugar 103

→ Hb/Hct 9.3/27.7

Urin output: daytime 동안(8hr) 90cc

Hemovac 800cc drainage

→ H/V fluid Hb/Hct

1.0/3.0

→ peritoneal fluid와 mix된 양상

→ Transame 12Ⓐ#6로 투여 시작

Albumine replacement

3.4 Cardioconsultation was done.

Isocket D/C

Monopril & Novasc D/C

Adalat D/C

→ Almarl 10mg#2로 투여 시작

(β－blocker)

plan) 1. BP & B－sugar check

2. SMA f/u

3. EKG & chest PA f/u

3.7 2cm 정도에 걸쳐 wound margin이 dirty하고 tenderness 없음

T.P/AIb 4.5/2.7

↓

Albumine 200ml replacement

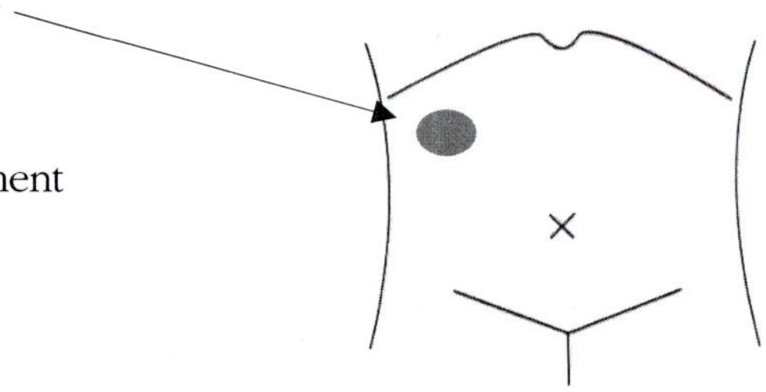

BP 190/100

→ cardioconsultation

Almanal 10mg ⎤
Novasc 5mg ⎦ # 투여 시작

Plan) consult to nephro $\bar{c}$ DM nephropathy

강일도

경 과 기 록

일 자	내 용	서 명
3.8 POD #8	Total I & O 2950/4340 (lasix 10mg 투여) wound site dressing was done. → partially stapler removal → full stich out was done. → mid portion에 wound margin이 uneven. Nephro consultation → ABR → Lasix 40mg#2 sig p.o → fluid restriction	강일도

등록번호	108 20 30	성별	M
성명	복 덩 이		
주민등록	781025－1234567		

협의진단기록
Consultation Record

심장내과　　　　정승상 선생님 귀하

의뢰구분: ☐ 응급 ☐ 보통　　환자상태: ☐ 외래진료가능 ☐ 외래진료불가

의뢰: Summary of Present Findings

본 38세 남환은 Renal tumor, Rt로 입원중입니다.
하기 분야에 선생님의 고진선처를 부탁드립니다.
감사합니다.

for Hypertension
pre－op. evaluation
(EKG상 supraventricular premature beat 관찰됩니다)

2016년 3월 4일 a.m.
Date Hour p.m

Prof. 양일수/백연교 M.D.
Sigature of attending physician

회신: Opinion and Recommendation

〈 Cardiology Note 16－3－4 〉

PHx: DM 10년전 Dx : Diamicron 1 Ⓣ/day
pulm Tbc ⊖ Hypertension ⊖
Smoking 30 p/y FHx of Hypertension ⊕
ROS : Chief pain ⊖ Dyspnea ⊖ DOE ⊖
Palpitation ⊖ Headache ⊖ Dizziness ⊖
P/E : BP 180/100 mmHg PR 82/min
Regular H.B $\bar{c}$ pansystolic ⓜ on LLSB & apex
thrill ⊖ Hearing ⊖

2016년 2월 27일 a.m.
Date Hour p.m.

정승상 M.D.
Sigature of attending physician

등록번호	108 20 30	성별	M
성명	복 덩 이		
주민등록	781025 - 1234567		

협의진단기록
Consultation Record

의뢰구분 : ☐ 응급 ☐ 보통　　환자상태 : ☐ 외래진료가능 ☐ 외래진료불가

의뢰: 민우식 선생님 귀하

본 38세 남환은 R/O ureter stone, Rt로 입원중입니다.
하기분야에 관한 선생님의 고진선처를 의뢰드립니다.
감사합니다.
For evaluation management plan of diabetic patient

2016년 2월 18일 a.m.
Date　Hour p.m.　　Signature 양일수/백연교 M.D.

회신

〈Endo. Note〉

현재 10년된 DM으로 oral agent로 well controlled status입니다. 현재대로 medication하시기 바랍니다. NPO 기간 중에는 glucose insuline - potassium solution으로 control하십시오.
감사합니다.

F/U consult 부탁드립니다.
감사합니다.

2016년 3월 2일 a.m.　　양일수/백연교
Date　Hour p.m.

등록번호	108 20 30	성별	M
성명	복 덩 이		
주민등록	781025－1234567		

수 술 기 록
Operation Record

Date: 2016. 2.28 Surgeon : P. K. Kim
1st Ass't: H. L. Jung 2nd Ass't: O. K. Park
Scrub nurse Circ. nurse

Preoperative diagnosis: Renal tumor, Right
GB polyp

Postoperative diagnosis: Same as above

Name of operation : Radical nephrectomy, Rt
cholecystectomy

Findings:

1. The right kidney was 10cm by 7cm by 5cm in size.
2. The right kidney was soft and smooth surfaced and grossly normal.
3. The tumor was located in upper pole of kidney and invasion to renal capsule was not suspected.
4. Adrenal gland was normal.
5. There was no adhesion around ureter and kidney
6. There was one renal artery and one renal vein.
7. There was no abnormal LN enlargement.
8. There was diffuse GB wall thickening.

Procedures:

Under the general endotracheal anesthesia, the patient was placed in supine position and the operative field was prepared and draped in the usual manners.

A right thoracoabdominal incision was made which was about 20cm in length and the subcutaneous tissue and fascia were incised. The external and internal oblique muscle were incised with electrical cutting. Two fingers were inserted into the paranephric space to push the underlining peritoneum forward. The transversus abdominal muscle was incised. The anterior rectus sheath, rectus muscle and posterior rectus sheath were incised.

Tissue to path. ☑Yes ☐No. Drains Yes Sponge count correct: ☑Yes ☐No

Dictated/Written by H. L. Jung Surgeon's Signature P. K. Kim

수 술 기 록

Operative Procedure

The peritoneum was incised as same length as skin incision. GS team was participated and cholecystectomy was done. Retroperitoneum was dissected around Treitz ligament. After confirming of IMV, right renal vein, renal artery, the renal vein and artery were dissected. The renal artery and vein were clamped with right-angle clamp and Satinsky clamp and cutted and then, they were ligated with 5 silk. The kidney was mobilized and the gonadal vein was ligated and cutted and, adrenal vein was ligated and cutted. Then the right ureter was dissected and ligated as distally as possible. The right kidney, two third of adrenal gland and ureter were extracted from operative field. There was no lymph node enlargement.

Then the LN dissection was performed from renal hilum to inferior mesenteric artery with sharp dissection. All bleedings were controlled and a hemovac was placed in renal fossa and retroperitoneal dependent position. The peritoneum was repaired with PDS and posterior rectus sheath was repaired with CCG continuously. The anterior rectus sheath with rectus muscle was closed with 1-0 Dexon. The transverse abdominis muscle was closed with 1-0 Dexon continuously and internal and external oblique abdominis muscles continuously. The fascia was closed with #4 silk and subcutaneous tissue with #2 silk interrupted. The skin was closed with #3 silk and a dressing was applied.

The patient was well tolerated during the above procedure and returned to the recovery room.

Dictated by H. L. Jung

등록번호	108 20 30	성별 M
성명	복 덩 이	
주민등록	781025－1234567	

조직병리검사보고
Pathological Report

병리접수번호(Accession No) : S－16－2536

검사물 접수일(Specimen received): 16/02/28

Organ and tissue received :

1. Gall bladder
2.
3.

Sent by ________

Pathological Findings and Diagnosis

Gross Description :

The specimen submitted for frozen section consists of a gallbladder, measuring 8x2cm. The serosal surface is pale pinkish and smooth. The opened specimen reveals a yellow velvety and partly eroded surface and a 0.5x0.5cm sized polypoid lesion on the fundus of the gall bladder. On cut section, it confines to the mucosal layer. The diagnosis of frozen section was polyp.

block ; 1, FSP FSX T－2 J. M. Lee

Pathological Diagnosis :

Gall bladder, cholecystectomy ; Tubular adenoma.

Date: 2016. 03. 03

Jun Soo Kim M.D.
Signature of Pathologist

등록번호	108 20 30	성별 M
성명	복 덩 이	
주민등록	781025－1234567	

조직병리검사보고
Pathological Report

Tissue received on the date of: 2016. 3. 2

Organ and location of specimen
1. Right kidney
2.
3.

Sent by ________ M.D.

Pathological Findings and Diagnosis

Gross Description

The specimen consists of a right kidney which is completely enveloped in irregular fibroadipose tissue. The specimen weighs 270gm and measures 13×7×4cm. Previous opening of the upper pole reveals a mass, covered by a smooth fibrous capsule. On section, the tumor mass, measures 5×6×4cm. It is composed of yellowish gray tissue with lobulated appearance, in which there are areas of cheesy necrosis with foci of hemorrhage. The lesion is relatively well demarcated from the renal parenchyme. A satellite nodule just below the main mass appears to bulge into the renal pelvis. The tumor does note appear to the invaded perinephrect fat. Adrenal gland measuring 2×1.3×0.3cm and weighing 10gm is separately sent. No gross evidence of tumor invasion. A ureter measuring 17cm is separately sent. It is essentially unremarkable.

K. H. Shin

Pathological Diagnosis :

Kidney, right, radical nephrectomy :

1. Renal cell carcinoma, clear cell type, confined to the renal capsule.
2. Tumor extension to the lumen of pelvis.

Ureter, right, separately sent: Epithelial hyperplasia without tumor extension.
Resection margin, ureter: Free from tumor.
Renal vessles: Free from tumor.
Lymph node, labelled as perirenal, separately sent (0/4): Free from tumor.
Adrenal gland, right, adrenalectomy: No pathological diagnosis.
H & E (14)

Date: 16. 03. 07

Youn il Kang M.D.
Signature of Pathologist

〈복 덩 이〉

★ 복덩이 차트를 보고 맞는 답에 O표 하시오.

1 상기 환자의 내용 중 맞지 않는 것은?

① 10년 전부터 당뇨병성 망막질환이 있었다. ② 타병원에서 전원되어온 환자이다.
③ 13년에 비골(종아리뼈) 골절을 당한 적이 있었다. ④ 응급실을 통해서 입원하였다.
⑤ 여동생은 신장결석, 작은 아버지는 죽상경화증이 있다.

2 주진단과 연관된 진단명과 수술명의 분류번호가 맞게 짝지어진 것은?

① C64,0 M8211/0, 55.4 ② C64.0, M8312/3, 55.51
③ C79.00, M8211/6, 55.4 ④ C79.09, M8312/3, 55.51
⑤ C64.1, M8312/2, 55.51

3 입원시 환자의 증상으로만 열거한 것은?

ㄱ. 혈뇨 ㄴ. 복통 ㄷ. 빈뇨 ㄹ. 설사 ㅁ. 전신쇠약

① ㄱ, ㄴ ② ㄴ, ㄷ ③ ㄱ, ㄷ ④ ㄹ, ㅁ ⑤ ㄴ, ㄹ

4 이 환자의 내용으로 맞게 기재한 것은?

① 전과(transfer)를 하였다. ② 수술 후 3일째의 섭취량은 2,229였다.
③ 입원당시의 소변검사에서 단백질과 당이 검출되지 않았다.
④ 실밥을 모두 뽑은 날은 수술 후 8일째였다. ⑤ 수술 후 7일째 복막내 Hemovac을 제거했다.

5 담낭(쓸개)과 연관된 진단명과 수술명을 분류한 것은?

① C22.1, M8211/3, 51.23 ② C22.1, M8211/0, 51.23
③ D13.5, M8211/0, 51.22 ④ D13.5, M8211/3, 51.22
⑤ D13.5, M8211/6, 51.23

6 상기 환자의 통계사항 중 틀린 것은?

① 재원기간은 30일이다. ② 수술건수는 1건, 생검수는 1건이다.
③ 마취방법은 전신마취이다. ④ 수술과는 외과 및 비뇨기과이다.
⑤ 응급실 경유하여 비뇨기과 입원했다.

7 상기 환자가 받은 검사로만 짝지어진 것은?

ㄱ. KUB ㄴ. CT ㄷ. Ultrasono ㄹ. MRI ㅁ. RGP

① ㄱ, ㄴ, ㄷ ② ㄴ, ㄷ, ㄹ ③ ㄷ, ㄹ, ㅁ ④ ㄱ, ㄴ, ㄹ ⑤ ㄱ, ㄹ, ㅁ

8 기타 진단 및 수술분류번호가 맞게 조립된 것은?

ㄱ. E14.9 ㄴ. E14.21+ ㄷ. N08.3* ㄹ. K90.8 ㅁ. I10.9 ㅂ. 07.29
ㅅ. 51.12 ㅇ. 55.23 ㅈ. 40.11

① ㄱ－ㄷ－ㅁ－ㅂ－ㅅ ② ㄱ－ㄷ－ㅂ－ㅅ－ㅇ
③ ㄴ－ㄹ－ㅁ－ㅂ－ㅈ ④ ㄴ－ㄷ－ㅁ－ㅂ－ㅅ
⑤ ㄴ－ㄷ－ㅁ－ㅇ－ㅈ

9 **수술기록지의 내용으로 맞지 않는 것은?**

① 오른쪽 신장의 크기는 10×7×5cm였다.
② 신장암은 위쪽 신장에 있었으며, 주변 림프조직까지 퍼져 있었다.
③ 부신은 정상이었다.
④ 절개방법은 우측 흉복부 절개이었다.
⑤ 담낭(쓸개) 벽은 두꺼워져 있었다.

10 **퇴원요약지의 내용이 맞는 것은?**

① 심계항진이 있었던 날은 3월 6일, 복강내 hemovac을 제거한 날은 3월 4일이다.
② 환자가 계속 복용 중인 당뇨병약은 Bithree이며 하루에 3알 먹는다.
③ 병기분류는 T2 No Mo이며, 퇴원 후 추후검사는 CT와 U/S이다.
④ 외래 추후 관리를 할 진료과는 비뇨기과, 안과, 심장내과 및 신장내과이다.
⑤ 고혈압이 있으며, 구토와 심계항진을 호소하였다.

02 담낭 결석 동반 췌장염
Pancreatitis c̄ gallbladder stone

1.1 췌장(이자, Pancreas)

구 성

▸ 두부(머리, head), 체(몸통, body), 미부(꼬리, tail)

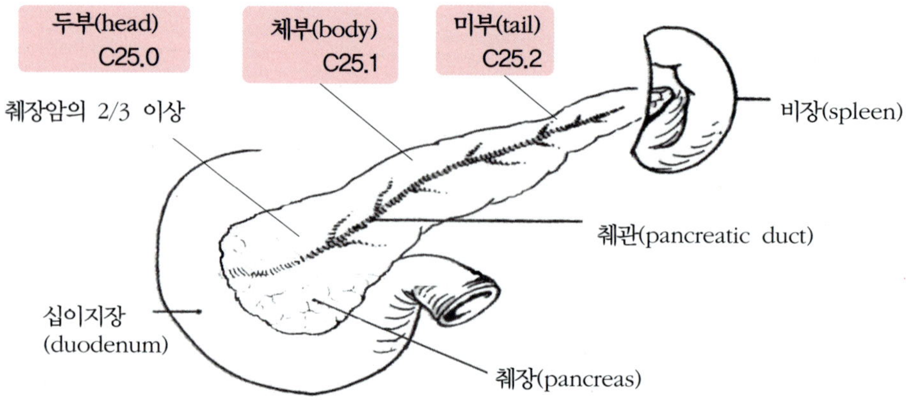

그림 1. 췌장(이자)의 구조 및 질병분류
췌장암(pancreatic cancer): C25.__

기 능

▸ 외분비(exocrine)와 내분비(endocrine) 동시 기능

- 외분비선
  - 전분을 소화시키는 효소(amylase)와 지방을 분해하는 효소(lipase) 생성
  - 췌장관을 통해 십이지장으로 보냄
- 내분비선
  - 인슐린(insulin) 분비: 내분비장기/췌장 → 과소분비
  - 당(glucose)을 혈액에서 세포로 전달

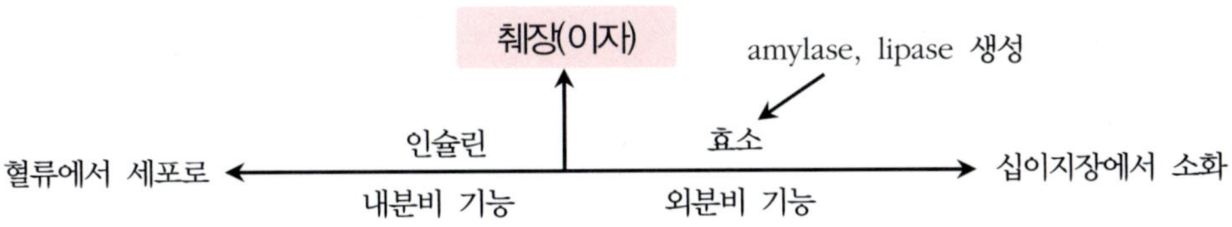

그림 2. 췌장(이자)의 기능

1.2 췌장염(Pancreatitis)

원 인

- 췌장(이자)의 염증
  - 소화효소가 췌장조직을 공격하여 선(gland)을 손상
  - 염증은 알코올중독증, 담석, 복부외상(trauma), 약물 때문에 발생

증 상

복통(abdominal pain), 압통(tenderness), 오심(nausea), 구토(vomiting)

치 료

통증을 완화하는 약물, 정맥내 수액주사, 식사 감시, 선(gland)의 부분절제

1.3 담석증(Cholelithiasis): 담석(Gallstones)

원 인

- 담낭(쓸개)과 담관에 담즙(bile)이 쌓여 딱딱하게 됨
- 결석은 담즙이 담낭에서 나와 담관을 타고 십이지장으로 가는 것을 막음

치 료

- Cholecystectomy(담낭/쓸개절제술)와 choledocholithotomy(총담관 절제술)
- Laparoscopic cholecystectomy(복강경을 이용한 담낭절제술)
- Chenodiol(약물치료): 간에서 콜레스테롤 합성 저하 및 결석 용해

1.4 담석의 위치 및 증상

- A. 담낭내 결석: 경미(mild) 또는 무증상
- B. 담낭관(cystic duct): 통증의 원인
- C. 총담관(CBD): 통증 및 황달의 원인
- D. 총담관 하부 및 췌장관을 막는 결석: 통증, 황달 및 췌장염의 원인

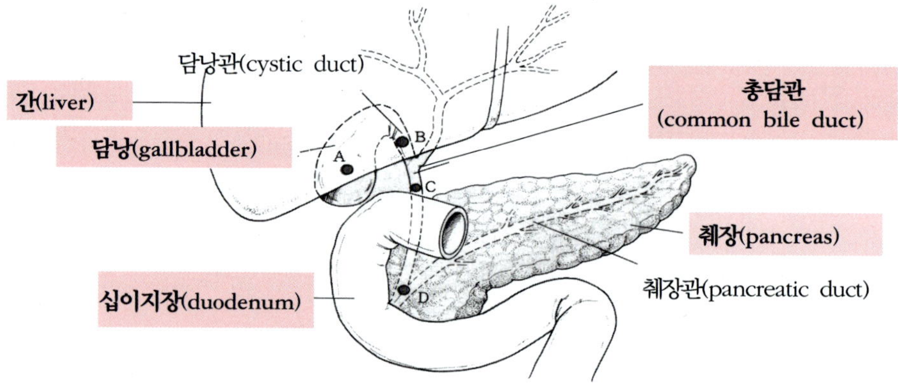

그림 3. 담석(Gallstones)

1.5 환자의 의식상태 순서

- 방심않는(alert) < 졸림(drowsy) < 혼미(stupor) < 혼수(coma)

2.1 재원일수(Length of Stay; LOS): 단입법(퇴원일-입원일)

∘

전과: transfer in(전입, 환자를 받는 과)
transfer out(전출, 환자를 보내는 과)
예) 입원일 '17. 6. 24: 내과 ⎤ 경과기록지
전과일 '17. 7. 16: 외과 ⎦
퇴원일 '17. 8. 27: 외과
☞ [풀이: 6. 30-24+16=22, 7. 31-16+27=42 → 답: 내과 22일 외과 42일]

2.2 재원일 찾는 방법

▸ 입퇴원기록, 경과기록, 의사지시기록, 간호기록, 퇴원요약 → 입·퇴원일

유사 용어

- 담낭(쓸개): Gallbladder(GB) = Cholecysto
- 총담관: Common bile duct(CBD) = Choledocho
- 결석: Stone = litho = calculus

  예) · GB stone = Cholecytolithiasis(담낭결석증)

  · CBD stone = Choledocholithiasis(총담관결석증)

2.3 약제

▸ 항생제(antibiotics): 미생물의 발육을 억제 또는 사멸시키는 약물

– claforan, sagacin, flagyl

– penicillin, streptomycin, tetracyclines, sulfonamides

차트 용어

· Chill	오한	· Constipation	변비	· Diarrhea	설사	· Dysuria	배뇨곤란
· Itching	소양증/가려움	· Nausea	오심/구역질	· Palpitation	심계항진 /두근거림	· Peri	주변
· Pseudocyst	가성낭	· Umbilical	제대의(배꼽의)	· Visual disturbance	시각장애	· Tinea pedis	족부백선/무좀

약 어	원 어	
BS	Breath sounds: chest	호흡음: 흉부
	Bowel sounds: abdomen	장(腸)소리: 복부
CBS	Clear breathing sound	깨끗한 호흡음
CT	Computed tomography	컴퓨터 단층촬영술
CVA(신체검진)	Costvertebral angle	늑골척추각
CVA(진단명)	Cerebral vascular accident	뇌혈관사고(뇌졸중=중풍) = stroke
CVAT	Costvertebral angle tenderness	늑골척추각 압통
DM	Diabetes mellitus	당뇨병
F/U	Follow-up	추적조사
GB	Gallbladder	담낭/쓸개
GEA	General endotracheal anesthesia	기관내 전신마취
HiBP, HNT	Hypertension	고혈압
ICS	Intercostal space	늑간강
Imp	Impression	의증
IV	Intravenous	정맥내(정맥내 마취: 전신마취)
LMCL	Left middle calvicular line	좌쇄골 중앙선
ⓜ	Murmur	잡음(심장)
MD	Moderatly developed	중등도 발달
MN	Moderatly nourished	중등도 영양
N-C	No complaints	불평없음
OR	Operating room	수술실
PMI	Point of maximum impulse	최대 박동점
PR	Pulse rate	맥박수(정상: 1분 60~80)
Rec	Recommend	권유
RHB	Regular heart beat	규칙적 심박동
ROS	Review of system	계통별 문진 소견
RR	Recovery room	회복실
SOW	Sips of water	물 한모금
U/S	Ultrasound	초음파
VDRL	Venereal Disease Research Laboratory (test for syphilis)	성병검사(매독검사) 예: reactive(+) 양성

등록번호	10811228	성별	F
성명	오 대 승		
주민등록	6412201－1234567		

입 퇴 원 기 록

Admission and Discharge Record

주 소:

출신지: 직 업: 전 화 :

연고자성명: 관 계: 주 소: 전 화:

	전과	
입원: 2016년 6 월 24 일 과 병동 호		20 년 월 일 과 병동 호
퇴원: 2016년 8 월 27 일 과 병동 호		20 년 월 일 과 병동 호
재원일수:		20 년 월 일 과 병동 호

최종진단명	분 류 번 호
주진단명 : Chronic pancreatitis $\bar{c}$ GB stone	
& pancreatic pseudocyst	
기타진단명:	
수술 및 처치명	
수술명: Cholecystectomy	
Op. cholangiogram	
기타수술 및 주요검사: ext. drainage of pseudocyst	

치료결과: 1. 완쾌 2. 경쾌 3. 호전안됨 4. 진단뿐 5. 가망없는 퇴원 6. 48시간내 사망 7. 48시간이후 사망

퇴원형태: 1. 퇴원지시후 2. 자의퇴원 3. 탈원 4. 전원

병원감염: 1. 수술후 2. 기타처치후 3. 비뇨기계 4. 호흡기계 5. 소화기계 6. 기타

원사인 : 부검: 예, 아니오

계속적 진료 계획

없음.있음 (약속일 2016 년 월 일 시)

담당 전공의 서명: 김안진	담당 전문의 서명: 이한운
의무기록 완성: 2016 년 월 일	의무기록사 서명 :

등록번호	10811228	성별	F
성명	오 대 승		
주민등록	6412201－1234567		

퇴 원 요 약 지

Discharge Summary

Admission date: 2016. 6. 24.

Discharge date: 2016. .

Final Dx: 1. Chronic pancreatitis c̄ GB stone
& pancreatic pseudocyst

C.C: 1. Abd pain
2. Radiating Lt CVA tenderness
D: 3days

PHx: 08년 Acute pancreatitis: local에서 management

FHx: none

Imp) Acute pancreatitis

Tx: Preop Dx: Chronic pancreatitis c̄ GB stone & pancreatic pseudocyst

Op: Cholecystectomy
Op. cholangiogram
Ext. drainage of pancreatic pseudocyst

서인구

등록번호	10811228	성별	F
성명	오 대 승		
주민등록	6412201－1234567		

신체검진기록

Physical Examination

'16. 6. 24 CC: Abd. pain

Radiating Lt. CVA pain

D : x 3 days

PHx: '08. pancreatitis로 local clinic에서 입원 치료

FHx: N－C

ROS: general weakness (＋) fever (＋) chill (－) headache (－)
dizziness (－) nausea (＋) vomiting (＋) abdominal pain(＋)
constipation (－) diarrhea (－) dysuria (－) polyuria (－)
dyspnea (－) palpitation (－) visual disturbance (－) wt. loss(－)

P/E	V/S	B.P 110/80
		P.R 110/min
		B Temp 37。5′
	G/A	acute ill looking
		M/D, M/N
		alert mental state
	Skin	warm & dry
		No petechiae
		No skin rash
	HEENT	Normocephaly
		Not anemic conjunctiva
		anicteric sclera
		Not dehydrated tongue
		Not injected tonsil

임혁후

신 체 검 진 기 록

일 자	내 용	서 명
'16. 6. 24	Neck Supple Not palpable L/N Chest CBS $\bar{s}$ rale No wheezing No external deformity Heart RHB $\bar{s}$ murmur No thrill PMI at LMCL x 5th ICS Abd. Flat & rigid Not palpable mass decrease BS Epigastric & peri−umbilical: pain & tenderness Back & Ext Lt. CVA pain & tenderness No pitting edema Imp) Acute pancreatitis Plan) Gomco suction $\bar{c}$ V−tube insertion Foy mixed to fluid Anti−ulcer medication	임혁후

등록번호	10811228	성별	F
성명	오 대 승		
주민등록	6412201－1234567		

경 과 기 록

Progress Notes

일 자	내 용	서 명
	〈Admission Note〉	
6.24	본 53세 여자 환자는 C.C: 1. Abdominal pain esp) epigastric D: for 3days 를 주소로 본원 ER 경유 내과 G－I part에 입원하였다. 환자는 평소 hunger pain과 intermittent epigastric discomfort가 있었으며 내원 4일 전 저녁에 빵을 먹고 잔 후 다음날 epigastric pain develop되어 Home medication했으나 Sx improve되지 않아 안양 병원 방문 후 management 받다가 more aggrevation되어 본원 ER로 transfer되어 내과 G－I part에 입원하였다. PHx: 8년 전 췌장염으로 개인 local clinic에 Adm.하여 Tx 받음 No DM No HIBP No pul tbc No hepatitis FHx: none ROS: General weakness (＋) Fever (＋) Chill (－) Headache (－) Dizziness (＋) Nausea (＋) Vomiting (＋) Abd. pain, esp) Epigastric Constipation (－) Diarrhea (－), Dysuria (－) Polyuria (－) Polydypsia (－) Cough (－) Sputum (－), Dyspnea (－), Palpitation (－), Visual disturbance (－) Hearing disturbance (－), Wt. loss (－) P/E GA : Acute ill－looking app. alert mentality Skin: Warm & dry No petechiae No skin rash	서인구

경 과 기 록

일 자	내 용	서 명
6.24	HEENT: Normocephaly Not anemic conjunctiva No icteric sclera Not dehydrated tongue Not injected tonsils Neck: Supple Not palpable LNs Chest: CBS $\bar{s}$ ⓡ No wheezing No external deformity Heart: Rapid heart beat $\bar{s}$ ⓜ No thrills PMI at LMCL x 5th ICS Abdomen: Flat & rigid Not palpable mass Decreased BS Epigastric & periumblical pain & tenderness Back/Ext.: Lt. CVA pain & tenderness No pitting edema Anus genitalia: N－S Imp) Acute pancreatitis Plan) 1. L－tube Gomcosuction 2. Foy mixed fluid 3. Antiulcer medication	서인구

경 과 기 록

일 자	내 용	서 명

6.25 S : Abdominal pain
fever
O : V/S BP 120/70mg
BT 39°C
PR 90/min

Lab) amylase 125mg
CBC WBC (10600)
Hb (9.2 → 10.0)
PLT (228K)
Electrolyte (135 / 3.8 / 98 / 211)
A : Acute pancreatic
Pan. pseudocyst

P : Abd U/S
amylase/lipase, follow－up 서인구

〈 Off Service Note 〉

6.29 본 53세 여자 환자는
Dx : Acute pancreatitis
Pseudocyst formation으로 입원 중입니다. 내원 당시 amylase(5.24)에서 6.26일 amylase/lipase (81/137)로 normalized 되었습니다. 현재 problem도 fever(39.5°C)와 aggrevated leukocytosis, pseudocyst formation으로 abd U/S와 abd. CT를 시행하였습니다. Abd U/S상 liver 내 air density 보였으나 CT상 liver에 abd echogram lesion이 없으며 GB stone, pseudocyst formation pancreas내 decreased density 소견 보이고 있습니다. 현재 Anti는 claforan, sagacin flagyl로 cover하고 있습니다. fever control 및 pseudocyst에 대한 operability를 고려해 보아야 될 것으로 사료됩니다. 현재 medication은 L－tube $\bar{c}$ Gomco로 NPO 상태로 Milid zauta Foy mixed fluid Antibiotics입니다.

수고하십니다.

서인구

경 과 기 록

일 자	내 용	서 명
	〈 On Service Note 〉	
6.30	본 53세 여자 환자는 Dx : Acute pancreatitis Pseudocyst formation 내원 당시 amylase 524 → 81로 감소되었습니다 high fever, leukocytosis, pseudocyst formation으로 abdo u/s상 liver에 multiple increased density CT상 pseudocyst formation pancreas내 decreased density 있습니다. anti는 claforan, sagain, flagyl 사용중 fever down 되는 상태이고 abdo pain 감소 추세입니다. NPO. L−tube $\bar{c}$ Gomco suction milid Zautar Flaly mix 중 vital closely observation 하겠습니다.	서인구
7.3	S : mild periumbilical pain 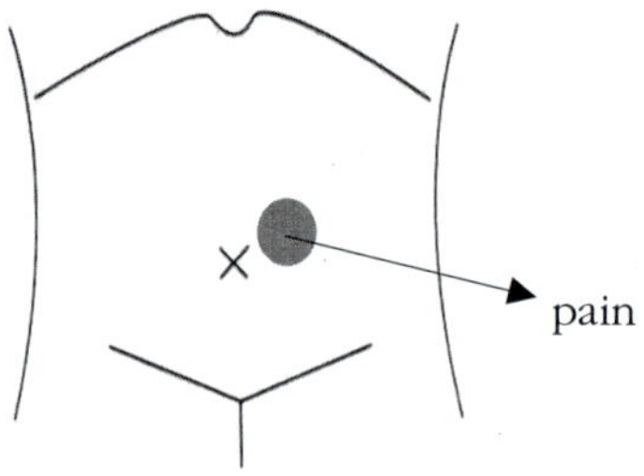 O : audible B.S gas passing, defecation (loss stool) mild fever (37.5˚C) Gomco suction remove state A : Acute pancreatitis pseudocyst formation P : 1. antibiotics 2. SOW 3. V/S close observation 4. pain control 5. pancreatic rest 6. F/U abd U/S	서인구

경 과 기 록

일 자	내 용	서 명
7.8	S : mild periumbilical discomfort afebrile O : audible B.S Abd F/U: no interval change pancreatitis c̄ fluid collection Gall stone in GB c̄ chronic cholecystitis WBC: 6900 Hb: 10.7 S－electro: 131/4.9/97/24 VDRL (+) A : 1. Acute pancreatitis 2. Pseudocyst formation P : 1. SD 2. Pain control	서인구
7.13	S : Mild periumbilical discomfort mild fever O : Audible B.S Abd U/S F/U: fluid collection (No interval change) Gall stone in GB RHB s̄ ⓜ CBS s̄ ⓡ BT: 37°C A : Acute pancreatitis c̄ pseudocyst formation P : 1. U/S guide aspiration 2. Antibiotics 3. Conservative management	서인구

경 과 기 록

일 자	내 용	서 명
7.16	〈 Transfer Out Note 〉 본 53세 여환은 Acute pancreatitis pseudocyst formation으로 입원 중인 환자로 abdo U/S상 interval change 없고 U/S guided aspiration도 고려 중인 환자입니다.	서인구
7.16	〈 Transfer In Note 〉 본 53세 여환은 acute pancreatitis, pseudocyst로 입원 중으로 금일 transfer되었다.	서인구
7.24	S : Mild itching sensation on IV site O : BP 110/70 mmHg afebrile state CBS $\bar{s}$ rale RHB $\bar{s}$ ⓜ Mild abd. discomfort A : Acute pancreatitis $\bar{c}$ pseudocyst formation P : 1. Antihistamin 2. F/U abd U/S 3. Antibiotics therapy	
7.29	S : Mild abdo. discomfort O : CBS $\bar{s}$ rale RHB $\bar{s}$ ⓜ afebrile state BP : 120/80 mmHg A : Acute pancreatitis $\bar{c}$ pseudocyst formation P : 1. Abdo CT 2. dermatology consult 3. conservative manage	서인구

경 과 기 록

일 자	내 용	서 명
8.3	S : Mild abdo. discomfort O : Afebrile state BP: 110/80 mmHg CBS s̄ rale RHB s̄ ⓜ abdo CT: Lesser sac fluid → removal A : Mild pseudocyst formation → decreased Acute pancreatitis pseudocyst formation P : oral GB	서인구
8.6	S : N-C O : Abd. CT: pancreatic psedocyst (site: mild decreased) lesser sac의 fluid: decreased CBS s̄ rale RHB s̄ ⓜ A : Acute pancreatitis c̄ pseudocyst formation gall stone P : 1. consult to GS 2. oral GB 3. Chest PA. EKG F/U	서인구
8.9	S : Nonspecific complaints O : Oral GB: gallstone CBS s̄ rale EKG : R/O myocardial ischemia R/O nonspecific T change Chest PA : No active disease A : Pancreatitis c̄ pseudocyst formation GB stone	서인구

경 과 기 록

일 자	내 용	서 명
	〈 OR Note 〉	
8.12	Preop Dx : Pancreatic pseudocyst $\bar{c}$ GB stone Postop Dx : Same Op. name : Cholecystectomy Op cholangiogram External drainage Op. findings : 1. The 7x5x3cm sized cystic lesion was noted on the pancreatic head portion. 2. It was aspirated with needle 3. Its amout was about 70cc serous chocholated colored fluid. 4. The liver was slightly fatty changed and light brownish colored. 5. The other intraperitoneal organ was grossly normal. OP. procedures : 1. Under GEA 2. Supine position 3. Skin prep $\bar{c}$ drap 4. Great omentum was divided. ligated. 5. GB was removed. 6. Op. cholangiogram was done. 7. Ext. drainage. 8. Pt. send RR in good condition.	김안진
8.12	〈 Immediate Post－op 〉 Pt was full awaken state Pt was EKG monitoring state : Normal EKG rhythm	

경 과 기 록

일 자	내 용	서 명
8.12	EKG was done Control tube insertion state Drain site color & amount : relatively bloody: 4 x 4 x 20 sheet pad Semifowler's position CBC: 11.5/33.7 Pancreatic fluid pathology sent S－amylase: 70 Cold steam inhalation state ABG: 7.338/237/46.3/24.1/1.7 Pancreatic op에 대한 drain site close observation & sugar level check	김안진
8.13	POD#1 abd pain complaints drain color: Sl. bloody. CBC follow up: No active bloody P) fluid therapy drain color closed obser Conservative tx	김안진
8.14	Abd. pain complaint Abd. site: color & amount : Sl. watery chocholate color Lt: 4 x 4 x 20 sheet Rt: 4 x 4 x 15 sheet (Lt 〉 Rt) P) Aseptic dressing	김안진
8.15	Ambulation good drain site amount & color: sl watery chocholate color Lt. 4 x 4 x 10 sheet Rt. 4 x 4 x 7 sheet V/S: stable	김안진

등록번호	10811228	성별	F
성명	오 대 승		
주민등록	6412201-1234567		

협의진료기록
Consultation Record

Request For Consultation To　　　　To 한장수 선생님

Summary of Present Findings

For skin problem on both hand & pruritus
본 53세 여자 환자는 Acute pancreatitis & pseudocyst formation으로 입원중입니다. 상기 분야에 관한 고진선처 부탁드립니다.

감사합니다.

2016. 07. 19　　a.m.　　　　홍준부 / 이조승 M.D
Date　　Hour p.m.　　　　Signature of Attending Physician

Report of Consultation

Opinion and Recommendation

〈 Skin Note 〉

D: 1wk
그전부터 pruritus가 있었으며 주사놓은 자리에 특히 심하며 lesion migration하며 itching
Skin finding: rice to bean sized erythematosis papule & plaque on trunk esp. abdomen inner thigh
Imp) Drug eruption
Drug reaction일 가능성이 크나 oral antihistamines + Avil injection 후 현재는 병변이 거의 소실된 상태입니다. 현재의 medication 계속 쓰면서, oral anti-histamines (# 161) 투여하고 follow up 해 보는 것이 좋겠습니다. 감사합니다.

2016. 7. 21　　　　한장수 M.D.
Date　　Hour p.m.　　　　Signature of Attending Physician

등록 번호	10811228	성별 F
성명	이 행 운	
주민 등록	461201－1234567	

협의진료기록
Consultation Record

Request For Consultation To　　　Dr. 피부과 김우익 선생님

Summary of Present Findings

For Tinea pedis

본 53세 여자 환자는 acute pancreatitis로 입원 치료 중입니다. upper ext.와 back에 itching sensation이 있습니다.
상기분야에 관한 선생님의 고진선처를 부탁드립니다. 감사합니다.

1998. 07. 27　a.m.　　　양진구 / 최동부 M.D.
Date　Hour p.m.　　　Signature of Attending Physician

Report of Consultation

Opinion and Recommendation

〈 Skin Note 〉

Imp: Tinea pedis
D: 7days
P/E: whitish scaly patchs on soles & toe webs
P.I: Mycospor 2회 도포⊕
Fungus study (Neg)
Rec) 현재 바르는 약을 사용하는 것이 좋겠습니다.
(자가용 Mycospor)

감사합니다.

2016. 7. 29　　　강수목 M.D.
Date　Hour p.m.　　　Signature of Attending Physician

등록번호	10811228	성별	F
성명	오 대 승		
주민등록	6412201－1234567		

협의진료기록
Consultation Record

Request For Consultation To Dr. 황달희 선생님

Summary of Present Findings

Follow－up consult 부탁드립니다.
감사합니다.
(for discharge plan)

2016. 08. 24 a.m.
Date Hour p.m.

지승독 / 전복승 M.D.
Signature of Attending Physician

Report of Consultation

Opinion and Recommendation

〈 F/U Note 〉

Echo상 significant한 wall motion abnormality 없고 환자가 angina가 없는 점으로 보아 현재로서는 management가 필요한 ischemia는 없어 보입니다.

Rec) Wait & See

감사합니다.

2016. 08. 26
Date Hour p.m.

원교학 / 임성인 M.D.
Signature of Attending Physician

등록번호	10811228	성별	F
성명	오 대 승		
주민등록	6412201－1234567		

수 술 기 록
Operation Record

날짜: 2016년 8월 12일　　집도의: H.U. Lee M.D
제 1 보조의: Q.S. Shin M.D.　제 2 보조의: A.J.Kim M.D.
참여간호사:　　순환간호사 :

Preoperative diagnosis : Pancreatic pseudocyst with GB stones

Postoperative diagnosis : S/A

Name of operation : Cholecystectomy, Operative cholangiogram
External drainage

Findings :

There was minimal amount of ascitic fluid collection in the peritoneal cavity. The GB was dilated and it was measured about 8x6cm in size and contained 0.5x1.0cm sized small multiple black pigmented stones. The GB wall was slightly thickened and edematous and was 0.3cm in thickness. The CBD was not enlarged and was about 0.6cm in diameter. The 7x5x3cm sized cystic lesion was noted on the pancreatic head portion, and it was aspirated with needle and its amount was about 70cc serous chocholated colored fluid. The liver was slightly fatty changed and light brownish colored and there was not palpable nodule and not cirrhotic change. The other intraperitoneal organ was grossly normal.

Procedures :

Under the general endotracheal anesthesia, the patient was supine position on the operative table. The operative field was prepared and draped as usual manners The Rt. upper paramedian skin incision was made about 15cm in length and deepened to the SQ layer and the rectus muscle was splitted along the its fiber direction. After the peritoneum was opened, the above examined throughly and the GB was exposed to the incision wound. The hepatoduodenal ligament was sharply dissected and the cystic duct was hooked using the #3 silk to prevent the stone passage. The cystic artery was identified and clamped, divided and ligated. Next, the serosa of GB was incised along avascular plane from the liver bed and the cystic duct was ligated with #4 silk. The operative cholangiogram was taked and stone was not noted on the CBD.

Tissue to path. ☑Yes ☐No　Drains 1 silastic　Sponge count correct ☑Yes ☐No
Dictated/Written by H.U. Lee　Surgeon's Signature Q.S. Shin

수 술 기 록

Operative Procedure

The needle was intoduced on the pancreatic pseudocyst and 70cc fluid was drainage and sump drain was inserted. All bleeder was controlled and one silastic drain were introduced into the subhepatic space via a new stab wound on the right flank. The peritoneum was closed with 1-0 Vicryl continous suture and the fascia was closed with #5 silk interrupted sutures. The SQ layer and skin were approximated with #3 silk interrupted sutures in each layer. The patient well tolerated during all procedure and was sent to the recovery room in good condition.

Dictated by H. U. Lee

등록번호	10811228	성별	F
성명	오 대 승		
주민등록	6412201 – 1234567		

병리검사 보고서
Pathological Report

접 수 일: S – 16 – 2553
의뢰의사: 김원민

Organ and tissue received
1. Gallbladder
2.
3.

Sent by __________M.D

Pathological Findings and Diagnosis

Gross Description

The specimen consists of three compartments. The first one is a gallbladder, measuring 8x3cm. Its outer surface is pinkish gray and smooth with focal ragged area. The opened specimen reveals qreenish bile tinged velvety mucosa. The wall is not thickened and gall stone is not found. The second one is a small piece of pinkish gray soft tissue, clinically from the cystic duct, measuring 1cm in length.

The third one consists of samll amount of gray brown friable material, clinically from the pancreas, measuring less than 0.5cc in toto.

W.M.Kim

Pathological Diagnosis :

Gallbladder, cholecystectomy: Chronic cholecystitis
Cystic duct, excision: Chronic nonspecific inflammation
Tissue from pancreas: Enzymatic fat necrosis

2016. 08. 14

Kang Jin, M.D.
Signature of Pathologist

〈오 대 승〉

★ 오대승 차트를 보고 맞는 답에 O표 하시오.

1 최종진단명의 분류번호로 맞게 조립된 것은?

가. K80.10	나. K86.3	다. K86.1	라. K85.9
마. K80.50	바. K80.41	사. K80.00	아. K80.21

① 나, 다, 라 ② 다, 마, 아 ③ 라, 바, 사 ④ 가, 나, 다 ⑤ 가, 마, 아

2 환자의 상태를 나타낸 것 중 틀린 것은?

① 복통을 주소로 응급실을 통해 입원하였다. ② 입원 당시에 감염이 있었다.
③ 과거력상 췌장염으로 수술받은 적은 없으나 CVA가 있었다.
④ 발백선으로 피부과 타과의뢰를 하였다. ⑤ 상복부 통증이 있었다.

3 상기 환자의 재원일수로 맞는 것은?

① 외과 64일 ② 내과 22일, 외과 42일, 총재원일수 64일
③ 내과 23일, 외과 42일, 총재원일수 65일 ④ 내과 65일
⑤ 내과 42일, 외과 22일

4 신체검진에 대한 설명이 맞는 것은?

① 하복부와 제대(배꼽) 주위의 통증이 심하다. ② 심계항진이 있다.
③ 열이 있다. ④ 눈에 황달기는 없었으나 체중감소가 있었다.
⑤ 목에 림프절이 촉진되었다.

5 상기 환자가 사용하고 있는 항생제로 맞는 것은?

① afloxan ② aldactone ③ cibacen ④ sagacin ⑤ sulpyrin

6 주수술명에 대한 분류번호는?

① 51.22 ② 51.32 ③ 51.59 ④ 51.91 ⑤ 51.23

7 수술지의 내용이 아닌 것은?

① 췌장의 가성낭은 췌장 머리쪽에 위치하고 있었다.
② 담낭, 총담관은 모두 약간 커져 있었다.
③ 담낭에는 여러 가지 작은 검은 색소 돌들이 있었다.
④ 흡인한 거짓낭은 초콜릿색을 띠고 있었다.
⑤ 복막내 기관은 정상이었다.

8 상기 환자가 시행한 검사로 짝지어진 것은?

가. cholangiogram	나. abd. U/S	다. MUGA	라 abd. MRI	마. abd. CT	바. ECG

① 가, 나, 마 ② 가, 다, 바 ③ 가, 라, 바 ④ 나, 다, 마 ⑤ 나, 라, 바

9 의식상태를 나타내는 다음 용어 중 그 정도가 가장 명료한 것은?

① coma ② alert ③ stupor ④ drowsy ⑤ hazy

10 경과기록지에서 VDRL(+)의 분류번호는?

① A51.0 ② A52.9 ③ A53.0 ④ A53.9 ⑤ A51.9

03 위암 및 악성 림프종
Stomach cancer and malignant lymphoma

1.1 악성림프종(Malignant lymphoma): 혈액암(Hematologic malignancy)

호지킨스병(Hodgkin's disease): Hodgkin's lymphoma

- **특 징**: 림프절(lymph nodes), 비장(지라, spleen) 등 림프조직의 악성종양
- **원 인**: 불명
- **증 상**: 비장·간 비대, 빈혈, 복수, 황달, 발열, 권태, 쇠약, 창백, 소양증, 청색증, 체중 감소
- **진 단**: 림프절의 악성세포인 Reed-sternberg cell 발견
- **치 료**: −국소적인 질환 - 방사선요법
  −광범위한 침윤 - 화학요법 및 방사선요법 또는 화학요법

비호지킨림프종(Non−Hodgkin's lymphoma; NHL)

- **유 형**: −Lymphocytic lymphoma: 림프구로 구성
  −Histiocytic lymphoma: 조직구 또는 큰 대식구와 유사한 큰 림프구로 구성

예) ① Malignant lymphoma, diffuse large B-cell
미만성 대 B-세포(조직세포형) 악성림프종
② Malignant lymphoma, diffuse histiocytic type
→ C83.3

- **특 징**: Hodgkin's disease와 유사한 림프절의 악성종양
- **증 상**: 초기부터 사방 침범 및 침윤된 림프절은 커지고 조직 파괴
  −진행속도: NHL 빠름, Hodgkin's disease 느림 → 생존기간 차이 큼
- **치 료**: 화학요법, 방사선요법
- **일 명**: 림프육종(lymphosarcoma), 세망세포육종(reticulum cell sarcoma)
  Burkitt's lymphoma, stem cell lymphoma

림프절의 주요 용어

· cervical nodes	경(목)부림프절	· axillary nodes	겨드랑이절
· mediastinal nodes	종격림프절: 폐사이	· inguinal nodes	샅타구니(서혜) 림프절
· tonsil 편도	목뒤의 림프조직 덩어리	· adenoids	아데노이드: 목의 비인두 (nasopharynx)

1.2 림프종(Lymphoma)의 기원: 림프구(lymphatic cell)

① **Nodal lymphoma(75%)**: 림프절(lymph node C77.__), 편도(tonsil), 비장(지라, spleen), 흉선(가슴샘, thymus)

Extranodal lymphoma(25%): 위(stomach), 장(창자, intestine), 유방(breast)

② **T세포(T cells): 흉선(가슴샘, thymus)**

B세포(B cells): Fabricus의 bursa

표 1 • 호지킨병 및 비호지킨 림프종의 필수 약물

약 물	종 양
· Adriamycin	· 림프종
· L-Asparaginase	· 혈병-급성 림프구성
· Bleomycin	· 호지킨병, Kaposi 육종-활동성
· Chlormethine	· 호지킨병
· 2-Chlorodeoxyadenosine	· 모발상세포 백혈병
· Cyclophosphamide	· 비호지킨 림프종, 유방, 유잉육종
· Cytarabine	· 백혈병-급성 림프구성/비림프구성 비호지킨 림프종
· Dacarbazine	· 호지킨 림프종
· Daunorubicin	· 백혈병-급성 비림프구성 또는 골수성
· Doxorubicin	· 호지킨병, 비호지킨 림프종, 골육종
· Mercaptopurine	· 백혈병, 급성 림프구성
· Methotrexate	· 백혈병, 급성 림프구성, 골육종
· Prednisone	· 호지킨병, 백혈병, 급성 림프구성, 다발성 골수종, 비호지킨 림프종
· Procarbazine	· 호지킨병
· Vinblastine	· 생식세포, 호지킨병, 카포시 육종-활동성
· Vincristine	· 호지킨병, 백혈병, 급성 림프구성, 신경아세포종

2.1 위암(Stomach cancer): 고형암(Solid tumor)

특징: 한국 사망원인 1위

- 1/3 예방, 1/3 조기진단 완치, 1/3 고식적 치료

원인: 45세 이상의 흡연 남자, 식습관, 가족력, 과거력 보유자

- 고농도 전리방사선 폭로 경험자

증상: 초기에는 무증상

- 상복부 통증, 팽만감, 허약, 구토, 상복부 덩어리 촉진, 위출혈, 부종, 체중감소, 복수(ascites)
- 호발부위: 위 유문(날문, pylorus)

병리: Adenocarcinoma(선암종) 90% → diffuse type

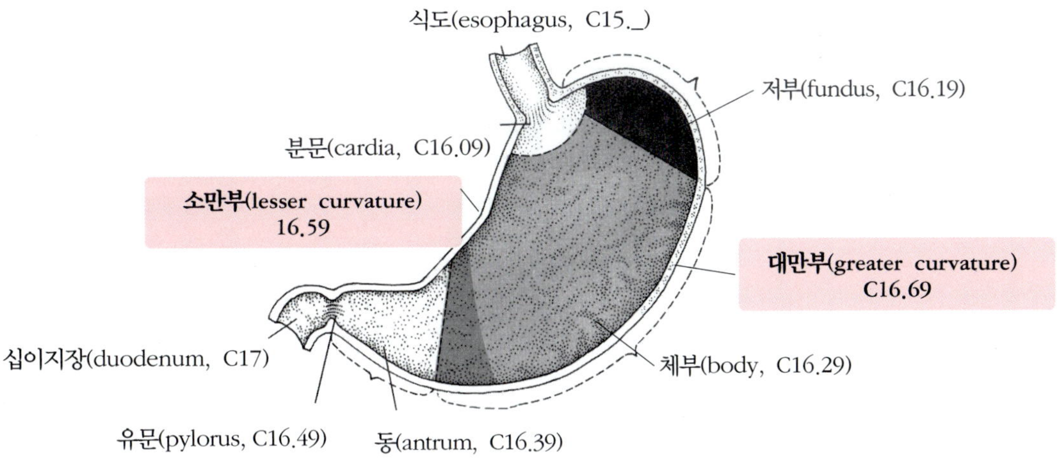

그림 1. 위(stomach)의 구조 및 질병분류(위암: C16._)

진 단

- 상부위장관조영술 Upper gastrointestinal series(UGI)
- 위내시경 Fiber gastroscopy(FGS)
- 조직생검(확진) Biopsy(Bx)
- 전산화 단층촬영술 Computed tomography(CT)
- 조기집단검진 Mass screening

치 료

- 초기 발견 시: 완치율 80%
- 장기 국한: 근치수술
- 전이: 화학요법, 방사선요법

중요 질병분류

- FGS(위내시경): 44.13
- FGS(위내시경) + Bx(생검): 44.14

2.2 조기암 및 진행암: 층(layer)의 깊이

점막(mucosa) ➡ 점막하(submucosa) ➡ 근육(muscle) ➡ 장막(serosa)
↓ ↓ 시작
조기암(early cancer) 진행암(advanced cancer)

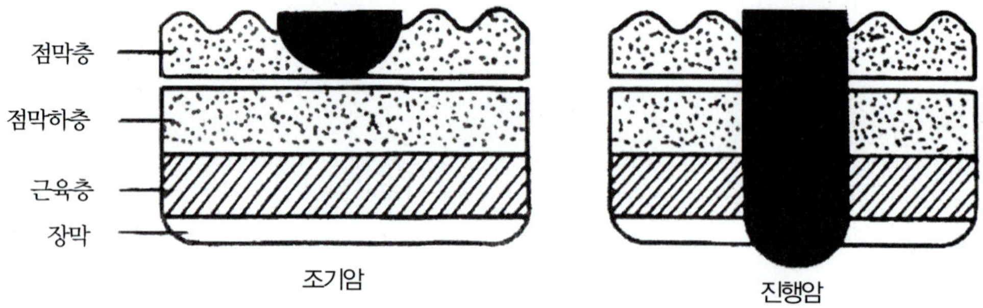

그림 2. 조기암과 진행암

2.3 수술요법

근치수술(Curative surgery): 완치 목적

- 위절제술(Gastrectomy): 위의 부분적 또는 완전 절제
  - Billroth I: gastroduodenostomy(남은 위와 십이지장 연결)
  - Billroth II: gastrojejunostomy(남은 위를 빈창자에 연결/주로 십이지장 궤양 시)
- 문합술(Anastomosis)
  - 측부의 통로로 두 개의 관을 연결
  - 2개의 다른 공간 또는 기관(organ) 사이에 외과적으로 형성된 개구부
    → 결장조루술(colostomy)

고식적 수술(Palliative surgery): 전이암 시 생명연장, 증상완화 목적

2.4 화학요법

▸ 일차적 화학요법(Primary chemotherapy)

−근치목적

▸ 유도 화학요법(Induction or Neoadjuvant chemotherapy)

−수술 전 암덩어리(mass)를 줄여 수술 가능 유도

▸ 부가적 화학요법(Adjuvant chemotherapy)

−수술 후 추가 시행

▸ 완화적 화학요법(Palliative chemotherapy)

−진행된 암의 증상완화

▸ 구제적 항암화학요법(Salvage chemotherapy)

−항암제 투여 후 재발 또는 효과가 없을 경우 부수적 시행

표 2 • 퇴원 시 약 처방

종 류	약 제
· Narcotic analgesics(마약성 진통제)	Mogadon
· Sedatives and hypnotics(진정제 및 수면제)	Codein phosphate
· Antacids(제산제)	Normo, Amphogel
· Digestives & enzymes(소화제)	Pancreon F
· Antispasmodics(진경제)	Buscopan

한국 암등록 조사서 주요 항목

① 번호: 병원지정번호(암등록본부 지정번호) ② 환자등록번호 ③ 주민등록번호

④ 직업: 경제기획원 직업분류표 ⑤ 초진년월일: "암"으로 처음 진단받은 날

⑥ 원발장기명: ICD-O-3판 → 원발장기가 2개 이상인 경우 각각 입력

⑦ 조직학적 진단명 : ‣ 조직학적 형태(Morphology) + 행태(Behavior) = M___/__

‣ 행태: /2 (정상소재암), /3 (악성+원발성)만 사용

⑧ 사망년월일 ⑨ 생존기간: 사망일-초진일 → 개월수 ⑩ 병기분류: stage

⑪ 암의 최종진단방법: 전이암 시 → M__/3 + (6번) 전이부위의 조직학적 검사

‣ 임상적 방법

− 검사 없이 임상만/임상검사/조직검사 없는 진단적 수술부검/특수 생화학적·면역학적 검사

‣ 현미경적 방법

− 세포학적·혈액학적/전이부위 조직검사/원발부위의 조직생검/조직검사 시행한 진단적 수술부검

⑫ 치료방법: 수술, 화학요법, 방사선요법, 면역요법, 기타

표 3 • 암의 화학약제 및 생물학적 제제

화학약제(Chemotherapeutic agents)	생물학적 제제(Biological agents)
• 알킬화약(Alkylating Agents)	• Colony-stimulating factors(CSFs)
Carmustine(BCNU)	Interferon
Cisplatin, carboplatin	Interleukins(IL-1, IL-2, IL-3)
Cyclophosphamide(Cytoxan)	Monoclonal antibodies
Melphalan(Alkeran)	
Nitrogen mustard	• 식물 유도체(Plant Derivatives)
Chlorambucil	Vinblastine sulfate(Velban)
	Vincristine sulfate(Oncovin)
• 항생제(Antibiotics)	VP-16(etoposide)
Actinomycin D	VM-26(teniposide)
Bleomycin sulfate	Taxol
Daunorubicin hydrochloride	
Doxorubicin hydrochloride(Adriamycin)	• 스테로이드
Idarubicin	Dexamethasone(Decadron)
Mitomycin C	Diethylstilbestrol(DES)
	Flutamide
• 항대사약(Antimetabolites)	Leuprolide
Cytosine arabinoside(ara-C)	Prednisone
5-flurouracil(5-FU)	Tamoxifen citrate
Methotrexate(MTX)	Testosterone
6-thioguanine(6-TG)	
Fludarabine	
Pentostatin	

차트 용어

· Conjunctiva	결막	· Dypspnea	호흡곤란	· Discharge	흐름/퇴원	· Divorce	이혼
· Lower back pain	하부 요통	· Neck stiffness	경부(목) 강직	· Obstruction	폐색	· Palpable	촉진
· Pea-size	땅콩 크기	· Palpable	촉진할 수 있는	· Palliative operation	고식적 수술	· Submandibular	하악밑/턱밑
· Supraclavicular	쇄골 위의	· Engogement	충혈(혈액의 축적에 의한 기관, 혈관 및 조직의 과잉충만)				

약 어	원 어	
Bx	Biopsy	생검
DAA	Discharge against advice	자의퇴원
FGS	Fiber gastroscopy	위내시경
LN	Lymph nodes	림프절
LROM	Limitation range of motion	운동범위 제한
OB	Occult blood	잠혈
UGI	Upper gastrointestinal series	상부위장관조영술

등록번호	111 35 67	성별 F
성명	이 천 운	
주민등록	701201－1234567	

입 퇴 원 기 록
Admission and Discharge Record

<table>
<tr><td colspan="4">주 소: 경기도 안양시 안양동 12－1</td></tr>
<tr><td colspan="4">출신지: 직 업: 전 화 :</td></tr>
<tr><td colspan="4">연고자성명: 백만수 관 계: 주 소: 전 화:</td></tr>
<tr><td>입원: 2017년 1 월 20 일 과 병동 호</td><td rowspan="3">전과</td><td colspan="2">20 년 월 일 과 병동 호</td></tr>
<tr><td>퇴원: 2017년 1 월 31 일 과 병동 호</td><td colspan="2">20 년 월 일 과 병동 호</td></tr>
<tr><td>재원일수:</td><td colspan="2">20 년 월 일 과 병동 호</td></tr>
<tr><td colspan="3">최종진단명</td><td>분 류 번 호</td></tr>
<tr><td colspan="3">주진단명 : Stomach adenocarcinoma</td><td></td></tr>
<tr><td colspan="3">기타진단명: Metastatic right supraclavicular LN</td><td></td></tr>
<tr><td colspan="3">Malignant lymphoma</td><td></td></tr>
<tr><td colspan="3"></td><td></td></tr>
<tr><td colspan="3"></td><td></td></tr>
<tr><td colspan="3"></td><td></td></tr>
<tr><td colspan="3">수술 및 처치명</td><td></td></tr>
<tr><td colspan="3">수술명 : Chemotherapy</td><td></td></tr>
<tr><td colspan="3">기타수술 및 주요검사: Abd U/S</td><td></td></tr>
<tr><td colspan="3">Mammography</td><td></td></tr>
<tr><td colspan="3">FGS with bx</td><td></td></tr>
<tr><td colspan="3">Rt. supraclavicular LN bx</td><td></td></tr>
<tr><td colspan="3"></td><td></td></tr>
<tr><td colspan="4">치료결과: 1. 완쾌 2. 경쾌 3. 호전안됨 4. 진단뿐 5. 가망없는 퇴원 6. 48시간내 사망 7. 48시간이후 사망</td></tr>
<tr><td colspan="4">퇴원형태: 1. 퇴원지시후 2. 자의퇴원 3. 탈원 4. 전원</td></tr>
<tr><td colspan="4">병원감염: 1. 수술후 2. 기타처치후 3. 비뇨기계 4. 호흡기계 5. 소화기계 6. 기타</td></tr>
<tr><td colspan="4">원사인 : 부검: 예, 아니오</td></tr>
<tr><td colspan="4">계속적 진료 계획</td></tr>
<tr><td colspan="4">없음·있음 (약속일 20 년 월 일 시)</td></tr>
<tr><td colspan="2">담당 전공의 서명: 박인황</td><td colspan="2">담당 전문의 서명: 민주지</td></tr>
<tr><td colspan="2">의무기록 완성: 20 년 월 일</td><td colspan="2">의무기록사 서명 :</td></tr>
</table>

등록번호	111 35 67	성별 F
성명	이 천 운	
주민등록	701201－1234567	

퇴 원 요 약
Discharge Summary

1. 진단명
2. 주소 및 진찰소견
3. 검사소견
4. 치료 및 효과
5. 향후 치료계획
6. 퇴원약
7. 서명

Final Dx: 1. Stomach ca.(adenocarcinoma, poorly differentiated)
2. Malignant lymphoma (Diffuse large B-cell type)

C.C: For chemotherapy
Lower back pain

P/Ex: Neck: a few pea－sized LN, bilateral mass

Lab. & X－ray Findings
CBC 6200 (DC 45－16－9－13－15) Hgb/Hct 13/38
ESR 50 Eosinophil leukocyte 1050/mm^3
Serum amylase 84 Serum K 5.3 Alkaline phosphatase 115
FBS 88 Stool OB (＋＋)
U/A: WNL
Chest P－A: Mild pleural thickening in left lower lobe
Abdomino－sonography: Known malignant lymphoma
No evidence of liver metastasis or stone
Rt. supraclavicular LN bx: Metastatic adenocarcinoma
FGS $\bar{c}$ bx: Adenocarcinoma of cardia, poorly differentiated

Therapeutic Procedures
1. CHOP with Bleomycin
2. Pain control
3. Antacids
4. Condition of discharge is not improved

Plan of Therapy and F/U
DAA because of economic difficulties

퇴 원 요 약

Discharge Medication and Signature

1. Codeine Phosphate	0.06	#3 tid p.o×7 days
Mogadon	1.0	
Norumo	2.0	
Pancreon F	6T	
Buscopan	3T	
2. Amphogel	210 cc	#3 tid. p.o×7 days

Park

등록번호	111 35 67	성별 F
성명	이 천 운	
주민등록	701201－1234567	

병 력 기 록
History

C.C : Lower back pain
Epigastric tenderness and palpable mass on epigastrium

P.I : 상기 48세 old female patient는 상기 C/C로 OPD를 경유하여 IM으로 본원에 들어왔다. 환자는 2014년 1월부터 Mal. lymphoma가 있었으며 RT와 Chemotx를 4번 받았고 5번째 chemo.를 위해 본원에 재입원하였다.

P.H : Tbc (－), DM (－), HTN (－), Febrile disease (－)
Malignant lymphoma ('14. 1) → chemo ＋ RT

F.H : N－S

P.H : divorced (2011)

ROS : General weakness (＋) Headache (＋)
Eyes: visual loss (－) discharge (－) pain (－)
Ears: discharge (－) pain (－)
Nose: discharge (＋) obstruction (＋)
Neck: sore throat (－) neck stiffness (－)
Cardiorespiratory : dyspnea (＋) chest pain (－)
palpitation (－) cough (＋) sputum (－) hemoptysis (－)
Gastrointestinal : epigastric tenderness (＋) anorexia (＋)
constipation (－) diarrhea (－)
nausea (＋) vomiting (－) melena (－)
Genitourinary : free
Extremities : free
Neuromuscular : lower back pain (＋)

Choi

등록번호	111 35 67	성별	F
성명	이 천 운		
주민등록	701201－1234567		

신체검진기록
Physical Examination

G/A : chronic ill looking appearance
Emaciated, pale

M/S : clear

H/N : Normocephaly
Palpable a few pea－sized lymph nodes on bilateral cervical lesion
No vein engorgement

Eyes : L/R (+/+) c̄ isocoria
Not icteric sclera
Not anemic conjunctiva

ENT : Nose discharge (+) Obstruction (+)
No pharyngeal injection
No hearing disturbance

Chest : Symmetric expansion RHB s̄ ⓜ
CBS s̄ ⓡ

Abdomen : Soft & flat
Slight distention & palpable mass on epigastrium
No palpable L/S/K
Epigastric tenderness

Extremities : No pitting edema
No LROM
Imp) Malignant lymphoma
R/O Recurrence in abdomen

Choi

등록번호	111 35 67 　　성별 F
성명	이 천 운
주민등록	701201－1234567

경 과 기 록
Progress Notes

1. 자세한 경과(특수검진, 처치, 수술, 전과 등의 사항 포함)를 기록할 것
2. 서명은 정확히, 알아보기 쉽게 할 것

	〈 Admission Note 〉	
1.20	See Intern note (Old chart review) admission date: 2014. 1. 11 discharge date: 2014. 1. 22 Dx : malignant lymphoma (submandibular LN biopsy), stage IV Tx : CHOP + Radiotherapy # Metoclopramide c̄ pain killing agent was given	Park
1.23	S : Upper abdominal fullness and lower back pain much subsided with pain killer agent. O : P/Ex － a few pea－sized LN were found in bilateral cervical region. Mammography － WNL P : 1. FGS c̄ bx 2. Abdominal sonography 3. LN biopsy	Park
1.24	S : Indigestion & Anorexia (+) Epigastric fullness & pain have much subsided. O : FGS c̄ bx was done It showed a large irregularly shaped ulcerating lesion on cardia of stomach P : Radiotherapy	Park
1.26	# Bleomycin was given	Park
1.27	S : Being well Abdominal discomfort has much improved Little back pain Reasonable oral intake # CHOP was bleomycin (anticancer chemotherapy) was given.	Park

경 과 기 록

일 자	내 용	서 명
1.28	FGS with biopsy finding: pathological dx : poorly differentiated, mucinous adenocarcinoma A : R/O Double primary cancer 1) Malignant lymphoma 2) Stomach ca P : LN biopsy GS consultation	
1.30	S : Lower back pain (+) Melena (−) O : Rt. supraclavicular LN biopsy was done under the local anesthesia in OR by GS doctor. P : 1) Palliative op. was recommended by GS doctor 2) GS transfer	
1.31	S : Patient refused palliative operation because of economic problem. She wanted DAA P : Discharge $\bar{c}$ medications	

등록번호	111 35 67	성별 F
성명	이 천 운	
주민등록	701201-1234567	

협의진단기록
Consultation Record

Request For Consultation To GS 강수부 선생님께

상기 환자는 2014년 1월 malignant lymphoma로 진단받고 radiotherapy와 cytotoxic chemotherapy를 받아 왔으며, FSG $\bar{c}$ bx 결과 stomach ca.로 나왔습니다. P/Ex상 bilateral cervical region에 a few pea-sized LN가 만져져 LN bx 의뢰드리오니 고진선처 부탁드립니다.

2017. 01. 29 — 민주지 / 박인황

Date Hour — Signature of Attending Physician

Report of Consultation

〈 Gs consultation report 〉

1/30 1. Rt. supraclavicular lymph node bx. was done under the local anesthesia in operating room
2. Findings: easily friable LN
3. Specimen was sent to pathology department.
4. Impression: Metastatic ca.

Recommend 〉 1) Palliative operation for stomach ca.
2) Transfer to our GS dept.

2017. 1. 31 — 강수부 M.D

Date Hour — Dr's signature

등록번호	111 35 67	성별 F
성명	이 천 운	
주민등록	701201 – 1234567	

병리학적 검사보고

Pathological Report

Accession No. S – 2885

Specimen received 2017. 1. 24

Organ and location of specimen

1. stomach
2.
3.

Sent by ________ M.D.

Clinical diagnosis

Malignant lymphoma, metastatic

Clinician: Jang/Min M.D.

Pathological findings and diagnosis

Gross description : Received in fresh consists of 2 pieces of gray white soft tissue measuring 0.3cm, each.
Entirely embedded.

Microscopic description : There is ulcerating & fibrosed mass on cardia of stomach

Pathological dx : stomach, cardia, endoscopic biopsy: mucinous adenocarcinoma poorly differentiated.

2017. 1. 28

Signature of Pathologist Seo M.D

등록번호	111 35 67	성별 F
성명	이 천 운	
주민등록	701201 − 1234567	

병리학적 검사보고

Pathological Report

Accession No. S − 2889

Specimen received 2017. 1. 30

Organ and location of specimen

1. Rt. supraclavicular LN
2.
3.

Sent by Kang M.D.

Clinical diagnosis

1) Malignant lymphoma
2) Stomach ca

Clinician: Han M.D.

Pathological findings and diagnosis

Gross : The specimens consist of several fragments of pinkish yellow soft tissue, measuring 0.1 ml in volume.
Entirely embedded.

Pathological Dx. : LN, supraclavicular, right, excision :
Metastatic adenocarcinoma, poorly differentiated
(diffuse large B-cell type)

Comment : Review of the previous endoscopic biopsy slides reveals the same as the present biopsy.

2017. 2. 3

Signature of Pathologist Kim M.D

〈이 천 운〉

★ 이천운 차트를 읽고 맞는 것에 O표 하시오.

1 악성 림프종에 대한 질병분류번호가 맞는 것은?

① C83.0 ② C83.3 ③ C83.5 ④ C83.9 ⑤ C85.1

2 상기 환자의 차트 내용이 맞게 기재된 것은?

① 악성 림프종이 위로 전이된 상태이다.
② 흉부 방사선 검사 결과 확인된 진단명의 분류번호는 J92.0이다.
③ 환자는 남편과 일시적으로 별거 중이다.
④ 고식적인 수술을 권했으나 환자는 경제적인 어려움으로 거절하였다.
⑤ 눈에 빛의 반사는 즉각적이었으며 결막에 충혈이 있었다.

3 주소(C.C.) 중 화학요법에 대한 분류번호가 맞는 것은?

① 99.25 ② Z51.1 ③ Z51.2 ④ Z51.5 ⑤ Z51.9

4 진료통계 내용 중 옳은 것은?

① 전과 건수: 1건 ② 협의진단 시행과: 흉부외과
③ 퇴원 시 결과: 사망 ④ 퇴원 시 형태: 퇴원지시 후
⑤ 위 조직검사: 1건

5 임상검사 결과가 옳게 기재된 것은?

① 한쪽 목부분에 완두콩만한 크기의 림프절 덩어리가 촉진되었다.
② 방사선 검사상 오른쪽 하엽 흉막에 짙게 나타났다.
③ 위암은 이번 입원기간 동안 새롭게 확인된 진단명이다.
④ 위내시경 생검결과 위의 분문에 염증성 병변의 불규칙한 모양이 나타났다.
⑤ 복부 초음파검사 결과 간의 전이 또는 돌이 발견되었다.

6 약물명 중 퇴원 시 처방된 것은?

① Mogadon ② Interleukins ③ Tamoxifen citrate ④ Diethylstilbestrol ⑤ Inhibace

7 위암에 대한 질병분류번호가 맞는 것은?

① C16.99, M8140/3 ② C78.8, M8460/3 ③ C16.09, M8480/3
④ C16.19, M8140/6 ⑤ C78.8, M8460/6

8 확인된 전이 부위의 질병분류번호가 맞는 것은?

① C78.6 ② C77.0 ③ C77.3 ④ C77.2 ⑤ C78.5

9 림프종에 대해 '한국 암등록 조사서' 작성 시 ICD-O에 대한 분류번호는?

① Stomach, unspecified, C16.99 ② Stomach, cardia, C16.09
③ Submandibular LN, C77.0 ④ Supraclavicular LN, C76.0
⑤ Stomach, metastasis, C78.8

10 입원기간 동안 받은 검사 및 치료에 대한 분류번호로 연결된 것은?

① 40.11, 44.14, 99.25 ② 44.11, 44.13, 99.25 ③ 40.3, 44.14, 99.25
④ 40.3, 44.13, 44.14 ⑤ 40.11, 44.14, 99.29

04 복부 대동맥류
Abdominal aortic aneurysm

1.1 동맥류(Aneurysm)

원 인: 죽상경화증(atherosclerosis)으로 동맥벽이 약해지거나 깨어짐에 따라 동맥이 부분적으로 넓어짐

증 상: 심장, 대동맥 또는 동맥의 벽이 이완되거나 돌출되어 나옴
그 안에 혈전이 생겨 깨어지면 embolism(색전증) 초래

발생 부위: 보통 대동맥에 발생

▶ **동맥류 파열(aneurysm rupture)**

- 동맥류의 위험성은 동맥벽이 바깥쪽으로 밀려나가, 점차 얇아지고 터질 수 있음

▶ **심실 동맥류(ventricular aneurysm)**

- Coronary atherosclerosis(관상 죽상경화증), myocardial infaction(심근경색증)의 합병증으로 발생

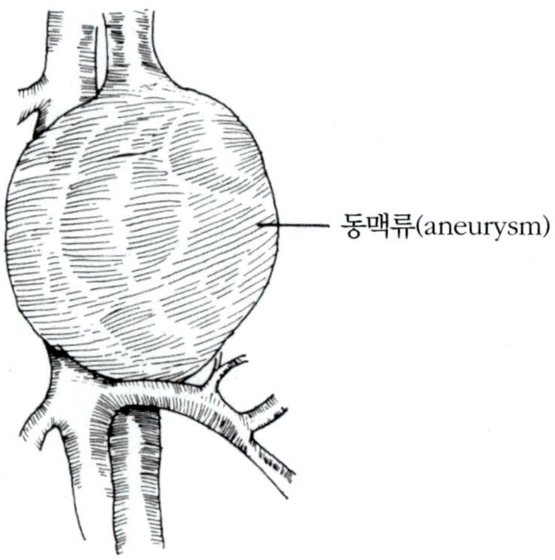

그림 1. 대동맥의 동맥류(Aneurysm of the aorta)

치 료

- 침범한 환자의 혈관, 부위, 환자건강에 달려 있음
- 뇌의 작은 동맥류: 작은 클립(clip)으로 혈관 폐색
- 큰 동맥의 동맥류(대동맥): 합성이식(synthetic graft)

1.2 골밀도 검사(Bone densitometry; BDM)

- 뼈의 치밀도 검사
- 골다공증을 진단하기 위해 시행

1.3 골다공증(Osteoporosis: 뼈의 치밀도 감소)

- 폐경기에 에스트로겐(estrogen)의 결핍 때문에 나이든 여성에게 발생률 높음
- 쉽게 골절(골반 등)되고, 키가 줄며, 척추후만증(kyphosis) 발생

치 료

- 에스트로겐 보상요법(estrogen replacement theraphy)
- 칼슘섭취 증가
- 매일 체중부하 운동프로그램 중요

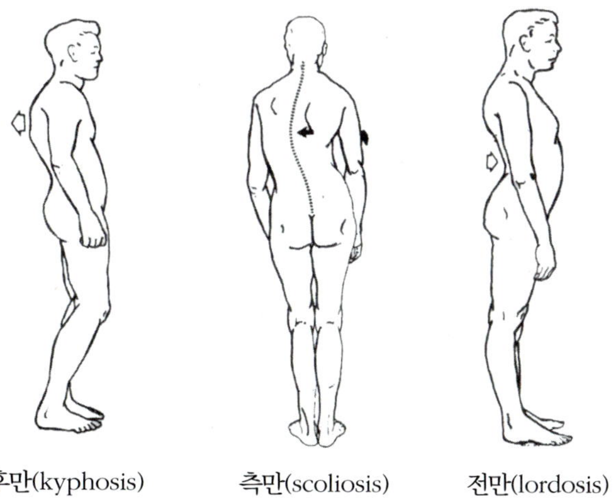

그림 2. 근골격 기형

혈압 강하제(Antihypertensive drugs)			
· Capoten	· Inderal	· Minipress	· Renitec

2.1 백혈병(Leukemia)

- 비정상 백혈구(white blood cells)의 과잉 생산
- 적혈구(red blood cell), 혈소판(platelets) 감소

증 상

- 빈혈, 호흡곤란, 감염, 출혈

원 인

- 불명, 방사선 조사, 감염, 약물 및 유전적 소인

치 료

- 항암제, 방사선치료

백혈병의 종류	의 미
· Myelogenous leukemia	**골수성 백혈병**
· Acute myelocytic leukemia(AML)	급성 골수성 백혈병
· Chronic myelocytic leukemia(CML)	만성 골수성 백혈병(=granulocytic)
· Lymphatic leukemia	**임파성 백혈병** ▸ 림프증식이 발생, 어린이에게 발병률 높음
· Acute lymphocytic leukemia(ALL)	급성 림프성 백혈병
· Chronic lymphocytic leukemia(CLL)	만성 림프성 백혈병
· Monocytic leukemia	**단구성 백혈병**
· Acute monocytic leukemia(AML)	급성 단핵구성 백혈병
· Chronic monocytic leukemia(CML)	만성 단핵구성 백혈병

2.2 추간판탈출(Herniation of intervertebral disc; HIVD)

원 인

▸ 추간원판(intervertebral disc)의 수핵(pulposus nucleus)이 척추관으로 이탈(HNP)

– 척수신경근 압박

증 상

▸ 허리 통증, 목 통증, 좌골신경통 발생

▸ 심한 경우 신경에 손상을 주기도 함

발생부위

▸ 가장 흔한 발생 부위

– L_4–L_5(요추/허리뼈 4-5번째), L_5–S_1(요추/허리뼈 5번째–천추/엉치뼈 1번째)

치 료

▸ 척추궁절제술(Laminectomy): 탈출된 수핵 제거

▸ 경피적 흡인 디스크절제술(Aspiration percutaneous diskectomy)

▸ 피부를 통해 관을 집어넣고 디스크 흡인(aspiration)

2.3 임상처치(Clinical procedures)

▸ 관절경 검사법(Arthroscopy)

– 내시경을 통해 관절의 내면을 시각적 검사

▸ 뼈스캔(Bone scan)

– 정맥주사로 방사선 인(radioactive phosphate)을 주입

– 뼈의 방사선 물질 흡수를 특수 스캐닝 기구로 측정

▸ 근전도검사(electromyography; EMG)

– 전기적 자극을 주고 근수축의 강도를 기록하는 과정

차트 용어

· Aggrevation	악화	· Fever	열	· Inguinal	서혜부의	· Replacement	교체
· Resection	절제술	· Trauma	외상	· Thrombus	혈전	· Weight loss	체중감소

약 어	원 어	
A/N/V/D/C	Anorexia, nausea, vomiting, diarrhea, constipation	식욕부진, 오심, 구토, 설사, 변비
AJ	Ankle jerk	발목반사
AML	Acute myelogenous leukemia	급성 골수성 백혈병
BM	Bone marrow	골수
BDM	Bone densitometry	골밀도 검사
DOE	Dyspnea on exertion	노력성 호흡곤란
DSA	Digital subtraction angiography	계수 공제 혈관조영술
DTR	Deep tendon reflex	심부건 반사
FFP	Fresh frozen plasma	신선 냉동 혈장
HNP	Herniated nucleus pulposus	수핵 탈출
5 DW	5% dextrose (in water) injection	5% 포도당 수용액 주입
GW	General ward	일반병동
KJ	Knee jerk	무릎반사
LBP	Low blood pressure	저혈압
L_4-L_5	Lumbar vertebrae	요추(허리뼈) 4-5번째
L_5-S_1	Lumbar vertebrae - Sacrum	요추(허리뼈) 5번째-천추(엉치뼈) 1번째
LE	Lower extremity	하지
LN	Lymph nodes	림프절
LSK	Liver, spleen, kidney	간, 비장(지라), 신장
PT	Physical therapy	물리치료
PVM	Paravertebral muscle	척추 방외근후
RT	Rebound tenderness	반사통
SLR	Straight leg raising	직하지 거상
T	Tenderness ‣ T/RT (+/−): 압통 있음/반사통 없음	압통
T.P.R.	Temperature, pulse, respirations ‣ 간호사 작성 = vital sign(V/S) 활력증후	체온, 맥박, 호흡
WB	Whole blood	전혈

등록번호	150 99 88	성별 F
성명	윤 달 인	
주민등록	681113－1234567	

입 퇴 원 기 록

Admission and Discharge Record

<table>
<tr><td colspan="4">주 소:</td></tr>
<tr><td colspan="4">출신지: 직 업: 전 화 :</td></tr>
<tr><td colspan="4">연고자성명: 이주인 관 계: 주 소: 전 화:</td></tr>
<tr><td>입원: 2017년 8 월 29 일 과 병동 호</td><td rowspan="3">전과</td><td colspan="2">2017 년 9 월 1 일 CS과 병동 호</td></tr>
<tr><td>퇴원: 2017 년 월 일 과 병동 호</td><td colspan="2">2017 년 월 일 과 병동 호</td></tr>
<tr><td>재원일수:</td><td colspan="2">2017 년 월 일 과 병동 호</td></tr>
<tr><td colspan="3">최종진단명</td><td>분 류 번 호</td></tr>
<tr><td colspan="3">주진단명 : Abdominal aortic aneurysm</td><td></td></tr>
<tr><td colspan="3">(Intrarenal saccular)</td><td></td></tr>
<tr><td colspan="3">기타진단명: Erythema nodosum</td><td></td></tr>
<tr><td colspan="3"></td><td></td></tr>
<tr><td colspan="3"></td><td></td></tr>
<tr><td colspan="3">수술 및 처치명</td><td></td></tr>
<tr><td colspan="3">수술명: Resection & Graft replacement</td><td></td></tr>
<tr><td colspan="3">(Hemashied 16)</td><td></td></tr>
<tr><td colspan="3"></td><td></td></tr>
<tr><td colspan="3">기타수술 및 주요검사:</td><td></td></tr>
<tr><td colspan="3"></td><td></td></tr>
<tr><td colspan="3"></td><td></td></tr>
<tr><td colspan="3"></td><td></td></tr>
<tr><td colspan="4">치료결과: 1. 완쾌 2. 경쾌 3. 호전안됨 4. 진단뿐 5. 가망없는 퇴원 6. 48시간내 사망 7. 48시간이후 사망</td></tr>
<tr><td colspan="4">퇴원형태: 1. 퇴원지시후 2. 자의퇴원 3. 탈원 4. 전원</td></tr>
<tr><td colspan="4">병원감염: 1. 수술후 2. 기타처치후 3. 비뇨기계 4. 호흡기계 5. 소화기계 6. 기타</td></tr>
<tr><td colspan="4">원사인 : 부검: 예, 아니오</td></tr>
<tr><td colspan="4">계속적 진료 계획</td></tr>
<tr><td colspan="4">☐없음 ☑있음 (약속일 년 월 일 시)</td></tr>
<tr><td colspan="2">담당 전공의 서명: 윤명석</td><td colspan="2">담당 전문의 서명: 이주명</td></tr>
<tr><td colspan="2">의무기록 완성: 2017 년 10 월 8 일</td><td colspan="2">의무기록사 서명: 양주자</td></tr>
</table>

등록번호	150 99 88	성별 F
성명	윤 달 인	
주민등록	681113 – 1234567	

퇴 원 요 약
Discharge Summary

Final diagnosis : Abd. aortic aneurysm (Intrarenal saccular)
Erythema nodosum

PI : 약 5개월 전부터 LBP developed.
PE : V/S 110/70 – 88 – 20 – 36.8°C

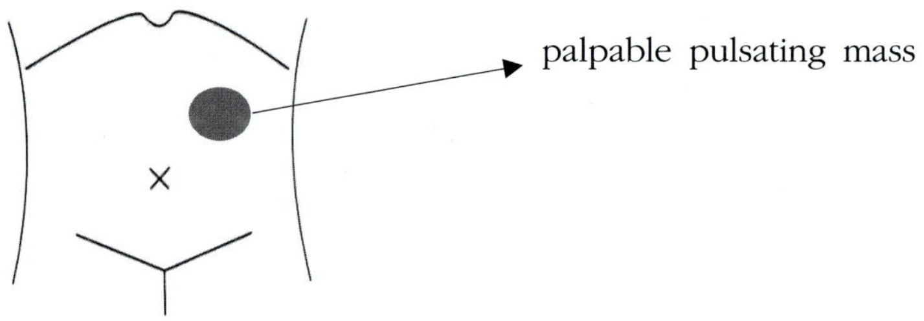

Abd CT (17. 9. 1)

1. 2.0 x 1.5 x 3.0cm sized saccular aortic aneurysm involves the ant. wall of abd. aorta at the level of Lt. lower renal a.
2. Mural thrombus (1.6cm in maximum thickness)

Aortogram (17. 9. 4)

Op : 17. 9. 7
Resection & Graft replacement (Hemashield 16mm)

17. 9. 11 L – tube remove
9. 18 Op wound clear: stich out
17. 9. 23 Discharge $\bar{c}$ med x 1wks
capoten 25mg p.o $\bar{c}$ 8h

Yoon

등록번호	150 99 88	성별 F
성명	윤 달 인	
주민등록	681113－1234567	

병 력 기 록

History

C.C : 1. LBP
2. Abd. mass: onset ┌remote: 5 Mo ago
└recente: 10 days ago

PI : 특별한 Trauma 없이 내원 5개월 전부터 LBP 있어 L/C에서 HNP Dx하에 conservative Tx해오던 중 최근 내원 10일 전부터 거동이 불편할 정도로 LBP aggrevation되어 OPD 통해 Adm.

PHx : TBC (－) DM (－) HBP (－) hepatitis (－)

FHx : 남편이 BM biopsy상에서 AML 진단받고 항암제 투여 중에 있음
모친은 심인성 위궤양으로 투약치료 중임

ROS : fever/chill (－ / －)
A/N/V/D/C (＋/＋/－/－/－)
Wt. loss: more than 1－2kg
General weakness (＋)

PEx : G/A : ch ill－looking app.
HEENT : anicteric sclera
not anemic conj.
Chest : RHB $\bar{s}$ ⓜ
CBS $\bar{s}$ ⓡ
Abd : soft & flat
palpable mass on LUQ
T/RT (＋/－)
Back & Ext : tenderness on $L_4－_5$, $L_5－S_1$ area
DTR : K/J (＋＋/＋＋)
A/J (＋＋/＋＋)

Imp) 1. Osteoporosis L－spine
2. R/O metastatic tumor of spine

Seo

등록번호	150 99 88	성별 F
성명	윤 달 인	
주민등록	681113－1234567	

경 과 기 록
Progress Notes

일 자	내 용	서 명
8.29	〈 Admission Note 〉 C.C : 1) LBP 2) Abdominal mass onse t: remote : 5months ago (LUQ) recent : 10days ago PI : 상기 환자는 별다른 trauma Hx 없이 약 5개월 전부터 LBP이 develop되어 L/C에서 X－ray check 후 HNP L_4 Dx하에 PT 및 po medication으로 치료 받았음. 그 뒤 intermittent back pain이 있어 약 1개월 전 L/C에서 다시 injection으로 치료받았음. 최근 약 10일 전부터 거동이 불편할 정도로 back pain이 심해져 OPD 통해 further evaluation위해 adm. # back pain : resting, motion 시에 차도 없이 지속적 pain 있고 back pain으로 잠을 자기가 힘들 정도임. # 현재 menstruation 중 PHx : Tb(－) DM(－) HBP(－) hepatitis(－) ROS : fever/chill (－/－) cough/sputum (－/－) A/N/V/D/C (＋/＋/－/－/＋) Wt loss (＋) : 1－2kg than 금년 봄 Indigestion(＋) General weakness (＋) Height : 161cm wt : 53.2kg P/Ex : V/S 110/70 －88 －20 －36.8 GA chr. ill app. HEENT not icteric not anemic no palpable LN Chest RH $\bar{s}$ ⓜ CBS $\bar{s}$ ⓡ	

경 과 기 록

일 자	내 용	서 명
	Abd. 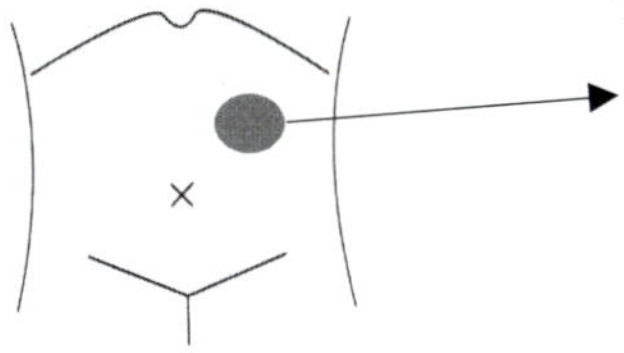 T/RT (+/−) ▶ palpable mass (+) not palpable L/S/K normoactive BS 〈 Back & lower Ext 〉 Maxicautery wound (3군데) at L_4-_5 bilat. PVMS : moderate ~ severe tenderness (+) on L_4-_5 L_5-S_1 area DTR : KJ (++/++) AJ (++/++) motor : intact sensory SLR : 90°/ 90° Lasegue (− / −) Path. reflex : Ankle clonus (−/−) babinski sg (−/−) multiple coin−sized. erythematous skin lesions on both legs esp. med. side 1~2군데 pustule (+) not palpable inguinal LN Ⓑ X−ray 1) L−S spine AP view: psoas buldging (−) ·normal axis ·clawing spur upper end plate L_4 Lt. & L_5 Rt. 2) L−S spine lat view ·saville classification상 Grade II의 osteoporosis ·L_4-_5 hypermobile ·L_4-_5, L_5-S_1, inter disc space에 convex scalloping (+) ·hypermobile L_4-_5 3) L−S spine both oblique : hypertrophy (+) on facet joint esp. L_4, L_5	

경 과 기 록

일 자	내 용	서 명
	·Problem list 1) back pain continuous 2) anorexia / nausea 3) abd. mass & tenderness 4) osteoporosis 심한 양상 특히 age에 비해 d/t malabsorption Dx 1) osteoporosis L－spine 2) R/O metastatic tumor of spine esp. G－I origin 3) abdominal mass R/O Gastric cancer Plan 1. B. scan d/t bone metastasis 2. BMD L－spine d/t osteoporosis 3. Abd. sonogram & GFS d/t R/O gastric ca. 4. if necessary L － spine MRI Abd － pelvic CT	*Park*
'17.9.1.	〈 Transfer in Note 〉 CC : LBP onset : remote : 5 months ago recent : 10 days ago PI : 상기 F/50 pt는 15년 9월 12일 Both L/E, below the knee, pain & swelling maculopapular rash로 본원 OS 방문하여 medication 처방받고 특별한 Tx 없이 지내시다 16년 가을부터 다시 갑자기 다리가 붓기 시작하여 걷기가 힘들 정도였으나 붓기가 점차 가라앉으면서 17년 3월경 처음엔 mild하게 양쪽 엉치 부위가 아파서 홍성의원에 들러 진통주사제와 po medication으로 증상이 완화되어 지내시다 다시 증상이 나타나며 점점 심해져 동네 사람들의 말을 듣고 local clinic을 다니며 L_{4-5} HNP 또는 vertebra의 곡선이 없어서 아프다는 말을 듣고 진통주사제, massage 등으로 지내시다 괜찮은 듯하여 15일 정도 Tx없이 지냈는데 내원 10일전 꼼짝하기 싫을 정도로 LBP이 더 심하게 develop되어 남편과 의논 후 본원 OS 방문	

경 과 기 록

일 자	내 용	서 명

'17.9.1

PHx 15년 9월 12일

OS : pain & swelling on both L/E below the knee

Derma : multiple erythema tender nodule

Uro : frequency nocturia

pul Tb (−) DM(−) HBP(−) Hepatitis (−)

FHx

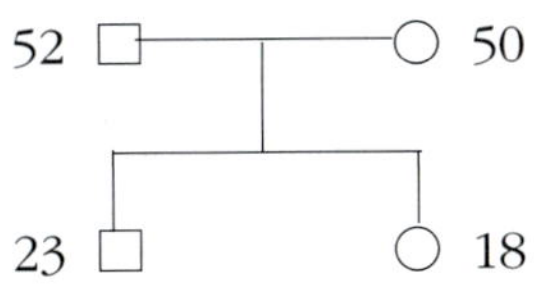

ROS : Ear Discharge (−) Dizziness (+): intermittent

A/N/V/D/C: (−/+/−/−/−): pain 있을 시

Dyspnea / cyanosis DOE (−)

Dysuria / Hematuria (−/−)

Headache (+): pain 있을 시

Fever/chill (+/−): pain 있을 시

PEx V/S 130/70 − 90 − 20 − 36.2°C

GA alert M/S

chr. ill looking app.

HEENT Not anemic conj

Anicteric sclera

No LAP.

Chest CBS $\bar{s}$ ⓡ

RHB $\bar{s}$ ⓜ

Abd

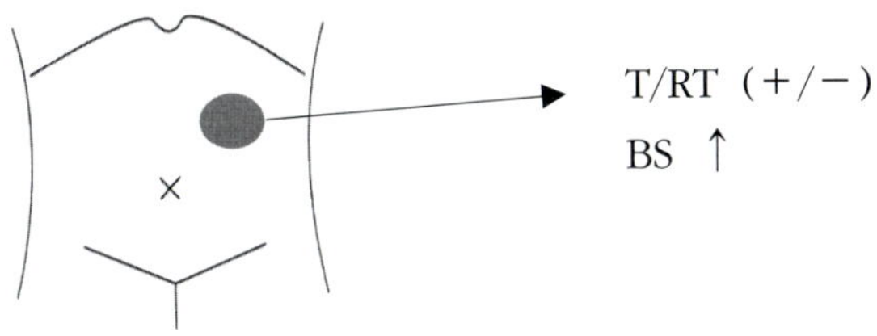

No palpable mass

B/ext. G−F

No pitting edema

Lab CBC 11.7−35−7000

é 138 − 4.1 − 107 BUN/Cr 1/0.8

Study US small saccular aortic aneurysm $\bar{c}$ mural thrombus

경 과 기 록

일 자	내 용	서 명
9.1	CT cardiac echo GFS superficial chronic gastritis imp) Abd. aortic aneurysm	*Choi*
	Abd CT 1. 2.0 x 1.5 x 3.0cm sized saccular aortic aneurysm involving the ant. wall of abdominal aorta at the level of left lower renal artery 2. Mural thrombus (1.6cm in maximum thickness) surrounds aortic aneurysm with no paraaorta & retroperitoneal hemorrhage 3. Hepatic cyst	
9.4	Aortogram	*Choi*
9.6	〈 ICU로 transfer하여 내일 Op 예정으로 Anti loading (R/O mycotic aneurysm 위해서) Teicoplain 400mg + 5% D/W 20cc IV Ceradolan 1.5gm + 5% D/W 20cc IV GN 80gm + 5% D/W 20cc HBP medication for subnormal BP Adalat 10mg po $\bar{q}$ 8h Widal test: negative	*Choi*
9.7	Op: Resection & Graft replacement (Hemashied 16mm) Post op CBC: 11.8 − 35 − 10100 ele: 133 − 33 − 109 BUN/cr: 6−1.2 G/U: 109 UA $\bar{c}$ ⓜ: protein + 1 Glu + 1 Op. field에서 W/B 1030 ┐ FFP 500 │ transfusion pentaspan 500 ┘ Post op로 CVP: 4 check V/S: 100/70 − 80 − 35 W/B: Remain 220 transfusion Post op로 volume expender 및 bleeding control 목적으로 FFP 10 ⓟ T/F하여 intake 4327/3777 output	*Yoon*

경 과 기 록

일 자	내 용	서 명
9.8	Dopa: 3μg/kg/min Niprile: D/C Anti: Teicoplain Ceradolan GM CBC: 11.3－34－10700 ele: 131－5.2－59 BUN/Cr: 6－0.6	
9.11	L－tube remove Dopa: D/C PT: 100% Blood culture: No growth 5days	
9.12	Transfer to G.W.	
9.13	V/S 150/90 － 70 － 20－ 36.8 Anti － HBP med. Adalat 10mg p.o $\bar{q}$ 8h	
9.14	V/S: 150/100 － 130/80	
9.15	Adalat 20mg po $\bar{q}$ 8h로 변경	
9.17	Anti → D/C	
9.18	Op. wound: stich out	*Yoon*
9.19	High fever(38.5°C) Facial flushing 있어 Adalat 20mg p.o $\bar{q}$ 8h를 Capoten 25mg po $\bar{q}$ 8h로 변경	
9.23	Discharge $\bar{c}$ med for 1wks Capoten 25mg po $\bar{q}$ 8h	*Yoon*

등록번호	150 99 88	성별 F
성명	윤 달 인	
주민등록	681113－1234567	

협의진단기록
Consultation Record

Request For Consultation To

Summary of Present Finding 피부과 황달군 선생님께

LBP을 주소로 내원한 환자입니다.
손등 및 lower ext에 rash 및 pustule이 있습니다.
evaluation 및 management 부탁드립니다.

Date 2017. 8. 30 Signature 김민오/고구만

Report of Consultation

Opinion and Recommendation

Papulo－nodule $\bar{c}$ central vesicle on U/E
purplish patch on L/E 2 years/2 days ago
'15 Erythema nodosum으로 치료
Itching
A) R/O Prurigo
Insect bite
$\bar{c}$ known E. nodosum
Rec) Cydraxine ($\frac{1}{2}$Ⓣ #3 p.o)
Esperson oint apply (tid)] thank you

Date 2017. 8. 30 Signature 황달군

등록번호	150 99 88	성별 F
성명	윤 달 인	
주민등록	681113 - 1234567	

협의진단기록

Consultation Record

Request For Consultation To

Summary of Present Finding 방사선과 이준구 선생님께

50세된 여자 환자로 abominal aorta에 saccular aneurysm이 있습니다.
DSA 부탁드립니다.
감사합니다.

Date 2017. 9. 2 Signature 안준후/한기준

Report of Consultation

Opinion and Recommendation

Dept. of Radiology

1. check chart & x - ray review
2. 실시일 : 2017. 9. 4 PM - on call
   DSA room
3. pre - angio order 참조하십시오.

Date 2017. 9. 5 Signature 이준구/양동추

등록번호	150 99 88	성별 F
성명	윤 달 인	
주민등록	681113-1234567	

위내시경 차트

Gastroscopy Chart

Name: 주어순 Sex: F Age: 50 Chart No. 1509988

Requested Dr. 전구주 Dept. OS Date: '17.8.31

1. Chief complaints and present illness

2. Radiological findings (Upper G.I Series)

3. Endoscopic findings (Endoscopic No. ________)

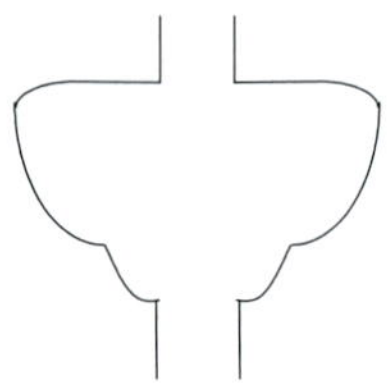

Photo. [+ ( ) / − ( )] Previous exam.________________________

Esophagus
Duodenum WNL

Stomach showed hyperemic patches on the antrum, body, and fundus

Impression : Superficial chronic gastritis

4. Histological findings : Slide. [+ ( ) / − ( )]

5. Remarks

Examined by Dr. 선두장

등록번호	150 99 88	성별	F
성명	윤 달 인		
주민등록	681113－1234567		

진단방사선처방전

Diagnostic Radiology Report

☑ Ambulatory ☐ X－ray ☐ Portable
☐ C－T ☐ Emergency ☐ U－S
☐ R－I ☐ New ☑ Old ☑ Others

환자연령	세	병 실	호		
방사선사		촬 영 일	년 월 일	과거촬영	유 무

Part & Type of Examination

BDM (예약) (Lumbar)

Findings

Bone mineral densitometry

The bone mineral density of L_2-L_4 is 1.008 g/cm^2 (90% for young adult and 91% for her age, normal range for both)

W. T. Lee

등록번호	150 99 88	성별	F
성명	윤 달 인		
주민등록	681113－1234567		

진단방사선 처방전

Diagnostic Radiology Report

☑ Ambulatory ☐ X－ray ☐ Portable
☐ C－T ☐ Emergency ☐ U－S
☐ R－I ☐ New ☑ Old ☑ Others

환자연령	세	병 실	호			
방사선사		촬 영 일	년 월 일	과거촬영	유 무	

Part & Type of Examination

Abd sono 예약

History & Clinical Findings

Palpable tender M.

GFS : superf. gastritis

Findings

A 2.0 x 1.5 x 2.2cm sized fluid sac is connected with the anterior wall of abdominal aorta by narrow neck.

This sac is surrounded by thickened wall (maximum thickness: 1.6cm) which is composed with inner hyperechoic and outer hypoechoic rims.

This sac is located just below the level of right renal artery (RRA).

SMA and celiac artery are intact.

On the doppler sonogram, whirling appeared color flow and abnormal pulsating doppler signal are noted in the lumen of this sac.

Liver is intact. Extrahepatic bile duct and MPV are not dilated.

Gallbladder is normal. Pancreas is intact.

Both kidneys are not remarkable. Splenic size is not enlarged.

No fluid is noted in peritoneal cavity.

Imp : 1. A small saccular aortic aneurysm with mural thrombus involving the anterior wall of abdominal aorta just below the level of RRA.
R/O Samll amount of periaortic hematoma.
2. Intact RRA, SMA and celiac artery.
3. Left renal artery cannot be evaluated.

Rec : Abdominal CT for further evaluation of LRA and the possibility of periaortic hemorrhage.

T. U. Kim/H. U. Seo

등록번호	150 99 88	성별 F
성명	윤 달 인	
주민등록	681113－1234567	

진단방사선 처방전

Diagnostic Radiology Report

☐ Ambulatory ☐ X－ray ☐ Portable
☑ C－T ☑ Emergency ☐ U－S
☐ R－I ☐ New ☑ Old ☐ Others

환자연령	세	병 실	호			
방사선사		촬 영 일	년 월 일	과거촬영	유 무	

Part & Type of Examination

Abd CT $\bar{c}$ Enhanced

History & Clinical Findings

R/O Abd. Aneurysm

Findings

Abdominal CT (Sep. 1. '17)

A 2.0 x 1.5 x 3.0cm sized saccular aneurysm involves the anterior wall of abdominal aorta at the level of left lower renal artery with no involvement of this left renal artery.

Mural thrombus(1.6cm in maximum thickness) surrounds the entire this saccular aneurysm with no periaortic hematoma.

Right renal artery is above this aneurysm and completely intact. Both kidneys show good usually nephrogram with no defect area of nephrogram.

Celiac artery and SMA are intact.

Liver, GB, pancreas and spleen are not remarkable except a minute cyst at S7 of liver.

Imp :
1. A 2.0 x 1.5 x 3.0cm sized saccular aortic aneurysm involving the anterior wall of abdominal aorta at the level of left lower renal artery.
2. Right renal artery and left renal artery (probable double left renal arteries) are preserved, although the left lower renal artery is at the level of aortic aneurysm.
3. Mural thrombus (1.6cm in maximum thickness) surrounds aortic aneurysm with no paraaortic and retroperitoneal hemorrhage.
4. A minute benign hepatic cyst at S7
5. Otherwise unremarkable on abdominal CT

W. B. Kim/I. H. Park

등록번호	150 99 88	성별 F
성명	윤 달 인	
주민등록	681113－1234567	

체온 · 맥박 · 호흡기록
T.P.R Sheet

ar 2017. 8	8/30		8/31		9/1		9/2		9/18		9/19	
Hosp. Days	HD #1		HD #4		HD #5		HD #6		HD #22		HD #23	
Op. Days												
Special medication												
Hour	AM	7PM	AM	2PM	6AM	1PM	AM	1PM	AM	2AM	5PM	2AM
R P T 190 41 170 40 150 39 130 38 60 110 37 T 50 90 36 P 40 70 35 30 50 34 20 R 10	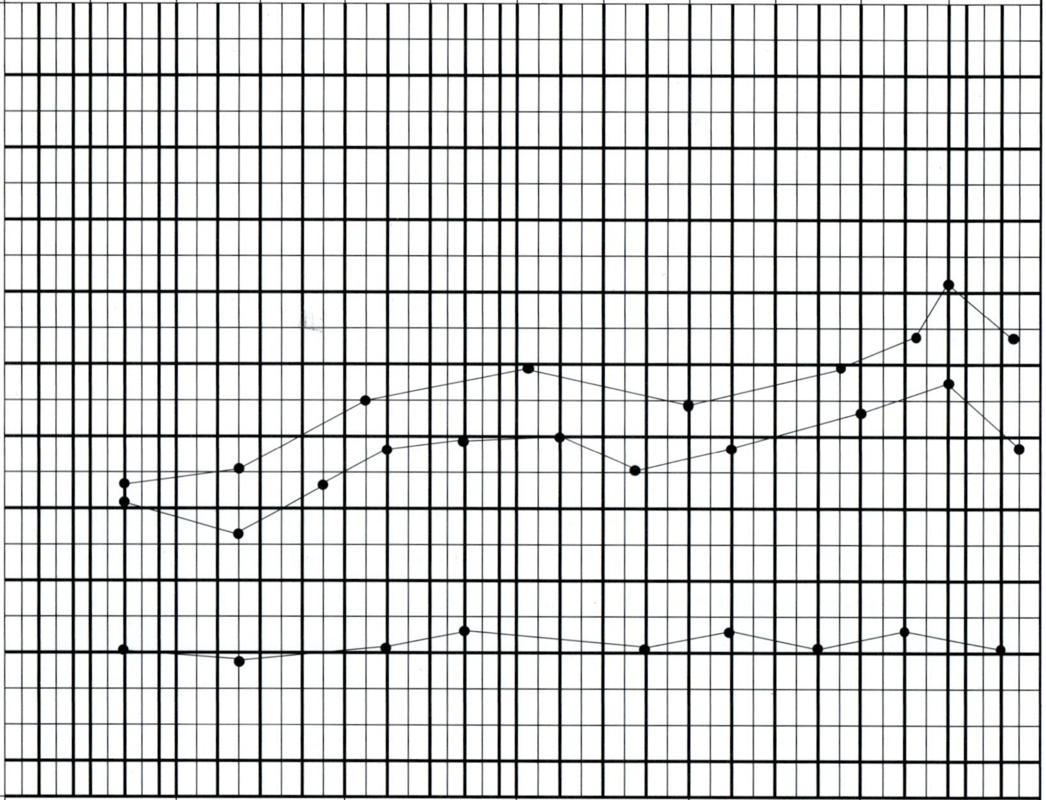											
Diet	NPO		SD		SD		SD		SD		RD	
Stool												
Urine												
Measurements Wt.	53.2kg		54.2kg		54.9kg		54.9kg		55.2kg		Unable	
Measurements Ht.	161cm										for weakness	
Measurements												
Other												

Head Nurse 양탁순 Resident Doctor

T.P.R

〈윤 달 인〉

★ 윤달인 차트를 읽고 맞는 것에 ○표 하시오.

1 입원과 → 퇴원과 → 중환자실의 재원일수 순서가 맞게 짝지어진 것은?
① 흉부외과 3일 – 정형외과 25일 – 중환자실 6일
② 흉부외과 2일 – 정형외과 23일 – 중환자실 5일
③ 정형외과 3일 – 흉부외과 22일 – 중환자실 6일
④ 정형외과 2일 – 흉부외과 23일 – 중환자실 5일
⑤ 정형외과 2일 – 정형외과 22일 – 중환자실 6일

2 상기 환자의 진단명 분류번호는?
① I72.5 ② I71.4 ③ I71.09 ④ I71.3 ⑤ I72.9

3 혈압조절을 위한 치료제로 사용한 약제는?
① Capoten ② Adalat ③ Dopa ④ Ciproby ⑤ Ronaben

4 가족력에 대한 분류번호로 맞게 짝지어진 것은?
① M9180/3, K25.91 ② 99.25, K25.91, F54 ③ C96.9, K25.31, F54
④ M9180/3, F59 ⑤ 99.25, K25.71, F59

5 Liver의 상태를 분류한 것 중 맞는 것은?
① R19.0 ② I21.9 ③ K76.8 ④ W.N.L ⑤ K75.9

6 피부과 진단 및 내시경 결과를 분류하면?
① A18.4, K29.3 ② L28.2, K29.3 ③ L52, C16.99
④ T14.0, K29.7 ⑤ L28.2, K29.0

7 BDM을 설명한 것 중 맞게 기재한 것은?
① 내시경을 통해 관절의 내면 검사
② 정맥주사로 방사선 인을 주입하고 뼈의 방사성 물질 흡수를 특수 스캐닝 기구로 측정
③ 전기적 자극을 주고 근수축의 강도 기록
④ 골밀도 검사로서 골다공증을 진단하는 데 사용
⑤ 피부를 통해 관을 집어넣고 디스크 흡인

8 상기환자의 수술분류번호가 옳은 것은?
① 35.22 ② 39.58 ③ 38.44 ④ 35.21 ⑤ 38.42

9 상기 환자의 차트 내용과 다른 것은?
① 환자는 본원에 처음 오는 신환이다.
② 체중이 1~2kg 이상 감소하였다.
③ 요추(허리뼈)수핵탈출증을 진단받고 치료받은 적이 있다.
④ 서혜부 임파선은 만져지지 않는다.
⑤ 요추 4-5번째, 천추 1번째에 압통이 있었다.

10 고열이 나타나기 시작한 날짜는 언제인가?
① 8월 30일 ② 8월 31일 ③ 9월 18일 ④ 9월 19일 ⑤ 9월 2일

05 간 전이 동반 직장암
Rectal cancer with liver metastasis

음식물 경로		Small intestine 소장/작은창자		Large intesine 대장/큰창자
1. Oral cavity 구강 2. Pharynx 인두 3. Esophagus 식도 4. Stomach 위	➡	5. Duodenum 십이지장 6. Jejunum 공장(빈창자) 7. Ileum 회장	➡	8. Cecum 맹장(막창자) 9. Ascending colon 상행(오름)결장 10. Transverse colon 횡행(가로)결장 11. Descending colon 하행(내림)결장 12. Sigmoid colon S상(구불)결장 13. Rectum 직장

그림 1. 음식물의 위장관계(digestive tract) 경로(1→13번 순서)

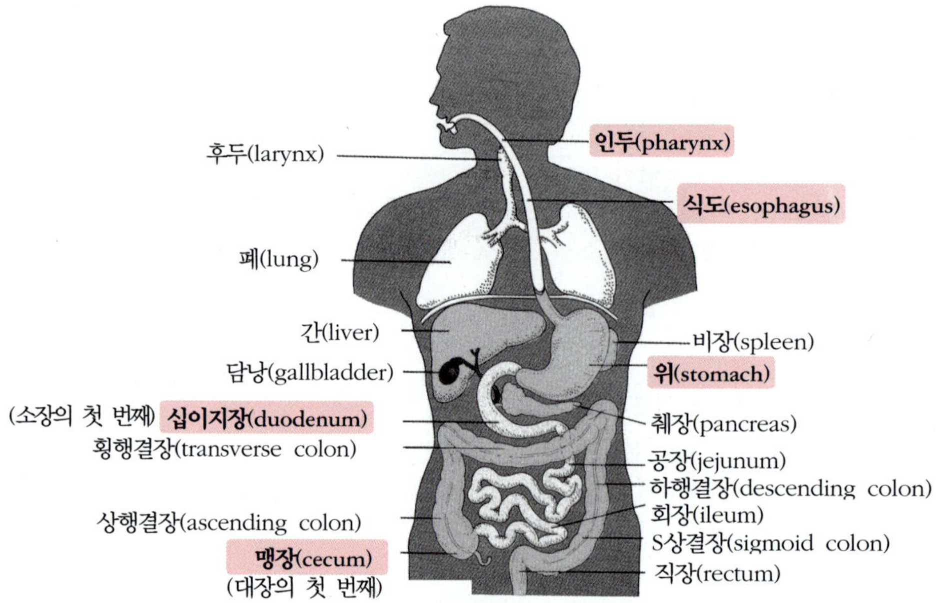

그림 2. 소화기관(gastrointestinal tract)

1.1 직장암

빈 도

- 대장암 발생률: 직장(54%) > S상결장(23%) > 맹장(12%) > 횡행결장(8%) > 하행결장(3%)
- 대부분 adenocarcinoma(선암종)

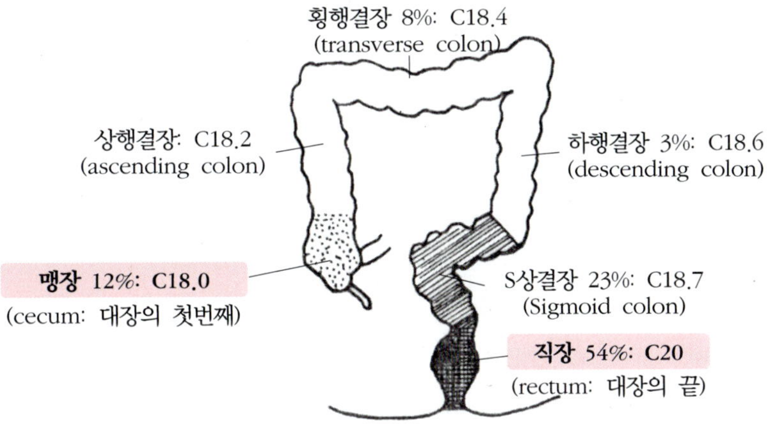

그림 3. 대장암 발생률 및 질병분류: C18._ (직장만 C20)

증 상

- 직장출혈, 혈변, 식욕부진, 빈혈, 동통, 장 습관 변화, 장폐색, 체중감소, 오심, 구토

원 인

- 궤양성 대장염, 크론병(Crohn disease): 10년 이후
- 약 10% 유전적 요인: 가족력(family history)
- 대장 직장암의 과거력, 대장 선종, 가족성 폴립증(polyposis)
- 저섬유소 식이, 고지방 음식 및 고정제된 음식(high-refined foods)과 관련

진 단

- 직장수지검사(rectal digital examination): 항문에 손가락 집어넣어 촉진
- 대변 잠혈검사(guaiac examination): 위장출혈 유무
- CEA(carcinoembryonic antigen): 대장암 발생 시 수치 상승 → 정상치: 5.0ng/ml 이하
- 직장경검사(proctoscopic examination): 50세 이상 성인
- 유연성 섬유광학 내시경검사(flexible fiberoptic scopes): 상행결장까지 진단, 생검(확진)

치 료

▸ 조기발견 및 조기치료: 효과적

① **수술**

- **수술 전 처치**
  - 저섬유식
  - 하제, 관장(enema), 세척 및 좌약 투여
  - 장내 살균제
  - 수술 전후 전신 항생제 투여
- **근치적 수술(curative surgery)**
  - Rt. hemicolectomy: 우측 결장
  - Lt. hemicolectomy: 좌측 결장
  - Anterior resection: 구불 결장
  - Low ant. resection: 항문에서 8cm 상방의 직장
  - Mile's operation: 항문에서 8cm 하방 직장
- **고식적 수술(palliative surgery)**
  - Resection and anastomosis, colostomy: 절제 및 문합술, 결장조루술

② **방사선요법**

- Stage B, C: 수술 후 보조요법

③ **화학요법**

- Stage B, C: 수술 후 보조요법
- Stage D: 고식적 치료(5-FU + leucovorin)

예 후(Prognosis): 치료가 성공하고 생존할 가능성 여부

▸ 근치수술 후 생존율

- 양성종양: 양호(대개 수술로 절제 가능)
- 악성종양: 불량[미분화, 전이(metastases) 시]

표 1 • 대장암의 진전도(Staging=Duke's Classification)

분 류	침범의 깊이
Duke's A(Stage I)	점막층(mucosal layer)에 국한
Duke's B1(Stage II)	장근층(muscularis propria)까지 침습했으나 림프절 전이 없음
B2	장근층을 뚫었으나 림프절 전이 없음
Duke's C1(Stage III)	장벽(serosal wall)을 뚫지는 않았으나 림프절 전이가 있음
C2	장벽을 뚫고 장주위 조직과 림프절 전이가 있음
Duke's D(Stage IV)	원격전이

유사 용어

- 장(창자): intestine = entero = bowel
- 출혈: bleeding = hemorrhage
- 뇌: brain = encephalo = cerebro
- 문합술: anastomosis = ~stomy

1.2 수술에 관한 용어

봉합(Suture, Stitch)의 종류

① **단속봉합(Interrupted suture)**

- 모든 봉합의 기본형
- 봉합의 코(suture)가 하나씩 완전히 독립되어 매듭지어지는 것
- 근막, 피부봉합에 이용
- Silk 봉합사를 사용하는 것이 효과적

▶ 종류

- 단순봉합(Simple interrupted)
- 수평석상 단속봉합(Horizontal mattress interrupted)
- 수직석상 단속봉합(Vertical mattress interrupted)
- 렘베르 단속봉합(Lembert interrputed)
- 홀스텟 단속봉합(Halsted mattress interrupted)

② **연속봉합(Continuous suture)**

- 봉합의 코(suture)가 계속적으로 연결
- 복막(peritoneum)을 봉합할 때 사용

▶ 종류

- 단순 연속봉합(simple continuous)
- 제륜봉합[Blanket(Looking) stitch]
- 피내 연속봉합(Subcurticular continous)
- 콘넬 연속봉합(Connel continous)

③ **쌈지봉합(Purse-string suture)**

- 관이나 개구부의 주위조직을 연속적으로 봉합한 후 실을 잡아당기면서 절단면의 끝의 조직을 함몰시켜 구멍을 막는 봉합법
- 창절 절단면이 주위 조직에 유착되는 것을 막음
- 충수돌기 절제술(appendectomy) 시 충수절단을 매몰할 때 사용
- 담낭, 방광의 배농관 삽입 시 사용

④ **유치봉합(Retention suture)**

- 복막, 근막, 피하, 피부를 한번에 봉합
- 복막을 1차적으로 닫고 근막, 피하, 피부를 한번에 봉합
- 피부봉합을 보통봉합으로 한 후 간격을 넓게 해서 근막, 피하, 피부를 한번에 봉합

1.3 수술을 요하는 기본사항

- 폐색(Obstruction), 봉쇄(blockage): 주로 동맥, 관(tubes), 도관(ducts)에 생김
- 천공(Perforation): 장기(organ), 동맥, 수포(bleb)의 파열
- 미란(Erosion): 계속적인 물리적 자극, 감염, 궤양 및 염증으로 조직의 표면이 소멸
- 종양(Tumor): 비정상적인 조직의 성장으로 악성

2.1 용어설명

배액술(Drain)

- **수술 후에 주로 Hemovac을 사용 → 절제부위 및 임파선 절제부위에 삽입**
- 매일 양과 내용물(증감) 관찰, 혈종 또는 염증의 유무 주의
- 일반적: 1일 배액량이 10～20cc 이하로 감소, 피판이 잘 부착, 혈종 또는 조직종이 없어질 경우 → Hemovac 제거

목 적

- **치료적: 기존에 존재하는 고름, 혈종 또는 장 내용물 등의 외부로의 배액**
- **예방적: 수술 후 출혈, 장 내용물 및 조직액 등이 고여서 합병증이 생길 경우**

종 류

- 배액관(drain)은 재질이 부드럽고, 조직에 상처 주지 않고, 이물질 반응이 적어야 함
- Silastic penrose, Tube drain, Hemovac(Closed suction drain), Penross-rubber penrose

2.2 재원일수 계산법

- 퇴원일-입원일

▸ 입퇴원기록, 경과기록, 의사기록에서 확인

예) 입원일: 2017년 4월 12일(4/30, 5/31, 6/30 등)

퇴원일: 2017년 5월 4일

[풀이: 30−12+4 = 22일]

2.3 층(layer)의 깊이

점막(mucosa) ➡ 점막하(submucosa) ➡ 근육(muscle) ➡ 장막(serosa)

점막(mucosa) ↓ 조기암(early cancer)

점막하(submucosa) ↓ 시작 진행암(advanced cancer)

차트 용어

· Adhesion	유착	· Adipose tissue	지방조직	· Aorta	대동맥	· Ascites	복수
· Constipation	변비	· Drain	배액관	· Fungal	진균의	· Stitch out	실밥제거
· Stool	대변	· Subserosa	장막하	· Swelling	종창, 팽윤		
· Tenesmus	뒤무직, 후중(배변 후 시원하지 않고 뒤무직하여 동통 지속)						

약 어	원 어	
Bx.	Biopsy	생검
GEA	General endotracheal anesthesia ‣ IV(정맥내), IM(근육내), endotracheal(기관내), endobronchial(기관지내), rectal(직장), inhalation(open drop, 개방점적식)	전신마취
HTN	Hypertension	고혈압
IM	Internal medicine	내과
LFT	Liver function test ‣ ALK, bilirubin, ASR(SGOT), ALT(SGPT)	간기능검사
LN	Lymph nodes	림프절
OPD	Out-patient department ‣ IPD inpatient department(입원)	외래
RT	Rebound tenderness	반사통
S-P	Silastic penrose drain	S-P 배액관
T	Tenderness	압통
Tx	Treatment, therapy	치료
TNM	Tumor, node, metastasis	종양, 림프절, 전이
USG	Ultrasonography	초음파
V/S	Vital signs	활력징후

등록번호	178 50 16	성별 M
성명	장 천 수	
주민등록	800708-1234567	

입 퇴 원 기 록
Admission and Discharge Record

<table>
<tr><td colspan="4">주 소 : 대전시 서구 복수동</td></tr>
<tr><td colspan="2">출신지 : 대전시 서구 도마동</td><td>직 업 :</td><td>전 화 :</td></tr>
<tr><td>연고자성명 : 민수석</td><td>관 계 :</td><td>주 소 :</td><td>전 화 :</td></tr>
<tr><td colspan="2">입원 : 2017년 4 월 12 일 과 병동 호</td><td rowspan="3">전과</td><td>2017 년 월 일 과 병동 호</td></tr>
<tr><td colspan="2">퇴원 : 2017년 5 월 4 일 과 병동 호</td><td>2017 년 월 일 과 병동 호</td></tr>
<tr><td colspan="2">재원일수 :</td><td>2017 년 월 일 과 병동 호</td></tr>
<tr><td colspan="3">최종진단명</td><td></td></tr>
<tr><td colspan="3">주진단명 : Rectal Ca. stage C-2 (Astler-Coller)</td><td></td></tr>
<tr><td colspan="3">stage IV (TNM classification)</td><td></td></tr>
<tr><td colspan="3">Liver metastasis</td><td></td></tr>
<tr><td colspan="3">기타진단명 :</td><td></td></tr>
<tr><td colspan="3"></td><td></td></tr>
<tr><td colspan="3"></td><td></td></tr>
<tr><td colspan="3">수술 및 처치명</td><td></td></tr>
<tr><td colspan="3">수술명 : Low anterior resection</td><td></td></tr>
<tr><td colspan="3">Colostomy closure</td><td></td></tr>
<tr><td colspan="3"></td><td></td></tr>
<tr><td colspan="3">기타수술 및 주요검사 : Colostomy wound : delayed closure</td><td></td></tr>
<tr><td colspan="3">(secondary suture)</td><td></td></tr>
<tr><td colspan="3"></td><td></td></tr>
<tr><td colspan="3"></td><td></td></tr>
<tr><td colspan="4">치료결과 : 1. 완쾌 2. 경쾌 3. 호전안됨 4. 진단뿐 5. 가망없는 퇴원 6. 48시간내 사망 7. 48시간이후 사망</td></tr>
<tr><td colspan="4">퇴원형태 : 1. 퇴원지시후 2. 자의퇴원 3. 탈원 4. 전원</td></tr>
<tr><td colspan="4">병원감염 : 1. 수술후 2. 기타처치후 3. 비뇨기계 4. 호흡기계 5. 소화기계 6. 기타</td></tr>
<tr><td colspan="3">원사인 :</td><td>부검 : 예, 아니오</td></tr>
<tr><td colspan="4">계속적 진료 계획</td></tr>
<tr><td colspan="4">없음 (있음) (약속일 2017년 5월 20일) 종양내과 외래에서 항암제치료 시작할 예정임</td></tr>
<tr><td colspan="2">담당 전공의 서명 : 이승리</td><td colspan="2">담당 전문의 서명 : 전승호</td></tr>
<tr><td colspan="2">의무기록 완성 : 2017 년 10 월 7 일</td><td colspan="2">의무기록사 서명 : 민용진</td></tr>
</table>

등록번호	178 50 16	성별	M
성명	장 천 수		
주민등록	800708-1234567		

퇴 원 요 약

Discharge Summary

Final diagnosis : Rectal cancer $\bar{c}$ liver metastasis

Brief History 2017년 3월 본원에서 stool caliber 감소와 constipation으로 sigmoidoscopic Bx 후 rectal Ca. imp하에 T-colostomy 시행하였음. 그 후 외래에서 암검사를 계속한 후 직장암수술을 위해 일반외과로 입원함.

C.C constipation (onset: 5MA)

P.I 상기 증상과 bowel habit change, tenesmus
→ A병원에서 colonoscopy상 R/O Rectal Ca. imp → 수술 위해 입원

PMHx DM/HT/Tbc(-/-/-)

S.R Wt. loss (-), small caliber frequent constipation

P.E Rectal exam : Anal verge 5cm 상방에서, 12시 방향으로, 직경 5cm 크기의 ulcerofungating mass

Lab CBC : 6000 - 13.7 - 39.5 - 264K
LFT : 191 - 7.4/4.2 - 1.4 - 67/24/25
CEA : 230

X-ray special study :
CT : rectal ca. $\bar{c}$ liver metastasis (S7, S8)

Pathology: Adenocarcinoma, moderately differentiated

Clinical course of hospital :
2017/04/12 : admission (외래를 통하여 GS 입원)
2017/04/21 : operation
2017/05/04 : discharge

Tx.(operation) : Low anterior resection

Postop Cx : None

Result : Improved

Plan of Therapy and F/U : 퇴원 후 외래를 통하여 암에 대한 검사와 치료를 계속할 예정임.

작성일 : 2017/05/10

전공의 : 이승리 수석전공의 : 장승구 담당교수 : 전승호

등록번호	178 50 16	성별 M
성명	장 천 수	
주민등록	800708－1234567	

경 과 기 록

Progress Notes

4/12 〈 Admission note 〉

S : Constipation

O : S/P transverse colostomy (2017. 3. 2)

3월 21일, 4월 6일 A병원 외과에서 시행한 암검사 결과

sigmoidoscopy $\bar{c}$ Bx : Rectal ca. adenocarcinoma

USG: S8, S7 (x3) : metastatic liver nodule

A : Rectal ca $\bar{c}$ liver metastasis

S/P transverse colostomy

P : preop－lab

LFT

Mile's op. and segmental hepatectomy

4/15 1. CEA 230 (3월 20일, CEA 193) *R1 Hong*

4/19 1. preop lab : OK

2. OP 고려 : rectal ca curative시 liver resection 고려 *R1 Hong*

4/21 〈 OP note 〉

Date of operation : 2017. 4. 21

Operator : Surgeon － Prof. 전승호 Assitants : CR 윤진훈/R1 이승리

Anesthesia : GEA

Preoperative diagnosis : Rectal ca $\bar{c}$ liver metastasis

Postoperative diagnosis : Rectal ca $\bar{c}$ liver metastasis

Name of operation : Low anterior resection $\bar{c}$ colostomy closure

Operative Findings :

1. Skin : low abd. midline incision
2. Skin to peritoneum : free
3. Peritoneal cavity : adhesion (+), ascites (－), seeding (－)

L/N swelling (+) para－aortic

iliac

para－rectal

경 과 기 록 지

4. Rectum
   AV 5cm 12시 방향에 직경 5cm sized ulcerating mass
   PRM 15cm (−)   DRM L5cm (−)
5. Low anterior resection was done c̄ colostomy closure
6. Bx (+)
7. Drain (+): S−P drain at pelvic cavity, penrose at anal canal
8. closure : layer by layer
9. colostomy site skin : delayed primary closure   R2 장민

4/21 〈 Postop. record 〉
V/S: stable
J−P drain: serosanginous   R1 *Hong*

4/22 〈 POD #1 〉
1. J−P drain : 152 cc

4/23 1. No fever
2. J−P drain : 65 cc
3. ambulation 중   R1 *Hong*

4/24 1. J−P drain : 179 cc
2. WBC 8300 alb 3.0

4/25 1. L−tube, Foley catheter : remove   R1 *Hong*

4/26 1. delayed 1' closure
2. No fever   R1 *Hong*

4/27 Therapeutic radiotherapy consult :
Palliative chemotherapy is recommended.
Radiotherapy는 benefit이 없음   R1 *Hong*

4/29 〈 POD #8 〉 〈 Off duty note 〉
Rectal ca c̄ liver metastasis (S7, S8)로 4월 21일 extreme low anterior resection 시행한 환자로 수술 후 8일째입니다.
Drain 모두 제거한 상태이고, 식사는 SFD start했으며, 내과에서 chemotherapy Tx 할 예정입니다. colostomy site wound의 stitch out은 늦게 하십시오 (4.26. repaired).

IF wound good
no fever
stitch out done
→ discharge 고려하세요.   R1 *Hong*

경 과 기 록 지

4/29 〈 POD #8 〉 〈 On duty note 〉

(Problem)

1. Rectal ca.
   1) colon obstruction으로 3월 2일 T-loop colostomy 시행
      liver USG상 metastasis in Rt. lobe (S7, S8)
   2) Low anterior resection 시행 후 Postop #8D state임
2. Drain은 all removal state
   Colostomy site wound는 4월 26일 delayed 1°closure 시행한 상태임.

(Plan)

1. Colostomy wound care & B.T check
2. Discharge 후 Chemo Rx 예정 (5월 23일) R1 *Park*

5/1 〈 POD #10 〉

S : Constipation
O : Wound - Clear
P : 1. NRD로 change
    2. Incision wound는 half stitch out 시행
    3. 5월 3-4일 쯤 discharge 고려 R1 *Park*

5/2 S : Stool (x 2회)
O : Wound - clear
P : 1. S/O was done (except colostomy site)
    2. 5/4 discharge 예정임. R1 *Park*

5/4 〈 Discharge Note 〉

Discharge 후 IM OPD를 통하여 chemotherapy 할 예정임.

1. Chemotherapy LV/5FU(pull) 4주간격 170cm 61kg
2. Lab. CBC, LFT, UGS, CEA

1차 #1 5. 23 LV/5-FU(pull)
   1) Levcorrin 33mg D1-5
      5-FU 600mg D1-5
   2) CBC, LFT, USG, CEA R1 *Park*

등록번호	178 50 16	성별	M
성명	장 천 수		
주민등록	800708 - 1234567		

협의진료기록
Consultation Record

협의진단을 위해 의뢰 치료방사선과 서준우 귀하

임상진단명 : Rectal ca $\bar{c}$ liver metastasis (S/P low ant, resection)

의뢰사유 : 상기 진단으로 수술(LAR) 시행 후 postop # 6일된 환자입니다.
Biopsy상 adenocarcinoma(m/d) with extension to perirectal adipose tissue clear resection margin, L/N 5/24 (+)로 나왔습니다.

liver내 segment(S7, S8): Rt. lobe에 3개의 metastatic nodule이 있습니다. Rectal ca. site에 귀과적 치료의 필요성에 대한 evaluation 및 plan 위해 의뢰드리오니 고진선처 앙망하나이다.

의뢰일자: 2017. 4. 27 의뢰의사서명: 이승리

회 신

Dx. : Rectal ca $\bar{c}$ liver metastasis S/P Mile's operation
Rectal exam : AV 5cm 상방 12시 방향 polypoid mass
Abd CT : perirectal soft tissue nodule → rectal ca perirectal invasion
Liver S7 segment에 2cm nodule & S8 seg 1.0cm nodule
Op. : 2017. 3. 2 transverse loop colostomy
2017. 4. 21 LAR
Op finding : AV 5cm 상방 12시 방향 ø5cm mass
Perirectal LN swelling (+)
S7 S8 in liver mass (+)

회신일자: 2017. 4. 27 회신의사서명 : Prof. 서준우

등록번호	178 50 16	성별 M
성명	장 천 수	
주민등록	800708 – 1234567	

협의진료기록
Consultation Record

협의진단을 위해 의뢰 치료방사선과 서준우 귀하

임상진단명 : Rectal ca $\bar{c}$ liver metastasis (S/P low ant, resection)

의뢰사유 : 상기 진단으로 수술(LAR) 시행 후 postop # 6일된 환자입니다.
Biopsy상 adenocarcinoma(m/d) with extension to perirectal adipose tissue clear resection margin, L/N 5/24 (+)로 나왔습니다.

liver내 segment(S7, S8): Rt. lobe에 3개의 metastatic nodule이 있습니다. Rectal ca. site에 귀과적 치료의 필요성에 대한 evaluation 및 plan 위해 의뢰드리오니 고진선처 앙망하나이다.

의뢰일자: 2017. 4. 27 의뢰의사서명: 이승리

회 신

Path #1. 4.5 x 3.5cm mass
#2. 6cm ulcerative lesion
#1. adeno ca M/D
1) extension to perirectal adipose tissue
2) clear RM
3) metastasis to 5/24 perirectal LN
#2. adeno ca. $\bar{c}$ extension to subserosa

Rec: Palliative chemotherapy is recommended
Radiotherapy는 benefit이 없습니다.

회신일자 : 2017. 4. 27 회신의사서명 : Prof. 서준우

등록번호	178 50 16	성별 M
성명	장 천 수	
주민등록	800708-1234567	

협의진료기록
Consultation Record

협의진단을 위해 의뢰 　　　　　　　　　　　　내과 민도사 귀하

임상진단명: Rectal ca $\bar{c}$ liver metastasis (S/P low ant. resection)

의뢰사유 : 상기 진단으로 수술(LAR) 시행 후 postop # 6일된 환자입니다.
Biopsy상 adenocarcinoma(m/d) with extension to perirectal adipose tissue clear resection margin, L/N 5/24 (+)로 나왔습니다.

liver내 segment(S7, S8): Rt. lobe에 3개의 metastatic nodule이 있습니다. Rectal ca. site에 귀과적 치료의 필요성에 대한 evaluation 및 plan 위해 의뢰드리오니 고진선처 앙망하나이다.

의뢰일자: 2017. 4. 27 　　　　　　　　　　의뢰의사서명: 이승리

회 신

Dx : Rectal ca $\bar{c}$ liver metastasis 　S/P Mile's operation

Rec : Pull chemotherapy가 indication되는 환자분으로
5월 23일 오전 10시 내과 OPD로 F/U 부탁드립니다.

회신일자 : 2017. 4 27 　　　　　　　　　　회신의사서명 : Prof. 민도사

등록번호	178 50 16	성별 M
성명	장 천 수	
주민등록	800708-1234567	

수 술 기 록

Operation Record

Date: 2017. 4. 21 Surgeon:
1st ass't: 전승호 2nd ass't: 이승리/조우
Scrub nurse: 김은용 Circ. nurse: 황은혜

Preoperative diagnosis: Rectal ca. with liver metastasis
Postoperative diagnosis: S/A
Name of operation: Low anterior resection with colostomy closure

Procedures and findings

Tumor mass was located at 5cm above anal verge and it was measured 4.5x3.5cm size. The tumor was ulcerating mass and located at anterior wall of the rectum.
On the liver, nodules was palpated at S7, S8 segment of Rt. lobe.
Peritoneal cavity: adhesion (+), ascites (−), seeding (−)
L/N swelling (+) para−aortic, iliac, para−rectal
The frozen report was metastatic adenoca. extension to perirectal adipose tissue. metastasis intrapelvic lymph node 5/24 (+)

Under the general anesthesia the patient was in supine position and the operative field was prepared and drapped in usual manner. A lower abd. midline skin incision was made and deepened to subcutaneous tissue. As peritoneum was opened above mentioned findings were noted.

1. Low anterior resection was done $\bar{c}$ colostomy closure
2. Bx (+)
3. Drain (+): S−P drain at pelvic cavity, penrose at anal canal
4. closure: layer by layer
5. colostomy site skin: delayed primary closure

Dictated/Written by: *Lee* Surgeon's signature: *Yoon*

등록번호	178 50 16	성별 M
성명	장 천 수	
주민등록	800708－1234567	

조직병리보고서
Pathological Report

병리접수번호: S－2017－3162

검사물 접수일: 2017년 4월 22일

임상소견: Rectal Ca.

채취 부위: rectum

Gross Description :

The specimen consists of a segment of rectum, measuring 24cm in length, Externally, the specimen is surrounded by shaggy fibroadipose tissue.
A 4.5x3.5cm sized (ulcerofungating tumor which partially involves the circum－ference of the rectum is located 1.5cm from the distal resection margin and 12cm from the proximal line of resection. Multiple cross sections reveal that the tumor infiltrates into the perirectal muscle tissue.
All lymph nodes are dissected from the perirectal adipose tissue. Also sub－mitted are two ovaries. labelled right and left and measuring 2.5x2.0x1.0cm in each size. Also submitted is an appendix, measuring 5.0cm in length.
A mucosal stip, measuring 4.0 cm in length, is also submitted and labelled "RM". Also submitted is lymphoid tissue, labelled "LN1" and measuring 1.0 cm in diameter.

Pathological Diagnosis:

Rectum (low anterior resection) :

1. Advanced ulceroinfiltrative carcinoma, rectum
   Adenocarcinoma, moderately differentiated
   with 1) extension to perirectal adipose tissue
   2) clear resection margins
   3) metastasis to 5 out of 24 intrapelvic lymph nodes
   (tumoral 2/6, proximal 3/18)
2. Adenocarcinoma, moderately differentiated, rectum (0.6cm)
   with extension to submucosa

Transverse colon, colostomy site, segmental resection :

Chronic nonspecific inflammation with submucosal and serosal fibrosis

보고일: 2017. 4. 26 병리의사: Jang

등록번호	178 50 16	성별	M
성명	장 천 수		
주민등록	800708－1234567		

외 래 기 록
Outpatient Record

5/21 ER로 내원하여 Tx.받음

C.C abd. pain (금일 오전 10경)

BHx 1. 2017. 4, Rectal ca $\bar{c}$ liver meta.로 본원 GS에서 4.21 LAR 시행 후
2017. 5.4 discharge함 (Bx.: A－C stage C－2)
2. 이후 abd. pain (－)
diet: tolerable
bowel habit : regular (x2～3/d) & gas passage: well로
problem 없이 지내오다 금일 오전부터 30min～1hr
간격으로 3～4min 지속되는 vague abd pain과 nausea
sense 있어 소화제 복용했으나 Sx. improve 없어 본원
ER visit.

P.E Abd: T/RT (＋/－)
Bowel sound : sl. decreased

Imp. #1. R/O intestinal obstruction

Plan 1. ER routine lab
2. simple abdomen (S/E)

Progress & disposition

5/22 Simple abd. : mild dilatation of small bowel & feces in colon
constipation (＋)
gas passage: well done
abd. pain : subsided되어 ER에서 discharge시킴.

외 래 기 기 록 지

5/22 두 번째 rectal ca. op.하고 discharge 후 chemotherapy 계속 중임.

Ht. : 170cm Wt. : 60kg

LV/5FU(pull) 4주간격 (CBC, LFT, USG, CEA)

Chemotherapy 1. 2017/5/23
1) Levcorrin 33mg D1－5
5－Fu 600mg D1－5
2) CBC, LFT, USG, CEA
2. 2017/6/20
3. 2017/7/20
4. 2017/8/22

CEA : 2017. 4. 12 230
2017. 6 . 5 18.6
2017. 7. 18 230
2017. 8. 22 17.4
2017. 10. 28 7.2

〈장 천 수〉

★ 장천수 차트를 읽고 맞는 것에 O표 하시오.

1 최종진단명의 분류번호가 맞게 짝지어진 것은?

① C20, M8140/3 C77.2, M8140/6
② C20, M8140/3, C77.5, M8140/6, C78.7
③ C22.9, M8140/6, C77.2, C78.5
④ C22.9, M8010/3, C77.5, M8010/6, C78.5
⑤ C20, M8010/6, C77.2, C78.7

2 상기 환자에 대한 설명으로 다르게 기재된 것은?

① 수술 후 활력징후는 안정적이었다.
② 2017년 5월 20일 종양내과 외래에서 치료할 예정이다.
③ 퇴원 후 복부의 압통이 있었으나 완화되어 응급실에서 퇴원했다.
④ 퇴원 후 화학요법과 방사선치료를 했다.
⑤ 퇴원 2일 전 결장조루술 자리를 제외하고 실밥을 제거했다.

3 상기 환자의 암등록 기재사항 중 진단방법에 해당하는 것은?

① 임상적 방법
② 전이부위의 조직학적 검사
③ 특수생화학적 검사
④ 원발부위 조직학적 검사
⑤ 혈액학적 검사

4 Colostomy 재형성을 위해 내원했다. 이때 부여할 수 있는 번호는?

① K91.4 ② Z43.3 ③ Z46.5 ④ Z93.3 ⑤ Z43.4

5 경과기록지에 대한 설명으로 다르게 기재된 것은?

① 4월 25일에 L-tube와 폴리카테터를 제거했다.
② 수술 후 8일째 배액관은 모두 제거된 상태였다.
③ 수술 후 10일째 상처부위는 깨끗했다.
④ 복강에는 복수가 차 있었다.
⑤ 방사선치료는 효과가 없어 고식적 화학요법을 권했다.

6 주진단명에 대한 주수술분류 번호로 맞는 것은?

① 45.25 ② 48.23 ③ 48.62 ④ 48.63 ⑤ 48.69

7 수술기록지에 내용과 다른 것은?

① 종양은 궤양성 덩어리로 직장 후벽에 위치했다.
② 항문관은 penrose, 골반강은 S-P 배액관을 했다.
③ 골반내 림프절 24개 중 5개가 전이되었다.
④ 대동맥 주변 림프절에 부종이 있었다.
⑤ 복막강에 seeding은 없었으나 유착은 있었다.

8 총재원일수와 입원과는?

① 21, 내과 ② 22, 일반외과 ③ 23, 일반외과
④ 24, 내과 ⑤ 24, 일반외과

9 입원기간동안 시행한 검사가 <u>아닌</u> 것은?

① CT ② Sigmoidoscopy ③ USG
④ EKG ⑤ LFT

10 상기 환자는 지난번 입원 시에 colostomy site가 puncture되었다. 이에 대한 분류번호는?

① T81.1, Y60.0 ② T82.0, Y62.0 ③ T81.2, Y60.0
④ T81.4, Y60.0 ⑤ T81.4, Y62.0

06 만성 신부전
Chronic renal failure

1.1 만성 신부전(Chronic renal failure; CRF)

원 인

- 신장의 요(urine)배설 부전
- 신장기능의 상실로 신장이 식사와 신체 대사작용으로부터 나온 질소성 노폐물과 산을 배설 못함

만성 신부전의 분류

- 급성: 과칼륨혈증, 폐수종을 동반하는 요독증, 핍뇨, 무뇨를 나타냄
- 만성: −만성 사구체신염(chronic glomerulonephritis)
  −만성 신우신염(chronic pyelonephritis), 고혈압(hypertension)
  −일명: 말기 신장질환(End-stage renal disease; ESRD)

치 료

- 혈액내 상승된 크레아틴(creatinine), 요소(urea), 질소(nitrogen) 등 노폐물을 제거하기 위한 투석(dialysis)
- 신장이식(kidney transplantation)
- 치료하지 않으면 치명적
- 적혈구 조혈제(erythropoietin) 사용 → 적혈구 및 에너지 증가

소변의 형성과정

glomerus(사구체) → Bowman's capsule(보우만 낭) → renal tubule(신장세뇨관) → renal pelvis(신우) → ureter(요관) → bladder(방광) → urethra(요도)

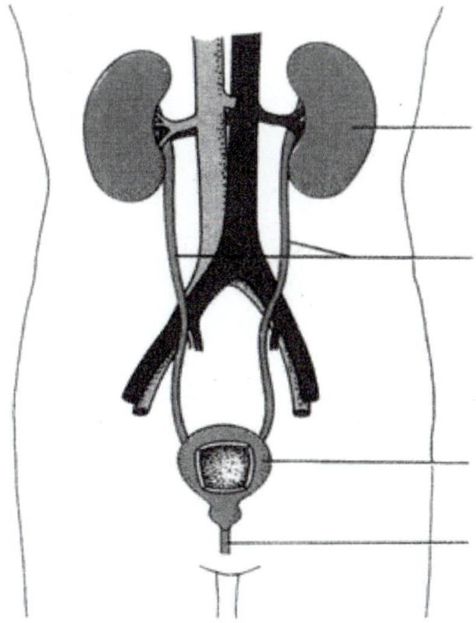

그림 1. 비뇨기계(Urinary system)

1.2 고혈압(Hypertension; HTN)

- 동맥의 높은 혈압
- 고혈압 수치: 140/90 mmHg 이상(성인)

정상혈압: 120/80 mmHg

· 120 : 수축기혈압(systolic blood pressure) · 80 : 이완기혈압(diastolic blood pressure)

고혈압의 분류

- **본태성 고혈압(essential hypertension)**
  - 혈압상승의 원인이 불명
  - 치료: 이뇨제, 베타차단제(beta blocker), 기타 약제
    몸무게 감소, 섭취하는 염(鹽)의 양 제한, 금연, 식사의 지방감소
- **이차성 고혈압(secondary hypertension)**
  - 혈압을 상승시킬 수 있는 사구체신염, 신우신염
  - 부신(adrenal glands) 질환과 연관된 병소

고혈압의 종류

- Hypertensive heart disease(고혈압성 심장질환): 심장에 영향을 주는 높은 혈압
- Renal hypertension(신장 고혈압): 신장질환으로 생긴 고혈압

1.3 흉막 삼출(가슴막 유출, Pleural effusion)

- 흉막강(가슴막강)으로 액이 새어 나옴
- 흉막 유출의 분류
  - 누출액(transudate): 막이나 조직을 통해서 나온 액
  - 삼출액(exudate): ① 혈관이나 상처로부터 스며나온 액으로 단백성분이 많음
    ② 포도상구균 감염으로 고름을 포함
    예) empyema(pyothorax, 농흉),
    hydrothorax(수흉), hemothorax(혈흉)

1.4 울혈성 심부전(울혈성 심장기능상실, Congestive heart failure; CHF)

원 인

- 심장이 신진대사에 필요한 만큼의 적절한 양의 혈액을 펌프할 수 없음
  → 많은 혈액이 동맥으로 나가기보다 정맥을 통하여 심장으로 들어오게 됨
- 혈류가 활발히 흐르지 못하므로 기관(organ)이나 조직에 울혈을 가져옴

증 상

- 부종(edema), 호흡곤란(dyspnea), 기과호흡(orthopnea)
- 폐부종(pulmonary edema), 피로, 발작성 야간성 호흡곤란
- 급성이 될 수도 있지만 보통 몇 년에 걸쳐 진전
- 폐안에 축적된 혈액(왼쪽 심부전)이 폐부종의 원인이 됨
  - 폐부종(pulmonary edema): 폐의 미세한 공기낭(sac)으로 모세혈관의 액이 새어 나옴

치 료

- digitalis: 심근의 수축력 강화
- diuretics(이뇨제): 체액손실(fluid loss) 촉진

1.5 내분비계(Endocrine System)

표 1 • 내분비계의 분류

외분비선(Exocrine glands)	내분비선(Endocrine glands): 9가지
• 한선(땀샘, sweat gland), 유선(젖샘, mammary gland) 타액선(침샘, salivary gland), 누선(눈물샘, lacrimal gland) • 분비관이 있어 체외로 분비	• 갑상선, 부갑상선, 부신, 췌장(이자), 뇌하수체 고환, 난소, 송과체(송방울샘), 흉선(가슴샘) • 분비관 없이 혈액 속으로 분비

표 2 • 내분비선의 비정상적인 상태

내분비선(endocrine gland)	과다분비(hypersecretion)	과소분비(hyposecretion)
갑상선(Thyroid gland)	• 안구돌출증(Exophalmic goiter) – Graves' disease – 갑상선중독증(thyrotoxicosis)	• 지방병성갑상선종(Endemic goiter) – 크레틴병(Cretinism): 소아 – 점액수종(Myxedema): 성인
부갑상선(Parathyroid gland)	• 부갑상선 기능항진증 (Hyperparathyroidism) – 낭성섬유성 골염(osteitis fibrosa cystic)	• 부갑상선기능저하증 (Hypoparathyroidism) – 근수축(tetany) – 저칼슘혈증(hypocalcemia)
부신피질(Adrenal cortex)	• 남성화(Adrenal virilism) • 쿠싱병(Cushing's disease)	• 에디슨병(Addison's disease)
부신수질(Adrenal medulla)	• 크롬친화종(Pheochromocytoma)	
췌장/이자(Pancreas)	• 고인슐린증(Hyperinsulinism)	• 당뇨병(Diabetes mellitus; DM)
뇌하수체(Pituitary): 전엽 (=Adenohypophysis, 선하수체)	• 선단거대증(Acromegaly) • 거인증(Gigantism)	• 난쟁이증(Dwarfism) • 범뇌하수체기능저하증 (Panhypopituitarism)
뇌하수체(Pituitary): 후엽 (=Neurohypophysis, 신경하수체)	• 부적절 항이뇨호르몬 분비 (Syndrome of inappropriate antidiuretic hormone; SIADH)	• 요붕증(Diabetes insipidus; DI)

1.6 투석(Dialysis)

▸ 신장의 기능이 불가능할 경우 혈류로부터 요소(urea) 등의 물질을 제거

혈액투석(Hemodialysis)

▸ 인공신장기(artificial kidney)를 이용

▸ 노폐물이 가득찬 혈류를 여과하여 투석된 피를 환자의 몸으로 돌려줌

복막투석(Peritoneal dialysis)

- 복강카테터(peritoneal catheter)를 이용
- 수액을 복강 속으로 삽입
- 이 액(fluid)은 복강의 모세혈관에 있는 노폐물질이 혈류에서 액으로 빠져나오도록 함
- 노폐물을 담은 수액은 복강카테터로 다시 나옴

복막투석의 종류

- 간헐적 복막투석(Intermittently peritoneal dialysis; IPD)
  - 기계장치의 도움으로 간헐적으로 수행
- 지속적 활동복막투석(Continuous ambulatory peritoneal dialysis; CAPD)

임상검사

- HBs Ag +, Anti HBs − → B형 간염 보균자; + + → 항체; − − → 간염 예방주사
- Hb(혈색소) 정상치: (남) 13.0~17.0 g/dl (여) 12.0~16.0 g/dl

2.1 차트 찾는 방법 및 진료통계

진단명 분류번호 찾는 방법

- 입퇴원기록의 최종진단명
- 퇴원요약의 진단명, 검사 후 진단명)
- 경과기록지의 O(객관적), A(평가)의 진단명
- 수술기록지의 수술 후 진단명
- 조직병리기록지의 진단명
- 임상병리기록지(감염, 빈혈, 매독, 감염 등)
- 협의진단 imp(의증), O(객관적)의 진단명

수술기록지가 생략된 경우 → 수술확인(경과기록, 퇴원요약, 의사지시기록)

- 경과기록지: 모든 내용 기재(입원일~퇴원일)
  → brief op. note(수술요약 기록)
- 퇴원요약지: 중요한 내용만 기재
  예) 진단명, 검사(CT, MRI…), 처치(bx. spinal tapping…),
  치료(colostomy, gastrectomy…), 약제 등

2.2 출제빈도 높은 건수 계산

수술건수

▸ 차트 찾는 방법: 입퇴원기록지, 수술기록지, 경과기록지

예) 수술기록지 계산 후 경과기록지 확인(brief op. note 또는 진단명, 마취 기재로 파악)

▸ 건수 계산:

- 동일한 날짜에 2개 이상 수술한 경우: 1건
- 다른 날짜에 각각 수술한 경우: 각각 건수 계산

예) ㉮ '17. 5. 12. Appendectomy(충수돌기절제술)
Tubal ligation(난관결찰술)
C/section(제왕절개)
수술건수: 1건

㉯ '17. 5. 12 Appedectomy(충수돌기절제술)
'17. 5. 30 Tubal ligation(자궁관결찰술)
수술건수: 2건

협의진료건수(consultation)

▸ 차트 찾는 방법: 협의진단기록, 경과기록, 의사지시기록

▸ 협의진단기록지 건수 계산 후 경과기록지 또는 의사지시기록지 확인

예) 경과기록지: repeat GS consult → 2건

▸ 임상과 또는 행정부서의 협의진료의뢰가 다른 경우: 각각 건수 계산

예) 외과, 산부인과, 영양과 협의진료의뢰 → 3건

차트 용어

· anteverted flexion	전경굴곡	· antrum	동	· bruise	타박상	· bruit	잡음
· dental caries	치아우식증	· dizziness	현기증	· erosion	미란	· femoral	대퇴골의(넙다리뼈의)
· foamy	거품성	· gum	잇몸	· impact	매몰	· incisior	견치
· insomnia	불면증	· molars	대구치(어금니)	· mucosa	점막	· pitting edema	함요부종
· radius	요골(노뼈)	· sore throat	인후통(목통증)			· uterus	자궁
· evaluation	평가/치료(예: further evaluation 더 나은 치료를 위해)						

약 어	원 어	
A/N/V/C/D	Anorexia, nausea, vomiting, constipation, and diarrhea	식욕부진, 오심, 구토, 변비 및 설사
AV	Arteriovenous	동정맥의
AVF	Anteverted flexion	전경 굴곡
BC	Blood culture	혈액배양
BR	Bed rest	안정/의사지시기록
BUN	Blood urea nitrogen	혈액뇨질소
CBC	Complete blood count (laboratory/hematology) ‣ CBC 8.9-3.7-128K → 8.9(빈혈)	전혈구검사(혈액검사) Hgb 헤모글로빈/혈색소 - 10g/dL 이하 → 빈혈
CHF	Congestive heart failure	울혈성 심부전(심장기능상실)
CRF	Chronic renal failure = ESRD	만성 신부전(콩팥기능상실)
CT	Computed tomography (procedure/x-ray)	컴퓨터 단층촬영술
CVAT	P/Ex.: Costovertebral angle tenderness	Physical examination(신체검사): 늑골척추각 압통
CVA	Dx.: Cerebral vascular accident(=stroke)	Diagnosis(진단명): 뇌혈관사고(=뇌졸중)
DOE	Dyspnea on exertion(excercise)	노력성 호흡곤란
DUB	Dysfunctional uterine bleeding	기능부전성 자궁출혈
ERSD	End-stage renal disease	말기 신장질환
G-F	Grossly free = free = intact = N-S = WNL = N-C	정상/육안
GFS	Gastrofiberscope	위내시경
HD	Hemodialysis	혈액투석
I/O	Intake and output	섭취량 및 배설량
L/S/K	liver, spleen and kidney	간, 비장(지라) 및 신장
LVH	Left ventricular hypertrophy	좌심실비대
OC	Oral contraceptive	경구용 피임제
qd	Every day	매일
PRBC	Packed red blood cells(transfusion)	농축 적혈구/수혈(pints)
RT	Rebound tenderness	반사통
T	Tenderness	압통
US, U/S	Ultrasound	초음파
VCUG	Voiding cystourethrogram	배뇨성 방광요도조영도

등록번호	210 68 78 성별 F
성명	유 수 호
주민등록	851012－1234567

입 퇴 원 기 록

Admission and Discharge Record

주　소 : 서울시 서초구 반포동 410				
출신지 : 대구시 남구 송현동 253		직 업 :	전 화 :	
연고자성명 : 이보람	관 계 :	주 소 :	전 화 :	
입원 : 2017년 3 월 8 일 IM 과 병동 호		전과	20 년 월 일 과 병동 호	
퇴원 : 2017년 3 월 21 일 IM 과 병동 호			20 년 월 일 과 병동 호	
재원일수:			20 년 월 일 과 병동 호	

최종진단명	분류번호
주진단명 : CRF	
기타진단명 : Hyperthyroidism	
Vaginal bleeding	
CHF $\bar{c}$ pleural effusion	
수술 및 처치명	
수술명 : Hemodialysis ($\bar{c}$ subclavian vein catheter insertion)	
AV fistula	
기타수술 및 주요검사 :	

치료결과 : 1. 완쾌 2. 경쾌 3. 호전안됨 4. 진단뿐 5. 가망없는 퇴원 6. 48시간내 사망 7. 48시간이후 사망	
퇴원형태 : 1. 퇴원지시후 2. 자의퇴원 3. 탈원 4. 전원	
병원감염 : 1. 수술후 2. 기타처치후 3. 비뇨기계 4. 호흡기계 5. 소화기계 6. 기타	
원사인 :	부검 : 예, 아니오
계속적 진료 계획	
없음있음 (약속일 년 월 일 시)	
담당 전공의 서명 : 이승길	담당 전문의 서명 : 박민일
의무기록 완성 : 2017 년 10 월 7 일	의무기록사 서명 : 서호기

등록번호	210 68 78	성별	F
성명	유 수 호		
주민등록	851012 - 1234567		

퇴 원 요 약

Discharge Summary

Final diagnosis : 1. ESRD, stage 5
2. Hyperthyroidism
3. Vaginal bleeding
4. CHF $\bar{c}$ pleural effusion

Admission record :

2010년	Proteinuria & hematuria detection (S병원 입원)
2016년 12월	Hypertension Sx (SBP: 220) - Y병원 입원하여
	CRF 진단받음 (kidney bx. 안함)
2017년 1월 이후	mens 양 ↑ duration ↑
2017년 3월 8일	CBC 8.9 - 3.7 - 128K
	BUN/Cr 151/14.8
	Emergency HD start & transfusion
	GFS: erosive gastritis

Operation & procedure :

2017년 3월 9일	Emergency HD start & transfusion
2017년 3월 16일	AV fistula Op.

Therapeutic procedures :

Kidney transplantation W/U 마치고 퇴원함.

Discharge medication and signature

ENAL	0.5T	po.	qid	× 2 wks
Prazosin	1mg	po.	qid	× 2 wks
CACA	2T	po.	tid	× 2 wks
Amphojel	1T	po.	tid	× 2 wks
Folic acid	1mg	po.	tid	× 2 wks
B - com	1T	po.	qid	× 2 wks

Plan of therapy and F/U : 박민일 선생님 OPD Follow up

기록일 2017/03/21 전공의 서명 DR1 *이승길* *Park*

등록번호	210 68 78	성별 F
성명	유 수 호	
주민등록	851012－1234567	

병 력 기 록

History

C.C : Vaginal bleeding (onset: 2017년 1월 말)
(recent: 2017년 1월 말)

P.I : 1. 2010년 URI Sx. 직후 gross total hematuria로 S병원 Adm. Hx.
: 당시 proteinuria & hematuria 있다고 들었음.
not specified origin [hypertension (－), edema (－)]
2. 이후에도 routine check에서, hematuria & proteinuria 지속됨
3. 2016년 11월 OB & GY 검진 시, cervicitis Dx 받고 2일 정도 po. med. 후, Nausea/vomiting 있어 내과 clinic 방문: SBP 220 detect되어 Y병원에 입원함. Kidney biopsy는 시행하지 않았고, ESRD로 진단받음.
4. 2017년 1월 말, mens할 시기에 규칙적으로 mens를 시작하였으나 mens 양이 평소에도 많았는데 양이 더 많고 18일간 지속됨: packed cell 2 pints를 수혈 받음.

P.H. : DM/Tbc/HT(－/－/－)
Allergy(－)

F.H & S.H. : Mother : HT(－), DM(－), kidney disease (－)
breast Ca & endometrial Ca. (－)
Alchol (－), Smoking (－)

ROS : G/A : fever/chilling(－/－) headache (－)
dizziness (＋) Wt. loss (－)
body itiching (－)

HEENT : hearing disturbance (－) sore throat (－)
visual disturbance (－)

Cardiovascular : palpitation (－) arrhythmia (－) pain (－)

Resp : cough/sputum/dyspnea (＋/－/－) chest pain (＋)
DOE (－)

Gastrointestinal : A/N/V/C/D (－/－/＋/－/－) melena (－)
fasting epigastric soreness (－)

Genitourinary : U/O↓(－) foamy urination (＋) edema (＋)
red urine (－)

Musculoskeletal : pain (－) weakness (－) numbness (－)

Neurological : insomnia (－) tremor (－) dizziness (＋)

Endocrine : temperature intolerance (－)

기록날짜 2017/03/08 인턴서명 : *Yoon*

등록번호	210 68 78	성별 F
성명	유 수 호	
주민등록	851012 - 1234567	

신 체 검 진 기 록

Physical Examination

G.A : Chronic ill appearance
Uremic face, uremic odor, pale, puffy

Skin/Head/HEENT : Severe anemia
PTH (−)
tongue: dehydration (−)
laceration on forehead due to accident (slip down/mountain)

Neck : L/N (−) V/E (−) T/E (−)

Chest/Lungs : Symmetric expansion
CBS $\bar{s}$ ⓡ

Cardiovascular : Systolic murmur grade IV/VI along LSB

Abdomen : soft & flat L/S/K (−) T/RT (−)
BS: OK

Bone/Joint/Muscles : CVAT (−) P/C/C (+/−/−) femoral bruise (+/+)

Imp :
1. ESRD: progressive of azotemia, Cr ↑
2. Vaginal bleeding of not specified origin (DUB)
   R/O Uremic bloody dysclasia
3. Normocytic normochromic anemia

Diagnostic plan :
1. ESRD W/U & emergency HD → 이후 long term plan 결정
2. anemia → if 고려
3. OB & GY consult for vaginal bleeding evaluation

기록날짜 2017/03/08 인턴서명 : *Yoon*

등록번호	210 68 78	성별 F
성명	유 수 호	
주민등록	851012－1234567	

경 과 기 록
Progress Note

〈 Admission note 〉

3/8

C.C Vaginal bleeding (onset: 2017년 1월 말)
(recent: 2017년 2월 말)

P.I
1. 2000년 URI Sx. 직후 gross hematuria가 있어 S병원 Adm Hx (＋)
: 당시 proteinuria & hematuria 있다고 들었으나
hypertension (－), edema (－)
2. 이후 수개월간 F/U 하다가 중단됨.
이후에도 1～2년마다 Routine check시에 proteinuria & hematuria 있다고 들었음.
3. 2017년 11월, 산부인과 검진 시 cervicitis Dx.받고 2일 정도 po. med. 후 Nausea/vomiting 있어 내과 local clinic 방문: SBP 220 detect되어 S병원에 입원하여 ESRD 진단받음 (신장 biopsy하지 않음).

(2017/11/07)	CBC	8.1－8100－220k	BUN/Cr	51/5.1
	é	148－5.7－118	TP/alb	5.9/3.4
	U/A	prot 300 ↑	glu (－)	
	24HU	prot 3.4	Ccr 10	
	C3/C4	52.6/31.5		

→ 당시 BP control 하면서 Mx.

(2017/02/08) BUN/Cr 119/8.6 → 148/10.1
(2017/01/27) CBC 7.2 － 9500 － 167k
(2017/02/08) CBC 4.3 － 16500 － 244k

4. 2017년 1월 말, mens할 시기에 규칙적으로 mens를 시작하였으나 mens양이 평소에도 많았는데 양이 더 많고 18일간 지속됨.
packed cell 2 pints 수혈받음.
→ 산부인과에서 oral pill rec 받고 2월 중순경부터 medication 시작하면서 vaginal bleeding 감소함.
→ 그러나 2월 말 다시 시작하면서 3월 8일 현재 입원 시까지 계속되고 있음.
OPD F/U 중 Cr 계속 증가하는 추세 보여 본원으로 입원함.

R3 *Kim*

경 과 기 록 지

P.H. DM/Tbc/HT(−/−/−)
Allergy(−)
F.H. Mother HT (−) DM (−) kidney disease (−)
breast Ca. & endometrial Ca. (−)
Alchol (−), Smoking (−)
ROS fever/chilling (−/−) HA/dizziness (−/+)
C/S/D (−) DOE (−) chest pain (+)
A/N/V/C/D (+/+/+/−/−) melena (−)
fasting epigastric soreness (−)
itiching (−) Wt. loss (−)
P/E G/A Chronic ill looking appearance
Uremic face, uremic odor
HEENT Severe anemia, anicteric
L/R (++/++)
PTH (−) PI (−)
tongue: dehydration (−)
laceration on forehead due to accident (slip down)

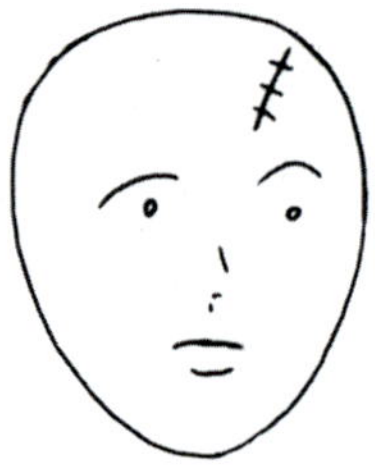

Neck L/N (−) V/E (−) T/E (−)
Chest Symmetric expansion
CBS $\bar{s}$ ⓡ
systolic murmur grade IV/VI along LSB
Abd soft & flat L/S/K (−) T/RT (−)
BS: OK abdominal bruit (+)
Back & Ext. CVAT(−/−) pitting edema(+/+) C/C (−) femoral bruise (+/+)

Problem
1. ESRD: progression of azotemia, Cr ↑
2. Hyperthyroidism
3. Vaginal bleeding
4. Anemia

Ass.
1. ESRD
R/O underlying IgAN
: 현재 Cr 상승은 bleeding에 의한 volume effect 있겠으나
long−term plan 결정해야 할 것임.
2. Vaginal bleeding
1) R/O underlying pathology
2) R/O uremic bloody dysclasia에 의한 menorrhagia
3. Anemia
1) ACD + volume loss

R3 *Kim*

경 과 기 록 지

Initial plan

1. anemia 심하므로 수혈 고려
2. emergency HD → 이후 long term plan 결정
3. ESRD W/U
4. 산부인과 consult for vaginal bleeding evaluation

3/8 C.C nausea, weakness
vaginal bleeding
- 7년 전 GN
- 2000. 11 S병원 ESRD, HT
  본원 OPD Lab: BUN/Cr 136/12
  CBC: Hb 4.5－Hct 15－Pt 124,000
  electro 137－3.4－102 Ca/P 5.4/8.1
  HBsAg(－)

Imp ESRD, HT, Anemia
Plan 내일 subclavian cath. & HD c̄ transfusion (emergency) R1 *Lee*

3/9 emergency HD c̄ transfusion (subclavian catheter) R1 *Lee*

3/10 S : Sx improved
vaginal bleeding 많이 줄었으나 지속됨.
(원래 mens 기간임)
O : CBC 9.5－99－6.3－115k
BUN/Cr 88/9.8
HD c̄ transfusion 후, CBC 16.2－3.3－10.6－140k
fever (－)
P : 1. Depo provera IM
2. Sx. 호전되면 long－term plan 결정 R1 *Lee*

3/11 O : CBC 10.2－2.94－9.2－26.4%－129k
é 139－38－106
BUN/Cr 44/6.7
Fe/TIBC 41/267
HBsAg/Ab (－/＋)
P : 1. anti → D/C
2. HD/PD long－term plan의 결정 R1 *Lee*

경 과 기 록 지		
3/12	S : vaginal bleeding 많이 줄었으나 여전히 bleeding. Transplantation하기 원함 P : Transplantation에 대한 F/E endoscopy 2017/03/15 abd. sono 2017/03/04 mammography HLA type HLA cross matching Lab 누락된 것 정리 24hr urine 모은 것 fail → 내일 다시 collection	R1 Lee
3/14	S : vaginal bleeding decreased but continue (x2 pad/day) P : Transplantation W/U (W/U sheet 작성) 치과 consult	R1 Lee
3/16	〈 OP note 〉 Operator : Pf. 장순철 Assistant : R2 안정한 Anesthesia : Local Op name : AVF (Lt. wrist) between radial artery and vein $\bar{c}$ prolene 6/0 side anastomosis 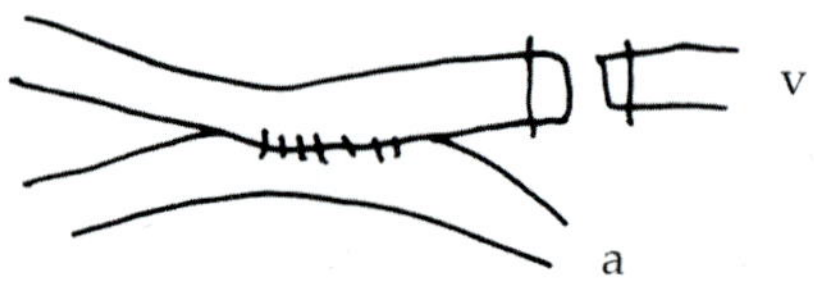 	R2 Ahn
	S : spotting (vaginal) 거의 안 나옴 O : VCU: no reflux residual urine (−) P : work sheet 작성 OB/GY reconsult 고려	R1 Lee
	cf : 현재 W/U 중 PSY consult ENT consult GY consult CPA, KUB 없음	
3/18	transplantation W/U 마친 후 3/21 퇴원 예정	R1 Lee
3/21	Discharge	R1 Lee

등록번호	210 68 78	성별 F
성명	유 수 호	
주민등록	851012－1234567	

협의진료기록
Consultation Record

Request For Consultation To 영상의학과 한효동 선생님 귀하

Summary of Present Findings

CRF 환자로 subclavian insertion 위해 자문드리오니 고진선처 바랍니다.

2017. 3. 9 a.m.
Date Hour p.m.

R3 김은호
Signature of Attending Physician

Rereport of Consultation

Opinion and Recommendation

2017년 3월 9일 시행하겠습니다.

2017. 3. 9
Date Hour

한효동 M.D.
Signature of Attending Physician

등록번호	210 68 78	성별	F
성명	유 수 호		
주민등록	851012 − 1234567		

협의진료기록
Consultation Record

Request For Consultation To　　　　산부인과 황금박 선생님 귀하

Summary of Present Findings

CRF 환자로 2017년 1월 말 18일간 지속되는 vaginal bleeding으로 pill po. Med 하였음. 이후 vaginal bleeding 지혈되었으나 2월 말부터 다시 시작되어 Hb. 3.7까지 떨어진 상태입니다. 이에 대한 귀과적 evaluation & Mx 위해 자문드리오니 고진선처 바랍니다. (금일 오후에 emergency HD 예정입니다.)

2017. 3. 9　　a.m.　　　　R3 김은호
Date　　Hour p.m.　　　　Signature of Attending Physician

Rereport of Consultation

Opinion and Recommendation

1. CRF
2. Uterine bleeding　2017/01/14부터 18일간
　　2017/02/말부터 현재까지

H/O　OC(1 cycle) :　WDB started since 2017/02/말
(since 2017/01/말)

Gyn Ex :　Ut : AVF
　Ad : (−)
　Cx : mild erosion around OS
　Vx : vaginal blood discharge ↑

Imp :　OC − WDB
　ESRD

Rec :　1. Depo − provera 150mg (1 vial) IM
　2. OPD F/U 3 weeks later　　감사합니다.

2017. 3. 9　　　　황금박 M.D.
Date　　Hour　　　　Signature of Attending Physician

등록번호	210 68 78	성별 F
성명	유 수 호	
주민등록	851012－1234567	

협의진료기록

Consultation Record

Request For Consultation To　　　　일반외과 주기적 선생님 귀하

Summary of Present Findings

CRF 환자로 vaginal bleeding을 주소로 입원한 환자입니다.
Kidney transplantation 위해 W/U 중입니다. 이 환자의 AVF 수술을 의뢰드리오니 고진선처 앙망하나이다.

2017. 3. 9　　　a.m.
Date　　　Hour p.m.

R1 이승길
Signature of Attending Physician

Rereport of Consultation

Opinion and Recommendation

2017년 3월 9일 OP 예정입니다.

2017. 3. 13
Date　　　Hour

주기적 M.D.
Signature of Attending Physician

등록번호	210 68 78	성별 F
성명	유 수 호	
주민등록	851012-1234567	

협의진료기록

Consultation Record

Request For Consultation To 정신과 이기쁨 선생님 귀하

Summary of Present Findings

CRF 환자로 kidney transplantation 예정입니다.
정신과적 problem은 없는지 고진선처 앙망하나이다.
(pre. post-psychiatric problem 가능성에 대한 고견 부탁드립니다.)

2017. 3. 13 a.m. 이승길

Date Hour p.m. Signature of Attending Physician

Rereport of Consultation

Opinion and Recommendation

S : "투석 후에 많이 좋아졌어요"
"동생에게 미안해요"
"투석(입원) 전에는 좀 힘들었어요"
O : 편안한 표정
Donor - 동생으로 결정됨/동생이 헌신적이었다고
moor : not depressive/not elated/not dysphoric
약간은 걱정스러운 모습 → tolerable
thought: WNL
perception & other cognitive finding : WNL
약간 recent memory disturbance만 호소함.
A : Stationary
P : 현재 큰 risk는 없는 것 같습니다. 이식 뒤 생기는
mood or behavioral change 있으면 reconsult 해 주세요.

2017. 3. 13 이기쁨 M.D.

Date Hour Signature of Attending Physician

등록번호	210 68 78	성별 F
성명	유 수 호	
주민등록	851012－1234567	

협의진료기록

Consultation Record

Request For Consultation To 치과 차회복 선생님 귀하

Summary of Present Findings

CRF 환자로 transplantation 위해 work－up 중인 환자입니다.
치과적 problem은 없는지 의뢰드리오니 고진선처 앙망하나이다.

2017. 3. 15 a.m.
Date Hour p.m.

이승길
Signature of Attending Physician

Rereport of Consultation

Opinion and Recommendation

C.C : Dental check－up for kidney transplantation

P.I : No specific history of dental pain
Cold sensitivity increased recently.

O.R : Gum－very white
Dental caries－G－F
Prosthesis for upper lateral incisiors
Others－G－F

PAN finding : Impacted lower 3rd molars are found.
But significant infection foci can not be found.

2017. 3. 15
Date Hour

차회복 M.D.
Signature of Attending Physician

등록번호	210 68 78	성별 F
성명	유 수 호	
주민등록	851012－1234567	

협의진료기록
Consultation Record

Request For Consultation To 이비인후과 구우승 선생님 귀하

Summary of Present Findings

CRF 환자로 transplantation 예정입니다.
ENT적 problem은 없는지 의뢰드리오니 고진선처 앙망하나이다.

2017. 3. 17 a.m.
Date Hour p.m.

이승길
Signature of Attending Physician

Rereport of Consultation

Opinion and Recommendation

A: ENT적 problem은 없습니다.

2017. 3. 17
Date Hour

구우승 M.D.
Signature of Attending Physician

등록번호	210 68 78	성별 F
성명	유 수 호	
주민등록	851012－1234567	

의사지시기록

Doctor's Order

〈 Admission order 〉

3/8

1. V/S check $\bar{c}$ 8hr.(BP $\bar{c}$ 4hr)
2. BR
3. CRFD
4. B. Wt. check
5. I/O qd check
6. Subclavian cath consult (영상의학과 한효동님)
7. Get HD permission & subclavian cath insertion
8. 2017/03/09－2 치료식 신부전식 상식 1500 0 0 0 0
   * salt 5g, prot≤40g, k≤40mEq, P≤800
9. Packed RBC 2 pints
   * during HD
10. Enalapril 10mg 12.500 mg 1ud
11. Prazosin 1mg 1.000 T 1ud
12. Ca. Carbonate 0.5g 2.000 T 3ud
13. Amphojel (r) 1.000 T 3 3P
14. FOLIC ACID 1mg 1.000 T 1ud
15. Bcomp (r) 1.000 T 1ud
16. Routine CBC/ESR/Chemistry Profile(11－23)/BUN/Cr
17. OB/GY consult
18. Lt. frontal area suture
19. Skull AP/Lat
20. N/S 1L IV $\bar{c}$ KVO (18GN)

등록번호	210 68 78	성별 F
성명	유 수 호	
주민등록	851012－1234567	

내시경 보고서
Gastroscopy Report

검사일자: 2017. 3. 15 검사명: Gastroscopy
진료과 : IM 시행의: 검사자:

Clinical 임상소견

Esophagus : Free

Stomach : Multiple mucosal erosions were noticed on the antrum.

Duodenum : Tiny numerous pale mucosal elevations were noticed on the duodenal bulb.

slide (－)
biopsy (－)
video (－)

Impression : 1. Erosive Duodenitis
R/O Brunner's gland hyperplasia
2. Acute erosive gastritis

M.D. 송기대

등록번호	210 68 78	성별 F
성명	유 수 호	
주민등록	851012 – 1234567	

임상병리과 보고서
Clinical Pathological Report

접수일자: 2017. 3. 8 진료과: IM
의뢰일자: 2017. 3. 8 보고일: 2017. 3. 8

L85 : 응급검사

WBC	8.9 x 103/μl	RBC	*1.22 x 1003/μl
Hb	*3.7 g/dL	Hct	*11.4 %
PLT	*128 x 103/μl	MCV	93.7 fL
MCH	30.1 pg	MCHC	32.1 g/dL
Na	*133 mmol/L	K	*3.3 mmol/L
Cl	106 mmol/L	T.CO2	*18.2 mmol/L
BUN	*151 mg/dL	Creatinine	*14.8 mg/dL

등록번호	210 68 78	성별 F
성명	유 수 호	
주민등록	851012－1234567	

HLA CROSSMATCH

접수일자: 2017. 3. 15 진료과: IM
의뢰일자: 2017. 3. 16 보고일: 2017. 3. 20

Clinical Indication of Study: evaluation for kidney transplantation

Donor
·Name : 최주미
·Age/Sex : 40/F
·Relation to Recipient : Sister

Result

T cell crossmatch	Warm	Positive
	Antiglobulin	Positive
B cell crossmatch (Warm)		Negative
Autocontrol		Positive

Remark : T cell crossmatch (warm, AHG)에서 autocontrol(patient serum＋donor cell)과 test(patient serum＋donor cell) well 모두에서 positive reaction이 관찰됩니다. (＞1:32) 환자 serum에 autoantibody가 존재할 가능성이 가장 크지만 이식수술 전에 반드시 HLA crossmatch의 재검사가 필요합니다.

등록번호	210 68 78	성별 F
성명	유 수 호	
주민등록	851012－1234567	

영상의학 보고서

접수일자: 2017. 3. 15　　진료과: IM
의뢰일자: 2017. 3. 16　　보고일: 2017. 3. 20

임상소견

No clinical information

2017/03/09

Right subclavian catheter placement

Clinical information : End－stage renal disease

Procedure & findings :

The patient's right upper chest was prepared and drapped in usual sterile fashion.

A puncture was made into the right subclavian vein with injection of contrast medium into the peripheral IV line, and the guide wire was inserted with into the superior vena cava.

A dural lumen hemodialysis catheter was inserted with it's distal tip at the junction of the right atrium and superior vena cava.

There was no immediate complications following the procedure.

Impression :

1. Successful placement of right subclavian hemodialysis catheter.

등록번호	210 68 78	성별	F
성명	유 수 호		
주민등록	851012-1234567		

영상의학 보고서

접수일자: 2017. 3. 15 진료과: IM
의뢰일자: 2017. 3. 16 보고일: 2017. 3. 20

임상소견

No clinical information

2017/03/13

Mammography routine-CR

Markedly dense breast이며, 양측 breast에 뚜렷한 mass 또는 micro-calcification 없음.
유두 퇴축이나 피부 비후의 소견 없음.
Axillary lymph node의 소견 없음.
이러한 breast density는 mammogram의 sensitivity를 감소시킴.

결 론 : Negative mammogram in dense breast.

요 망 : Ultrasonography if there are palpable abnormalities

판독의사

등록번호	210 68 78	성별 F
성명	유 수 호	
주민등록	851012－1234567	

영상의학 보고서

검사일자: 2017. 3. 18 검사명 :

진료과 : IM 검사자:

임상소견

No clinical information

2017/03/14

Abdomen & Kidney U.S.G. :

양측 kidney의 size가 작아져 있으며 (right kidney: 9.2cm, left kidney: 8.9cm) cortical echogenicity가 전반적으로 증가되어 있음.

Corticomedullary differentiation도 감소되었음. Left kidney midpole area에 약 1.2cm size의 cystic lesion이 관찰되고 simple cyst에 의한 것으로 생각됨. Liver나 spleen의 size는 정상범위 내이나 liver의 parenchymal echo가 약간 coarse한 pattern을 보임. Liver내에 focal lesion은 없으며, GB, CBD, portal vein, pancreas 등에 이상 소견 없음.

결 론 : Bilateral chronic renal parenchymal disease.
Slightly coarse liver echoes.

판독의사 최동민

등록번호	210 68 78	성별 F
성명	유 수 호	
주민등록	851012－1234567	

영상의학 보고서

검사일자: 2017. 3. 18　　검사명 :

진료과 : IM　　검사자:

임상소견

No clinical information

2017/03/16

V.C.U.G. :

Dilated contrast media를 poorly catheter를 이용하여 bladder에 400cc filling하였으며, filling 후 supine position에서 straining 시의 film에서 reflux의 evidence 없으며, 양측 oblique와 lateral view 및 voiding and post－voiding film에서 이상소견 없음.

결 론 : No evidence of reflux.
Negative V.C.U.G.

판독의사 오주영

등록번호	210 68 78	성별 F
성명	유 수 호	
주민등록	851012 – 1234567	

핵의학 보고서

접수일자: 2017. 3. 11 의뢰과: IM

처방일자: 2017. 3. 11 보고일자: 2017. 3. 4.

HBsAg	2017. 03. 11	2017. 03. 07.
	Negative	Negative
HBsAb	2017. 03. 11.	2017. 03. 07
	Positive	Positive
HBcAb(IgG)	2017. 03. 11.	2017. 03. 07.
	Negative	Negative
Anti HCV	2017. 03. 13.	
	Negative	
Ferritin	2017. 03. 13.	
(20 – 300)	*309	
PTH(intact)	2017. 03. 14.	2017. 03. 07.
(10 – 65)	40.4	414.3

등록번호	210 68 78	성별	F
성명	유 수 호		
주민등록	851012－1234567		

심장계 보고서

검사일자: 2017. 3. 18 검사명: 2－D Echocardiogram

진 료 과: IM 시행의: 검사자:

임상소견

Video No. : A62 1949 과거검사 여부 :

LV	IVS motion		WALL motion			LVPW motion		
	IVSd	9 mm	LVIDd		51 mm	LVPWd		9 mm
	LVSs	11 mm	LVIDs		35 mm	LVPWs		14 mm
	Excursion	mm	EF		53 %	Excursion		mm
	PE(Anterior)	mm	Subxiphoid		mm			
	PE(Posterior)	mm	LA/Ao		34/28 mm	RV EDD		mm
MV	Shape		EPSS		mm	MVA 2D		
	Motion		PHT		s	MVA DOPP		
	Excursion	mm	MR grade			Vmax		m/s
	EF slope	mm/s	LA		mm	Vmean		m/s
AV	Shape		Aortic root		mm	Vmax		m/s
	Motion		AR grade			Vmean		m/s
	Opening	mm		D. slope		PHT		s
PV	Shape		EF slope			Vmax		m/s
	Motion		PR grade			Vmean		m/s
TV	Shape		V_{max}		m/s	TR grade		
	Motion		V_{mean}		m/s			

Comments : 1. LV cavity size & contractility is WNL
2. IVS & LVPW thickness is WNL
3. Minimal TR & MR on C/D, TR PG = 23mmHg
4. Scant pericardial effusion (insignificant)

M.D. 민국선

등록번호	210 68 78	성별 F
성명	유 수 호	
주민등록	851012－1234567	

핵의학 보고서

접수일자: 2017. 3. 13 의뢰과: IM
처방일자: 2017. 3. 13 보고일자: 2017. 3. 13

상기 수술, 처치, 검사 및 마취의 위험 가능성 및 합병증 설명요약:
감염, 혈종, 출혈, 심부전 및 내출혈이 심하게 발생할 수도 있고,
의식소실, 사망

설명한 주치의사명:

본인은 본인(또는 상기환자)에게 행하여질 (수술, 처치, 검사, 마취)의 필요성, 내용, 예상되는 합병증과 후유증에 대하여 자세한 설명을 주치의사로부터 들었습니다.

따라서 불가항력적으로 또는 환자의 특이체질로 인하여 합병증 또는 우발적 사고가 발생할 수도 있다는 것을 충분히 이해하였으므로 불의의 사고 시 합리적인 절차에 따를 것임을 서약하면서 상기(수술, 처치, 검사, 마취)를 서면으로 신청합니다.

＊기 왕 증 : ☑ 없다 ☐ 있다
＊특이체질 및 질병 : ☐ 알레르기 ☑ 고혈압 ☐ 당뇨병 ☐ 심장병 ☐ 출혈소인
☐ 약으로 인한 사고 ☐ 마취사고 ☐ 기타________

2017년 3월 8일 8시 00분 오전
(오후)

상기환자 또는 대리인 조규진
주 소 : 서울시 송파구 잠실동
증 인 : 유신자
주 소 : 서울시 서초구 반포동

홍 도 우 **병원장 귀하**

등록번호	210 68 78	성별 F
성명	유 수 호	
주민등록	851012－1234567	

타 병 원 검 사

Flow Sheet

Indices \ Time		11. 17	11. 18	11.19	11.20	11. 21	11. 24
7300	WBC	8100	9500	11600		9600	11100
10.1	Hgb	8.1	7.2	7.4		7.3	8.1
	Hct	23.5	20.9	21.0		21.0	23.2
	PLT	220k	205k	194k		174k	216k
23.7/2.0	BUN/Cr	51/5.1	54/5.1	61/5.3	62/5.7	67/5.6	87/5.9
	Na/K	148/5.7	143/5.4	141/5.8	139/5.6	140/5.1	140/4.8
	Cl	118	117	114	103		112
6.6/	TP/Alb	5.9/3.4				5.3/3.0	6.0/30.4
83	FBS					84	91
	Bil 〈 TD					0.39/0.1	0.3/0.1
16/8	AST/ALT	19/10				14/8	21/14
	ALK, P.	43				35	38
	U. A.	8.2				8.0	9.5
	IP/Ca	42/8.2		/7.7	/8.1	3.3/8.4	5.2/8.2
	TG/HDL	121/				101/55	108/61
	T－Chol	229				169	248
3+/－	U/A(P/G)		300↑/(－)		300↑/－	300↑/－	
	(R/W)		M/3－5			20－30/3－5	20－30/1－3
	Stool(R/OB)			－/－			
	Urine VMA	－	－	－			
*Lipid B.		617		* 24 hr urine			
	HDL	51		3 Ccr 10, Pro 3.4g, Glu 192			
	Phospho lip	212		Na 121, K 67.8, Cl 129			
	Tchol	216		C3/C4/CH50 52.6/31.5			
	TG	81					

〈유 수 호〉

★ 유수호 차트를 읽고 맞는 것에 O표 하시오.

1 진단명에 대한 분류번호로 맞게 연결된 것은?

㉠ E05.00	㉡ N18.5	㉢ J93.9	㉣ K29.8	㉤ D64.9
㉥ K75.9	㉦ N93.9	㉧ K29.3	㉨ K29.1	㉩ I50.9

① ㉠-㉡-㉢-㉤-㉦
② ㉠-㉡-㉢-㉤-㉩
③ ㉡-㉤-㉥-㉦-㉩
④ ㉡-㉣-㉤-㉦-㉨
⑤ ㉡-㉢-㉤-㉥-㉧

2 환자에 대한 설명으로 맞게 기재한 것은?

① 오른쪽 손목의 요골(노뼈)동맥과 정맥사이를 prolene으로 양끝을 문합하였다.
② 여러가지 점막성 미란들이 위의 유문(날문)에서 보였다.
③ 하악 셋째 큰 어금니가 매복되어 있지만 특별한 이상은 없어 보였다.
④ 혈액투석 카테터를 우심방과 하대정맥의 연결부에 삽입했다.
⑤ 3주 후 외래방문을 권하였고 질 주변에 경미한 미란이 있었다.

3 수술·처치명에 대한 분류번호로 맞게 연결된 것은?

㉠ 44.13	㉡ 44.14	㉢ 39.27	㉣ 54.98	㉤ 45.23
㉥ 38.93	㉦ 38.95	㉧ 39.95	㉨ 93.08	㉩ 87.37

① ㉠-㉢-㉦-㉧-㉩
② ㉠-㉢-㉥-㉦-㉨
③ ㉡-㉢-㉥-㉦-㉩
④ ㉡-㉣-㉤-㉨-㉩
⑤ ㉡-㉣-㉤-㉥-㉩

4 입원당시 증상이 아닌 것으로 연결된 것은?

① 구토 – 가슴의 통증
② 빈혈 – 대퇴(넙다리)부 타박상
③ 함요부종 – 현기증
④ 거품성 배뇨 – 불면증
⑤ 흉통 – 식욕부진

5 신체검사상 사고로 발생한 사항에 대해 부여할 수 있는 번호는?

① S01.7, W01.8
② S01.8, W01.5
③ S01.8, W01.8
④ S00.99, W01.9
⑤ S00.99, W01.7

6 협의진단과 의사지시기록에 나타난 사항이 아닌 것은?

① 자궁의 전경이 굴곡되어 있었다.
② 잇몸은 매우 하얗고, 치아우식증이 있었다.
③ 입원기간 동안 농축 적혈구를 총 2pints 수혈받았다.
④ 섭취량과 배설량을 매일 체크하였다.
⑤ 지각과 인식은 정상이었고 기억력 장애만 호소하였다.

7 통계분석으로 맞게 연결된 것은?

	㉮	㉯	㉰
1) 퇴원상태	㉮ 완쾌	㉯ 경쾌	㉰ 사망
2) 타과의뢰	㉮ 5	㉯ 6	㉰ 7
3) 수술건수	㉮ 0	㉯ 1	㉰ 2
4) 마취	㉮ 전신	㉯ 척수	㉰ 국소
5) 퇴원과	㉮ 일반외과	㉯ 신장내과	㉰ 심장내과
6) 입원경로	㉮ 응급	㉯ 외래	

① 가-가-가-나-가-가
② 가-다-나-가-다-다
③ 나-다-다-다-나-나
④ 나-나-다-다-나-나
⑤ 나-나-나-가-나-나

8 BUN Cr은 어느 장기의 기능을 보기 위한 검사인가?

① 신장
② 방광
③ 심장
④ 갑상선
⑤ 자궁

9 의무기록에 기재된 약어의 의미가 <u>틀린</u> 것은?

① OC: oral contraceptive pill
② DUB: dysfunctional uterine bleeding
③ DOE: dyspnea on examination
④ BR: bed rest
⑤ BUN: blood urea nitrogen

10 상기 환자가 시행한 검사상 정상으로 나타난 것은?

① CT
② VCUG
③ GFS
④ USG
⑤ CBC

07 알코올성 간경변
Alcoholic liver cirrhosis

1.1 간경변(Liver cirrhosis)

정 의

- 간세포가 손상되어 섬유화되고 퇴행성 변화가 생기는 질환

증 상

- 콜 간염, 복수(acites), 간비대(hepatomegaly), 토혈(hematemesis), 황달(jaundice)
- 식도정맥류(esophageal varices), 섬망상혈관종(spider angioma), 출혈성 경향

원 인

- 일반적으로 영양실조를 동반하는 알코올중독증
- 알코올은 간세포에 중독효과로 지방세포 축적, 괴사, 섬유성 상흔 및 색깔의 변화초래
- 감염이나 독소도 간세포에 영향을 줌
- 간세포의 기능 저하로 빌리루빈이 체외로 배설되지 못할 때 황달(jaundice) 발생

간(liver)의 기능	비장(지라, spleen)의 기능
· 담즙(bile) 생성 · Glucose(당)의 양: 혈당량 정상 유지 · 혈단백 생성 · 오래된 적혈구 파괴 · 혈중의 독 제거하는 해독작용(detoxification)	· 임파양 기관(lymphoid organ) · 혈구 생산 · 혈구 파괴 · 혈액, 특히 혈소판(platelet) 저장

1.2 바이러스성 간염(Viral hepatitis): 바이러스에 의한 간의 염증

바이러스성 간염의 세 가지 유형

▶ **A형 간염(Hepatitis A)**

– A형 바이러스가 원인

– 과거에는 감염성 바이러스

– 감염된 물과 음식물에 의해 전파(바이러스는 대변으로 배설)

▶ **B형 간염(Hepatitis B)**

– B형 바이러스가 원인

– 일명 혈청성 간염(serum hepatitis): 5~10%가 만성간염으로 진행

– 혈액(수혈, 피하 주사바늘, 치과 또는 외과적 기구), 눈물, 침, 정액(semen) 등의 체액 통해 비경구적(parenteral)으로 감염되는 질환

▶ **C형 간염(Hepatitis C)**

– 혈액, 혈액제제 및 사람과의 접촉에 의한 전염

– 50%가 만성간염으로 진행

표 1 • 종양표지검사(Tumor Marker): 주로 암의 진단

검사항목	정상치	임상적 의의
AFP	20.0 ng/ml 이하	• 간경변, 만성간염, 간세포암, 암의 전이, 알코올중독
CEA	5.0 ng/ml 이하	• 소화기암, 폐암, 대장암, 흡연, 임신, 태아기형

간기능 검사

▶ 정의: 혈청(blood serum)내의 효소(enzyme) 수치 표시

▶ 간 손상 시 효소 수치 상승

– OT(serum glutamic oxalacetic transaminase or AST)

– SGPT(serum glutamic pyruvic transaminase or ALT)

– ALK(alkaline phosphatase)

혈액검사 결과

• HBs Ag (+)
• HBs Ab (−)
또는 Anti HBs] B형 간염 보균자   (+)/(−)] 항체 있음   (+)/(−)] 간염 예방주사

위장관 내시경(Gastrointesinal endoscopy)

▶ 굽어질 수 있는 굴곡성 튜브를 입 또는 항문으로 넣고 위장관 촬영

예) esophagogastroduodenoscopy(식도, 위, 십이지장 내시경검사)

colonoscopy(결장경 검사), proctoscopy(직장경 검사법) 등

원사인(Underlying cause of death)

- 직접 사망에 이르게 한 일련의 사건을 일으킨 질병이나 손상
- 치명적인 손상을 일으킨 사고 또는 폭력의 상황

차트 용어

· Alveolus	치조	· Cardiac arrest	심장마비	· Dysuria	배뇨곤란
· Engorgement	충혈	· Gingiva, gum	잇몸	· Hypokalemia	저칼륨혈증/K
· Hematemesis	토혈	· Hematochezia	혈변	· Melena	혈변
· Oliguria	핍뇨증	· Sclerotherapy	경요법	· Splenomegaly	비장(지라) 비대
· Tremor	진전(떨림)	· Varix	정맥류	· Venous	정맥

약 어	원 어	
ALK	Alkaline phosphatase	간기능 효소검사
ALT	Alanine transaminase	간기능 효소검사
A/N/V/C/D	Anorexia, nausea, vomiting, constipation and diarrhea	식욕부진, 오심, 구토, 변비 및 설사
AST	Aspartic acid transaminase	간기능 효소검사
CBS	Clear breathing sound	깨끗한 호흡음
CPR	Cardiopulmonary resuscitation	심폐소생술
CVAT	Costovertebral angle tenderness	늑골척추각 압통
é	Electrolyte 예) 131-3.7-100: 131/나트륨(Na); sodium	전해질
EVL	Esophageal varix ligation	식도 정맥류 결찰술
FB	Finger breadth 예) 2FB: 2개의 손가락 크기	손가락 폭
FFP	Fresh frozen plasma/transfusion	신선냉동혈장/수혈
Fx	Fracture	골절
GE	Gastroesophageal	위식도의
GFS	Gastrofiberscopy	위내시경
HCV	Hepatitis C virus	C형 간염 바이러스
IM	Intramuscular	근육내의(주사)
LC	Liver cirrhosis	간경변
LFT	Liver function test	간기능검사
LOS	Length of stay · 퇴원일－입원일=재원일수	재원일수
MICU	Medical intensive care unit	내과 중환자실
PRBC	Packed red blood cells/transfusion	농축 적혈구/수혈
RBC	Red blood cells(count)	적혈구(수)
RHB	Regular heart beat	정상 심박동
S-B tube	Small bowel tube	소장(작은창자) 튜브
SGOT	Serum glutamic oxaloacetic transaminase	간기능 효소검사
SGPT	Serum glutamic pyruvic transaminase	간기능 효소검사

등록번호	188 33 00	성별	M
성명	하 만 세		
주민등록	661201－1234567		

입 퇴 원 기 록
Admission and Discharge Record

<table>
<tr><td colspan="4">주 소 :</td></tr>
<tr><td colspan="4">출신지 : 직 업 : 전 화 :</td></tr>
<tr><td colspan="4">연고자성명 : 홍주미 관 계 : 주 소 : 전 화 :</td></tr>
<tr><td>입원 : 2017 년 2 월 27 일 과 병동 호</td><td rowspan="3">전
과</td><td colspan="2">2017 년 2 월 27 일 과 병동 호</td></tr>
<tr><td>퇴원 : 2017 년 3 월 26 일 과 병동 호</td><td colspan="2">2017 년 월 일 과 병동 호</td></tr>
<tr><td>재원일수 :</td><td colspan="2">2017 년 월 일 과 병동 호</td></tr>
<tr><td colspan="3">최종진단명</td><td>분류번호</td></tr>
<tr><td colspan="3">주진단명 : Alcoholic liver cirrhosis</td><td></td></tr>
<tr><td colspan="3">기타진단명 : Esophageal varix bleeding</td><td></td></tr>
<tr><td colspan="3">Alveolar bone Fx. in oral cavity</td><td></td></tr>
<tr><td colspan="3">Mandible bone Fx</td><td></td></tr>
<tr><td colspan="3">Sepsis</td><td></td></tr>
<tr><td colspan="3"></td><td></td></tr>
<tr><td colspan="3"></td><td></td></tr>
<tr><td colspan="3">수술 및 처치명</td><td></td></tr>
<tr><td colspan="3">수술명</td><td></td></tr>
<tr><td colspan="3">기타수술 및 처치명 : GFS</td><td></td></tr>
<tr><td colspan="3">Esophageal varix band ligation</td><td></td></tr>
<tr><td colspan="3">Sclerotherapy</td><td></td></tr>
<tr><td colspan="3"></td><td></td></tr>
<tr><td colspan="4">치료결과 : 1. 완쾌 2. 경쾌 3. 호전안됨 4. 진단뿐 5. 가망없는 퇴원 6. 48시간내 사망 7. 48시간이후 사망</td></tr>
<tr><td colspan="4">퇴원형태 : 1. 퇴원지시후 2. 자의퇴원 3. 탈원 4. 전원</td></tr>
<tr><td colspan="4">병원감염 : 1. 수술후 2. 기타처치후 3. 비뇨기계 4. 호흡기계 5. 소화기계 6. 기타</td></tr>
<tr><td colspan="4">원사인 : 부검: 예, 아니오</td></tr>
<tr><td colspan="4">계속적 진료 계획</td></tr>
<tr><td colspan="4">1. 없음 2. 있음 (약속일 년 월 일 시)</td></tr>
<tr><td>담당 전공의 서명 : 최인영</td><td colspan="3">담당 전문의 서명 : 서은국</td></tr>
<tr><td>의무기록 완성 : 2017 년 5 월 10 일</td><td colspan="3">의무기록사 서명 : 박한자</td></tr>
</table>

등록번호	188 33 00	성별 M
성명	하 만 세	
주민등록	661201－1234567	

응급실기록

Emergency Record

2017. 2. 27　　도착시간 7: 40 AM

환자주소	경기도 성남시 수정구 15－2				전화	0342) 40－2854	직업	장사
동행보호인	성명	홍주미	연령	45	성별	여	직업	무직
	주소	경기도 성남시 수정구 15－2			전화		관계	부인
내원 수단	☐ 구급차 119 (서초구)			☐ 경찰차		☐ 택시		
	☐ 도 보			☐ 늅는차		☐ 기타		
사고발생장소				발생시간				
사고발생경위	집 계단에서 Hemoptysis (≒150cc) abd pain 있는 것 발견하여 119 구급대 통해 내원함. 아파트 계단을 내려가다 넘어져 chin laceration (≒2cm) 됨							
사고발생보고	☐ 친척		☐ 경찰		☐ 기타			
내원당시 환자상태	활력증후 혈압 80/50 mmHg　맥박 /min　호흡 /min　체온 ˚C							
	의식상태: ☐ 명료　☐ 혼돈　☐ 반의식　☐ 무의식							
	기타: 내원당시 ascites 있으며 abd. pain							
응급처치후 처리	☐ 입원 과 호			☐ 외래의뢰		☐ 귀가		
	☐ 타병원			☐ 사망		☐ 기타		

작성자 RN 신향은

Brief History

C.C　Hematemesis

P.I　# Known alcoholic liver Ds

#2 어제 알코올 drinking

→ Develop되어 ER 방문

P.H　Alcoholic liver Ds

S.H　Smoking (－)

Alcohol Soju 2－3 bottle/day

ROS　Can not check

P/Ex　Acutely ill looking

Pale conjunctiva

Icteric sclera

Blood in mouth & nose

Chest CBS $\bar{s}$ ⓡ

RHB $\bar{s}$ ⓜ

Further exam can't

imp) UGI bleeding

R/O Varix bleeding　　Yoo

Req)　CBC $\bar{c}$ PLT　PT/PTT ┐ Stat

e'BUN/Cr　Glu　NH3 ┘

U/A

Chest PA　　Yoo

등록번호	188 33 00	성별 M
성명	하 만 세	
주민등록	661201－1234567	

퇴 원 요 약
Discharge Summary

Final Dx. : # Alcoholic liver cirrhosis
Esophageal varix bleeding
Alveolar bone Fx. in oral cavity
Mandible bone Fx. (open)
Sepsis

C.C Hematemesis Onset : '17. 2. 27 AM 6:00

P.I Known chr. alcoholism (2～3병 소주/day x 25 years)
Alcoholic L.C. (advanced) $\bar{c}$ ascites, portal HBP.
'16. 12월부터 abd. distension 있어 본원 외래 f/u
그 후 계속 alcohol drinking 하면서 지내다 금일 새벽 6시경 계단에서 slip down되어 ER 방문 후 varix bleeding imp하에 응급 EVL 시행하고 MICU로 admission

Lab. 2/27 GFS : E. varix bleeding (EVL 시행)
(F3 RC (＋) LS CB)
3/20 GFS : Sclerotherapy was done on the esophageal side of the GE junction (12cc = 7 + 5cc)
at ER(2/27) CBC : 7.4 － 24 － 5500 － 33000 PT : 14.7sec (54%)
e′ : 140 － 3.5 － 106 NH3 : 132
BUN/Cr : 8/1.0

LET.	OT/PT(3600/1233)	T.prot/alb(5.7/2.9)	ALP(167)
	Bil T/D(8.5/4.1)	Ca/P(7.3/2.1)	r－GTP(117)
	→ CT/PT(107/87)	T.prot(5.8/2.8)	ALP(91)
	Bil T/D(40.6/25.8)	Ca/P(8.2/5.8)	r－GTP(51)
	AFP(2.5)		

Blood culture : Streptococcus viridans group
입원하여 whole blood 3Ⓟ,
FFP 7 ⓤ, PRC 45 Ⓤ transfusion함.
→ '17. 3. 26 PM 5:30 expire 선언

Seo/Choi

등록번호	188 33 00 성별 M
성명	하 만 세
주민등록	661201－1234567

경 과 기 록
Discharge Summary

일 자	내 용	서 명

〈 Admission note 〉

2/27 C.C Hematemesis onset : 2.27 6:00 AM

P.I Known chr. alcoholism (하루 소주 2～3병)
& Alcoholic LC(advanced) & ascites
portal HTN, splenomegaly (sono상 15.3cm)
→ 평소 heavy drinking 하시던 분으로 별 문제없이 지내다 '16. 12월부터 abd. distension있어 본원 MED OPD f/u (OT/PT: 95/27 alb : 3.1 Bil T/D : 1.3/0.9 r－GTP : 259 ALP : 99) AFP : 5.2
→ HCV Ab(－) HBs Ag/Ab/Ig G－Ab(－/－/＋)/IgM(－)
GFS exam : check 못함.
그 후 계속 alcohol drinking 하면서 지내다 금일 새벽 6시경 집 계단에서 slip down(앞으로) 되어 보호자가 발견하여 ER 방문 후 varix bleeding imp하에 응급 EVL 시행 후 adm.

P.H HBP/DM/Tb (－/－/－) Hepatitis (＋)

S.H alcohol (＋): 소주 2～3 bottles/day x 25 yrs

F.H 08년 부친이 현재 정신병 증상은 없고 심한 우울증이 있는 양극성 정동장애로 정신과 치료도중 공원에서 할로겐화 살충제 먹고 자살시도한 적 있음.

ROS
Fever/Chill (－/＋) Headache/dizziness (－/－)
Neck pain(＋) Chest or severe abd pain (－/＋)
A/N/V/D/C (＋/＋/＋/－/－) Melena (＋) Hematochezia (＋)
Hematemesis (＋) Dysuria (＋) Oliguria (＋)

P/Ex
G/A Chr. ill looking c̄ drunken state, confusion
HEENT Not pale telangiectasia (＋)
Moderately icteric sclera
Neck Venous engorgement (＋/＋)
Chest Rapid heart beat s̄ ⓜ
CBS s̄ ⓡ
Abdomen Spider angioma
Distended abdomen rigid
Not palpable liver
No rebound tenderness

경 과 기 록

일 자	내 용	서 명
2/27	Back CVAT (−/−) Ext Pitting edema (−/−) Palmar erythema (+/+) Imp 1) Variceal bleeding(UGI) due to LC(alcohol) 2) Mandibular fx. 3) Alveolar bone fx.	*Lee*
2/27	Emergency EVL 시행 (내시경실) incisor 35∼36cm area active bleeding total 14개 시행 → F3 RC(+) L5 C8 varix on varix → No Re−bleeding P/Ex 상 위·아래 teeth incisor 1−4 Fx c̄ active bleeding 아래턱 deep skin laceration (bone → Repaired by PS. dept exposured) transfusion (PRC + FFP) antacid, Lamina−G, NPO 치과 consult Delirium tremens에 유의해서 보기	*Lee*
3/1	〈 Off−duty note 〉 *F3 LS CB RC(+) Dx; 1) Variceal (esophagus) bleeding → underlying alcoholic LC 2) Mandible & alveolar (oral cavity) bone Fx c̄ bleeding 3) Skin laceration (lower chin) Problem ; varix bleeding은 control되었다. * 현재 oral cavity 내에 oozing or bleeding 지속되고 있어 이에 대한 집중적 치료 요망됩니다. → CBC ↓의 원인 * I/O → +600 유지 Calorie → 최소한 1600 cal 이상 유지할 수 있도록 but ascites 있으므로 vol 되도록 줄이기 * '17. 3. 3 치과 꼭 연락 → Decision 내리기 * 필요하면 계속 transfusion (PRC & FFP) Hematuria에 대한 evaluation → Nephro consult, U/A f/u	

경 과 기 록

일 자	내 용	서 명
3/1	Plan) 1) 식사(LD부터) trial 2) 대변 색깔 잘 보기 계속 gauze packing in gum (upper) 3) CBC → routine으로 f/u (3/3/99) 4) 보호자에게 설명 * ICU 환자는 I/O balancing과 nutrition(calorie)이 생명입니다. 이에 대한 숙지가 필요합니다.	*Lee*
	〈 Duty on Note 〉 Dx. : 1. Alcoholic LC 2. E. varix bleeding (F3 RC(+) Ls CB) 3. Alveolar bone Fx. in oral cavity Mandible bone Fx. 4. Lower chin의 skin laceration Lab: GFS(2/27) : E. varix bleeding EVL 14 시행 Abd sono : 1. advanced L.C R/O alcoholic liver ds 2. portal HBP, moderate splenomegaly 3. a small gallstone LFT : OT/PT(3600/1233) prot/alb(5.7/2.9) ALP(167) Bil T/P(8.5/4.1) Ca/P(7.3/2.1) r−GTP(119) PT : 18.1 sec(31%) Problem list; 1. oral cavity bleeding (gum bleeding 발치 후) 2. hematuria 3. L.C. 4. alcoholism Plan : 1. Gum bleeding → Veselin gauze packing → 치과 consult 2. Check I/O : +600 유지 3. Cal : 1600 cal 4. Hematuria → Nephro consult U/A follow up 5. Alcoholism → thiamine IV 혹시 Delirium tremens 발생할 가능성 있기 때문에 DDx BEE(Basal energe expenditure) : 66+(13.7x68)+(5x172)−6.8x50 = 66+931.6+860−340=1517.6cal	Choi

경 과 기 록

일 자	내 용	서 명
3/3	S : Poor oral intake gum bleeding, mental alert O : Flapping tremor (−) CBC : 10.0−31−3700−21000 e′ : S−NH_3: 131 A : 1. 치과 consult 2. PS consult: packing하면 necrosis (chin의 suture site) 일어나기 때문에 loose packing 3. PRC 2Ⓟ transfusion 4. Check I/O : +600 보호자분에게 bleeding tendency가 있기 때문에 cerebral hemorrhage varix rebleeding, G−I hemorrhage에 대해 설명하였고 respiratory failure cardiac arrest가 오면 → intubation, CPR(+) → 본원 영안실 사용	Choi
	〈 Notify note 〉 S : Gum bleeding(+): continuous O : Fever(+): 39°C ↑ ← PRC T/F 이후 Subclavian self−removal하고 fever와 gum bleeding으로 힘들어 하고 IV therapy refuse(계속 설득했으나) → Flapping tremor(−/−) → Notify to 주치의 M/S: alert P : 1. Observation 2. 계속 Pt 설득 3. Compression of gum bleeding 4. Blood culture, CBC, e′ : S−NH_3] check	Choi
3/5	S : melena (+) gum bleeding O : mental alert flapping tremor (−) CBC: 8.3−25−5600−34000 Blood culture : Streptococcus viridance A : Gum bleeding에 의한 melena Blood culture 할 때 contamination Sepsis P : 1. PRC 4Ⓟ transfusion 2. FFP 5 units transfusion	Choi

경 과 기 록

일 자	내 용	서 명
3/7	S : Dark green color stool (+) gum bleeding ↓ O : CBC : 9.5−30−6000−48000 e′ : 131−3.1−100 A : 1. Sepsis 2. L.C. varix P : Gum bleeding severe하면 → PRC transfusion BP ↓ 소변 ↓ → FFP transfusion Check I/O → +600 유지	*Choi*
3/8	S : Mental alert, flapping tremor (−) O : CBC: 9.2−29−7900−46000 e′ : 131−3.7−100 B/Cr : 16/0.6 A : 1. L.C. $\bar{c}$ varix ascites 2. Alveolar bone Fx 3. Sepsis P : 1. Pt분이 irritable하면 → Demerol 50mg IM 2. I/O: +500 유지 3. BP: 80/60 ↓, urine out put 30cc/hr ↓ → FFP 2−3 units transfusion	*Choi*
3/12	S : Gum bleeding O : CBC : 9.5−28−5800−41000 e′ : 131−3.7−99 A : 1. L.C. $\bar{c}$ varix, ascites 2. Alveolar bone Fx 3. R/O sepsis P : 1. FFP PRC 2. Antibiotics 3. Hypokalemia가 되면 hepatic encephalopathy에 빠질 수 있으므로 electrolyte follow up	*Choi*
3/14	S : Melena (+) 200g O : CBC: 9.0−28−5600−56000 e′: 131−3.7−99 A : Liver cirrhosis Varix bleeding S/P EVL → Rebleeding으로 생각되어짐 P : 1. Sucralfate 2. FFP, PRC transfusion	*Choi*

경 과 기 록

일 자	내 용	서 명
3/20	S : Flapping tremor (+), Melena (+) O : CBC: 10.4－30－1099－62000 e′ : 131－4.4－101 B/Cr : 83/1.0 GFS : Sclero Tx was done on the esophageal side of the GE junction A : 1. L.C. $\bar{c}$ varix bleeding 2. Sepsis P : 1. FFP PRC transfusion 2. Electrolyte BUN/Cr CBC NH_3 3. Antibiotics 4. If active varix bleeding (hematemesis) → S－B tube: stomach에 300cc 정도만 ballooning함 (esophagus는 ballooning 하지 말기 바람) 5. lactulose enema $Ccr=\frac{(140-50)\times 68}{72\times 1.9}=\frac{6120}{136}=45$	*Choi*
3/25	S : Drowsy mentality O : CBC 9.6－28－17400－26000 e′ 141－5.1－109 B/Cr : 161/2.9 P : 1. Antibiotics 2. Lactulose enema 3. PRC FFP transfusion 4. BP ↓ (80/60) 정도 떨어지면 FFP 2Ⓟ transfusion 후 반응 없으면 → Dopa ↑ 5. 소변 urine out put ↓ 할 때 (30cc/hr ↓) 줄 때 → FFP 2Ⓟ transfusion	*Choi*
3/26	PM 5:30 cardiac arrest로 expire 선언 사후처치 후 내과 중환자실에서 안치실로 나감	*Choi*

등록번호	188 33 00	성별	M
성명	하 만 세		
주민등록	661201－1234567		

협의진단기록

Consultation Record

Request For Consultation To

Summary of Present Finding　　　　치과 한문진 선생님께

Dx. : 1) Advanced alcoholic liver cirrhosis with esophageal variceal bleeding(massive)
2) Alveolar bone Fx in oral cavity and bleeding (gingiva)
3) Deep laceration, mandible

C.C : Hematemesis & melena (2/27/'17 새벽)
식도 정맥류 출혈로 현재 ICU care중인 분으로(내시경 치료함) 상기 2번의 problem에 대해 귀과적인 management 부탁드립니다.
감사합니다.

Date 2017. 2. 28　　　　Signature 서은국/최인영

Report of Consultation

Opinion and Recommendation

〈 Dent note 〉

PE) 1. 2 1 | x x 3 brige 탈락
2. 2| retained root
3. 1| spontaneous exfoliation
(tooth avulsion)

Tx) 1. 2 1 | x x 3 bridge removal
2. 1| removal of teeth
2| retained root extraction

Date 2017. 2. 28　　　　Signature 한문진

등록번호	188 33 00	성별	M
성명	하 만 세		
주민등록	661201－1234567		

위 내시경 차트

Gastroscopy Chart

Name : 유주발 Sex : M Age : 51 Chart No. 188 33 00

Requested by Dr. : 전구주 Dept. MED Date : 17. 3. 20

1. Chief complaints and present illness : Melena (＋)

2. Radiological findings (Upper G.I Series)

3. Endoscopic findings (Endoscopic No. 1547)

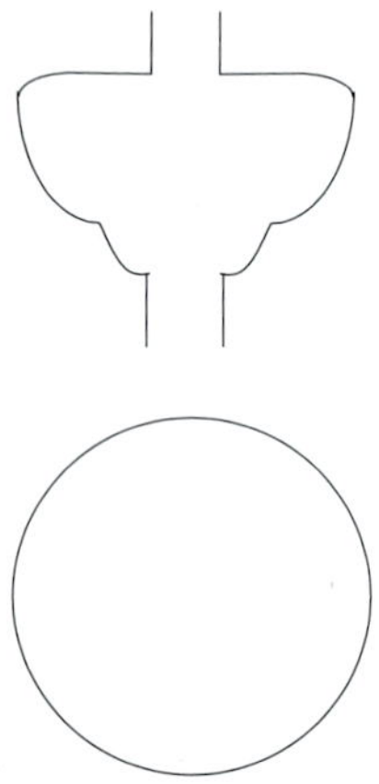

Photo. ＋ ( ) － ( ) Previous exam. ______

E/ multiple ulcerations were
S/ seen on the distal esophagus by the previous EVL. Active bleeding was not seen from the esophageal ulceration but suspicious clots were seen on the ulcer bases. There was active bleeding on the G－E junction, but it was not possible to identify the exact site, because a large blood clot was attached to the G－E junction, Woozing of blood was seen from the surrounding mucosa just out side the clot attached mucosa.

The sclero Tx was done on the esophageal side of the G－E junction(12cc: 7＋5 cc).

Impression: ______

4. Histological findings: Slide. ＋( ) －( )

5. Remarks

Examined by Dr. 양미준

〈하 만 세〉

★ 하만세 차트를 읽고 맞는 것에 O표 하시오.

1 진단명에 대한 분류번호로 틀리게 연결된 것은?

① K80.20, S02.691 ② A40.8, I10.9 ③ I85.90, R16.1
④ S02.82, S02.671 ⑤ K80.20, R16.1

2 경과기록지에 대한 내용과 다른 것은?

① 복부 초음파 결과 작은 담석과 간비대가 있었다.
② 혈뇨에 대해 신장내과 협의진료를 의뢰했다.
③ 3월 20일 전해질 검사 결과 나트륨이 131mEq/L이 나왔다.
④ 경화요법은 위식도 접합부의 식도면에서 시행되었다.
⑤ 짙은 녹색의 대변이 있었고 진전은 없는 것으로 나타났다.

3 입원당시 나타난 증상만으로 짝지어진 것은?

① 설사－오심 ② 두통－복부의 통증 ③ 목의 통증－오한
④ 핍뇨증－현기증 ⑤ 열－흉통

4 주진단명과 그와 관련된 분류번호로 짝지어진 것은?

① I98.1, K70.30, R17 ② I98.1, K74.6, R17 ③ I98.2, K74.6, R18
④ I98.3, K70.31, R18 ⑤ I98.3, K74.6, R17

5 의무기록 내용으로 틀린 것은?

① 토혈과 혈변을 주소로 내원하였다.
② 목의 정맥이 충혈되어 있었다.
③ 신선 냉동 혈장을 45pints 수혈하였다.
④ 간암여부를 진단하는 종양표지자는 정상치였다.
⑤ 늑골척추각 압통은 없었다.

6 상기 환자가 병원에 오게 된 경위에 대한 분류번호로 맞는 것은?

① S00.7, W10.0 ② S01.8, W10.0 ③ S01.8, W10.9
④ S01.48, W10.9 ⑤ S01.8, W10.3

7 간경변에 대한 내용과 다른 것은?

① 간세포가 손상되어 섬유화되고 퇴행성 변화가 생기는 질환이다.
② 감염이나 독소도 간세포에 영향을 줄 수 있다.
③ 간세포의 기능 저하로 빌리루빈이 체외로 배설되지 못할 때 황달이 온다.
④ 혈관 중간층에 퇴행성 변화로 섬유화가 진행되고 혈관의 탄성이 감소한다.
⑤ 만성적인 염증으로 인해 섬유화 조직으로 바뀌어 간의 기능이 저하된다.

8 가족력에 대한 분류번호로 맞게 짝지어진 것은?

① F31.5, T60.0, X48.8 ② F31.4, T60.0, X48.9 ③ F31.5, T60.1, X48.0
④ F31.4, T60.1, X48.8 ⑤ F31.4, T60.2, X48.9

9 **통계분석상 옳게 기재된 것은?**

① 협의진단의뢰는 1건이다.
② MICU 재원일수는 27일이다.
③ POD #7 이내 사망환자이다.
④ Total LOS 26일이다.
⑤ 자의퇴원환자이다.

10 **혈액검사상 다음과 같은 결과가 나왔다면 어떤 진단을 내릴 수 있겠는가?**

> HBs－Ag (＋)　　HBs－Ab (－)　　HBc－Ag (＋)
> GOT/GPT: 150/120

① B형 hepatitis
② C형 hepatitis
③ liver cirrhosis
④ fatty liver
⑤ A형 hepatitis

01 약물 중독 및 심방세동
Drug intoxication and atrial fibrillation

1.1 당뇨병(Diabetes mellitus; DM)

당뇨병(DM)의 원인

- 당뇨병은 내분비계 장기 중 췌장(이자)에서 인슐린 분비량 부족 시 발생 → 과소분비
- 혈중 포도당 농도가 높은 것이 특징
- 포도당은 우리 몸이 사용하는 가장 기본적인 에너지원

인슐린(insulin, β 세포)과 글루카곤(glucagon, α 세포)

- 혈액 속의 포도당 농도를 '혈당'이라고 함
- 혈당을 조절하는 2가지 호르몬 → 인슐린과 글루카곤
  - 혈당은 췌장에서 생산되는 인슐린과 글루카곤이라는 물질에 의해 일정 수준 유지

•인슐린: 혈당 낮추는 역할 → 췌장의 랑게르한스섬의 베타(β) 세포에서 만들어짐
•글루카곤: 혈당 높이는 역할 → 췌장의 랑게르한스섬의 알파(α) 세포에서 만들어짐

당뇨병 분류

- 소아: Type Ⅰ = E10._
  = Insuline-dependent diabetes mellitus(IDDM, 인슐린 의존성 당뇨병)
- 성인: Type Ⅱ = E11._
  = Non-insulin-dependent diabetes mellitus(NIDDM, 인슐린 비의존성 당뇨병)

표 1 • 당뇨병 중요 내용

· 당뇨병 원인: 췌장 인슐린 부족 · 혈당 조절 2가지 호르몬: 랑게르한스섬 – 인슐린: β세포에서 생성 – 글루카곤: α세포에서 생성	· 당뇨병 분류 – 소아: Type Ⅰ = E10._ = IDDM(인슐린 의존성 당뇨병) – 성인: Type Ⅱ = E11._ = NIDDM(인슐린 비의존성 당뇨병)

1.2 고혈압(Hypertension; HTN)

고혈압(HTN)의 분류

- 혈압(blood pressure; BP): 혈압이란 혈액이 혈관 벽에 가하는 힘
- 고혈압: 동맥(artery)의 높은 혈압 → 140/90 mmHg 이상(성인)

표 2 • 정상혈압: 120/80 mmHg
· 120 : 수축기혈압(systolic blood pressure; BP) = 최고 혈압 · 80 : 이완기혈압(diastolic blood pressure; BP) = 최저 혈압 · 맥압=혈관 탄력성=건강 상징: 수축기 혈압과 확장기 협압의 차 - 정상 맥압: 40 mmHg 전후 예) 120-80 = 40 mmHg

혈압 및 맥압

- 혈압의 분류
  - 수축기 혈압(Systolic blood pressure; SBP): 최고 혈압
    - 심장이 수축하면서 혈액을 내보낼 때 혈관에 가해지는 압력
  - 확장기 혈압(Diastolic blood pressure; DBP): 최저 혈압
    - 심장이 확장(이완)하면서 혈액을 받아들일 때 혈관이 받는 압력
- 맥압(pulse pressure): 혈관 탄력성 = 건강의 상징
  - 수축기 혈압(최고 혈압)과 확장기 혈압(최저 혈압)의 차를 맥압(脈壓)이라고 함
    예) 130/70 mmHg: 130 − 70 = 60 mmHg(맥압)
  - 성인의 정상 맥압: 40㎜ 전후
  - 맥압이 클수록 혈관 탄력도가 낮음 → 대동맥이 경화되면 맥압이 커짐
  - 운동 시: 수축기 혈압 > 확장기 혈압 → 맥압은 안정때 보다 커짐

표 3 • 살충제의 종류	
• 유기인계 살충제(organophosphous insecticides) 예) diazinon	• 카바메이트계 살충제(carbamate insecticides) 예) fenobucarb

2.1 심방세동(Atrial fibrillation) 및 심방조동(Atrial flutter)

심방세동(잔떨림, Atrial fibrillation): 심방 빠르고 불규칙적 심장수축

- 심장은 동방결절에서 시작된 전기신호가 전도계를 따라 규칙적으로 전달
  - 심방과 심실이 수축과 이완 반복
- 1분(분당)에 350번 이상 빠르고 불규칙한 맥박을 형성하는 부정맥(불규칙한 맥박) 질환
- 심방 내에 혈액이 정체되면서 뭉쳐져서 혈전 형성
- 좌심방 내 혈전은 일부 또는 전체가 떨어져 나가 뇌혈관 막으며 허혈성 뇌졸중 유발

심방조동(된떨림, Atrial flutter): 심방 빠르고 규칙적 수축

- 조동은 심방 또는 심실이 1분(분당)에 약 300회 정도로 빠르고 규칙적인 수축
- 심장 내부의 구조적 특성으로 부정맥이 형성되는 질환

표 4 • 심방 세동 및 조동: 정상 1분 60~80회	
• 심방세동(atrial fibrillation) – 심방 빠르고 불규칙한 심장 수축 – 1분에 350번 이상	• 심방 조동(atrial flutter) – 심방 빠르고 규칙적 수축 – 1분에 300번

2.2 부정맥(Arrhythmia)

부정맥(Arrhythmia): 심방세동, 심방조동

- 심방세동, 심방조동은 가장 흔한 부정맥
- 심장의 전기 자극이 잘 만들어지지 않거나 자극 전달이 잘 이루어지지 않음
  - 규칙적인 수축이 계속되지 않고 심장 박동이 빠르거나 늦어지거나 불규칙하게 됨

차트 용어							
• alert	명료(정상/의식상태)	• arrest	정지	• conjunctiva	결막	• engorgement	충혈
• enlarge	확대하다	• gastric lavage	위세척	• hematuria	혈뇨	• icteric=jaundice =hyperbilirubinemia	황달
• infusion solution	수액	• intoxication	중독	• intubation	기관내 삽관	• phototherapy	광선치료
• papable	촉진	• rash	발진	• persistent	지속적인	• isocoria	동공크기 동일
• recurrence	재발	• sclera	공막	• stone =calculus	결석	• pitting edema	함요부종
• ureter	요관	• ventilator	인공 호흡기	• weakness	약함	• thigh=femur • intact = free = G-F = WNL = N-S=N-C	대퇴(넙적 다리 정상

약 어	원 어	
ABGA	Arterial blood gas analysis	동맥혈가스분석
AF	Atrial fibrillation	세동
ALT	Alanine aminotransferase = LFT(liver function test) = OT/PT = GOT/GPT = SGOT/SGPT	알라닌 아미노전이효소 (간기능검사) – 정상수치: 40U/L 이하
AST	Aspartate aminotransferase = LFT(liver function test) = OT/PT = GOT/GPT = SGOT/SGPT	아스파르테이트 아미노전이효소 (간기능검사) – 정상수치: 40U/L 이하
BS	Breathing sound	호흡음
BUN	Blood urea nitrogen	혈액요소질소
CBC	Complete blood count	일반 혈액검사(전혈구계산)
D/C	Discontinue	중단
CVA	Diagnosis(Dx) 진단명: Cerebral vascular accident Physical examination(P/Ex) 신체검진 : Costovertebral angle	뇌혈관 사고 늑골척추각
DM	Diabetes mellitus	당뇨병
d/t	due to	~로 인한
DTR	Deep tendon reflex	심부건 반사
Echo	Echography = sonography	초음파 검사
EKG = ECG	Electrocardiography	심전도 검사
HTN	Hypertension	고혈압
HB	Heat beat	심박동
Hgb = Hb	Hemoglobin	헤모글로빈=혈색소 – 빈혈: 10 mg/dL 이하
IV	Intravenous	정맥내: 정맥 통해 투약 또는 처치
MICU	Medicine intensive care unit	내과 중환자실 – 중환자실: ICU, CCU
LA	Left ventricle	좌심실
PLR	Prompt light reflex	즉각 빛 반응
LLF	Left lower field	왼쪽 아래 부분
ⓜ	Murmur	잡음 → ⓡ rale 수포음
NPO	Nothing per os = Nothing by mouth	금식
$\bar{s}$	Without	$\bar{s}$ = 동반없이($\bar{c}$ = 동반)
Tbc	Tuberculosis	결핵
T/f	Transfer	전과
USG	Ultrasonography(U/S)	초음파 검사
V/S	Vital signs	활력징후

장 만 복 요약 차트

등록번호 : 26 84 75　　　이름 : 장만복
입원일 : 2017. 12. 11　　　퇴원일 : 2017. 12. 28　　　퇴원과 : IM

Diagnosis : Drug Intoxication
Type ll DM
Essential HTN
Persistent AF
R/O Bladder tumor
Alcoholic fatty liver

C.C : Diazinon, fenobucarb

P.I : 52세 남환으로 11년 전 DM 2004년 Pul. Tbc. 2015년 pul. Tbc recur. AF, 2017년 10월 R/O CVA (Rt. side weakness)로 입원 치료받았던 자로 내원 3개월 전 사업실패로 빚에 쪼들려 오다가 내원 당일 공원에서 소주 2병과 함께 종이컵 1컵 정도의 상기 농약(살충제) 마시고 서울 K병원에서 G. Lavage 10ι, 1-PAM 2g, Charcoal 50g, BUN 2 Ⓐ mix 처치 후 T/f.

P.Hx : DM(+): MxP3 32u/16u, ACBA
HTN(−), AF(+), Pul Tbc(+), '04, '13
Rt. side weakness − 현재 intact
OP Hx (+) − appendectomy ('08년)
Depression − 현재 improved

P/Ex.
G.A) Alert consciousness
Skin) No rash
H/Neck) No neck vein engorgement
E/ENT) Isocoria $\bar{c}$ PLR(+/+)
Not pale conjunctiva
Not icteric sclera
Thorax) irregular HB $\bar{s}$ ⓜ
decreased BS at LLF

Choi

1

장 만 복 요약 차트

등록번호 : 26 84 75 이름 : 장만복
입원일 : 2017. 12. 11 퇴원일 : 2017. 12. 28 퇴원과 : IM

Abd) soft & flat
Normoactive to ↓ BS
No abdo tenderness
Not palpable abdo. mass
B/Ext) No CVA tenderness
No thigh pitting edema
Neurology) DTR (++/++)
Imp) Drug intoxication
Plan) Atropine IV till secretion dry up
PAM IV (antidote)
supportive care

Lab.

CBC	9.8 / 39.4 / 343k
Bil(T/D)	0.43 / 0.12
ALP/ r GT	21 / 32
AST/ALT	26 / 35
BUN/Cr	23 / 1.3
Na/k/Cl	140 / 3.9 / 99

Treatment and Results

#1 Drug intoxication
adm 후 Respiratory arrest 발생하여 ICU care 후에 증세 호전되어
General ward에서 약물치료 시행함

#2 Type 2 DM
IV with infusion solution due to NPO
HbA1c = 10.3%로서
1-MxP3 split dose (28 u / 14 u)로 조절되지 않는 상태이나 환자 퇴원하여
외래에서 조절하기로 하고 퇴원시킴

#3 HTN c̄ AF.
Echo) enlarge LA (4.83cm)

Choi

2

장 만 복 요약 차트

등록번호 : 26 84 75　　　이름 : 장만복
입원일 : 2017. 12. 11　　　퇴원일 : 2017. 12. 28　　　퇴원과 : IM

〈 Progress notes 〉

12/11 #1

S & O) Chilling, dyspnea 호소하며, sudden respi. arrest 발생
→ EKG상 HR 70회/min
Intubation & Ambu bagging was done
Atropine 1Ⓐ IVSS x 2회
→ HR 160회/min & femoral a. pulse 확인됨.
ABGA (O_2 15ι, ambu bagging)
7.11-59.6-174.6-98.6%
→ Bivon 3Ⓐ IVSS
ICU arrange하여 내림.

A) Respiratory arrest
d/t organophosphate and carbamate intoxication

P) Ventilator care
SIMV
RR 16회/min
TV 500ml
PAM IV 계속

#2. Hematuria
처음 Foley catheter 꽂을 때 Hematuria (+)
→ F/U 시 hematuria (−)
Catheter injury 가능성도 없고 그 전에 Ureter stone →
ESWL한 Hx 있음 → F/U 해보고 Sono 내일 Check 할 것

Choi

〈진단방사선 보고서〉

12/11

Chest AP :
No abdominal bowel gas pattern
No evidence of ascites or organomegaly.
Mild spondylosis of L-spine.　　*Park*

장 만 복 요약 차트

등록번호 : 26 84 75　　　이름 : 장만복
입원일 : 2017. 12. 11　　　퇴원일 : 2017. 12. 28　　　퇴원과 : IM

12//17
EKG :
Atrial, Fibrillation
Left Axis Deviation Abnormal, ECG　　　*Choi*

12/18
Abd. kidney sonogram
Imp) Tiny GB stone.
Left renal stone　　　*Choi*

〈Physician's Orders〉

12/11 1. Check V/S $\overline{q}$ 6hrs. I/O
2. O_2 4L / min via NP
3. frequent suction → D/C
4. NPO except med.　　　*Lee*

12/11 추) 1. Blood culture X2 (호, 혐) → MICU
2. Foley catheter insertion
L/T insert $\overline{c}$ drainage

12/13 1. SIMV - TV 300ml
RR 16회/min
FiO2 0.24
2. 1hr 후 ABGA

12/28 Discharge　　　*Lee*

〈장 만 복〉

★ 장만복 차트를 읽고 맞는 것에 O표 하시오.

1 환자에 대한 설명으로 옳지 않은 것은?

① 결핵이 과거에 재발되었다.
② 당뇨는 조절이 잘 되지 않았다.
③ 입원 후 호흡정지가 발생하였다.
④ 입원시점에 중환자실로 배당되었다.
⑤ 뇌혈관 사고로 약해진 우측은 현재 정상이다.

2 정상소견을 보인 검사로 옳은 것은?

① Hgb
② EKG
③ OT/PT
④ Sonogram
⑤ Chest X-ray

3 환자에 대한 질병분류번호로 옳지 않은 것은?

① I48.1
② I60.4
③ E11.9
④ K70.0
⑤ T60.0, X68.8

4 환자가 과거에 앓은 질환으로 옳지 않은 것은?

① 골절
② 충수염
③ 우울증
④ 심방세동
⑤ 요관결석

5 환자에게 행해진 처치로 옳지 않은 것은?

① 타병원에서 위세척 및 활성탄을 투여받고 전원되었다.
② 호흡정지가 있어 Atropine과 Pam을 정맥내 투여하였다.
③ 호흡곤란으로 기관내 삽관 및 심장마사지를 시행하였다.
④ 당뇨병은 금식 때문에 수액에 섞어서 정맥내 투여하였다.
⑤ 입원당일 폴리 카테터(foley catheter) 삽입 시 혈뇨가 있었다.

6 입원 시 환자의 신체상태로 옳은 것은?

① 복부에 압통이 있었다.
② 피부에 발진이 있었다.
③ 복부의 덩어리가 촉진되었다.
④ 늑골척추각 압통은 없었다.
⑤ 대퇴의 함요부종이 있었다.

02. 외 과 계

Surgery

I. 전체 차트 (Full Chart)

II. 요약 차트 (Summary Chart)

MEDICAL RECORD PRACTICE

01 좌 상완골 원위부 골절
Lt. distal humeral fracture

1.1 골절(Fracture; Fx)

▸ Closed fracture(폐쇄성 골절): 뼈는 부러졌으나 외상(open wound)이 없는 상태

▸ Open fracture(개방성 골절): 뼈는 부러졌으나 외상이 있는 상태

표 1• 골절의 분류

개방성 골절(open fracture)	폐쇄성 골절(closed fracture)
· 복합골절(compound fx.)	· 단순골절(simple fx.)
· 감염성골절(infected fx.)	· 분쇄골절(comminuted fx.)
· 총탄성골절(missle fx.)	· 함몰골절(depressed fx.)
· 천자골절(puncture fx.)	· 약목골절(greenstick fx.)
· 이물질골절(foreign body fx.)	· 매복골절(impacted fx.)

치 료

① **정복(reduction):** 뼈를 정상위치로 회복

- Closed reduction(비관혈적 정복): 절개하지 않고 손으로 복원
- Open reduction(관혈적 정복): 골절부위에 절개(incision) + 내부 고정도구 추가

→ 내부고정(IF): 금속판(plate), 나사(screw), 핀(pin), 못(nail)

② **고정(fixation)**

- 관혈적 정복 및 내부고정(OR c̄ IF; open reduction and internal fixation)
- 비관혈적 정복 및 내부고정(CR c̄ IF; closed reduction and internal fixation)

1.2 추간원판 탈출(Herniated intervertebral disk; HID)

▸ 추간원판의 수핵이 척추관으로 이탈되어(HNP) 척수신경근을 압박하여 통증

- 좌골신경통(sciatica): 허리에서 다리 아래 사이로 뻗치는 좌골신경의 통증
- 요통(허리 통증, Low back pain)
- 목의 통증(Cervical pain)

▸ 심한 경우 신경에 손상

▸ 가장 빈번한 발생 부위는 L_4-L_5, L_5-S_1[HLD, herniated lumbar disc(추간판 탈출)] → M51.2

치 료

① **추궁절제술(laminectomy)**

- 돌출된 디스크에 여유를 줄 수 있도록 추궁의 부분을 외과적으로 절제

② **경피적 흡인 디스크절제술(aspiration percutaneous diskectomy)**

- 피부를 통하여 관을 집어넣고, 디스크를 흡인(aspiration)

③ **화학적 수핵분해(chemonucleolysis)**

- 탈출된 디스크 중심을 디스크 용해효소(chymopapain) 주사

1.3 수핵탈출증(Herniated nucleus pulposus; HNP)

▸ 디스크 안쪽 부분에 수핵(nucleus pulposus)이 빠져나와 척수신경을 누름

표 2 • 혈액학적 검사(Hematology)

검사항목	정상치	임상적 의의
헤모글로빈, 혈색소 Hemoglobin(Hgb)	남: 13.0-17.0 g/dl 여: 12.0-16.0 g/dl	↑ 적혈구증다증 ↓ 빈혈
적혈구 용적 Hematocrit(Hct)	남: 36-54 g/dl 여: 36-47 g/dl	↑ 구토, 하리, 선천성 심질환 ↓ 철결핍성 빈혈, 빈혈, 부종

예) Hb/Hct (13.1/40): 정상, Hb/Hct (9.7/35): 빈혈

1.4 염좌(Sprain; 삐는 것)

▸ 관절 상해로 인해 인대(ligament), 건/힘줄(tendon), 인접조직의 손상으로 심한 통증

2.1 심전도(EKG) 및 부정맥(arrhythmia)

심전도(Electrocardiogram, EKG = ECG)의 정의

▸ 심박동 주기 중 발생하는 심장의 전기적 활동상태를 그래프상 나타낸 것

심전도의 전기적 변화: 5개의 파

① P파: 심방의 흥분으로 인한 최초의 전기파

- SA node(sinoatrial node, 동방결절)로부터 AV node(atrioventricular node, 방실결절)로 전기적 흥분이 지나갈 때 발생

② QRS파: 심실이 흥분하여 활동 전압이 생길 때 발생: 수축기

③ T파: 전기적 회복기로 심실이 이완될 때 발생

▸ 순서: P파 → QRS파 → T파

부정맥(arrhythmia)의 의미

▸ 부정맥: 비정상적인 심장의 리듬

- 리듬이 불규칙적이며 너무 빠르거나 너무 느린 박동수
- 즉 맥박이 빠르고 느린 것: 맥박 정상치 1분당 60~80회
- 부정맥의 대표적인 증상은 심장이 자주 쿵쾅거리거나 참기 힘든 가슴 통증

표 3 • 뼈의 돌기 및 함요

뼈의 돌기(Bone process)	뼈의 함요(depression)
• 골머리(Bone head)	• 구(고랑, Sulcus)
• 결절(Tubercle)	• 동(굴, Sinus)
• 전자(넙다리돌기, Trochanter)	• 와(오목, Fossa)
• 조면(거친면, Tuberosity)	• 구멍(Foramen)
• 과(Condyle)	• 열(Fissure)

2.2 입원 경로 및 질병분류 시 주의점

입원 경로 찾는 방법: ER(응급실), OPD(외래) local 경유 등

▸ 경과기록지, 퇴원요약지, 병력기록지 → PI(present illness, 현재질병)

▸ 응급실은 응급기록지 첨부됨

금기증(contraindication): 처치 → 실행되지 못함 → 금기

▸ Z53.0: KCD 1권 / 금기증 때문에 수행되지 못한 처치

예) 골절수술 위해 입원, OT/PT(간기능검사) 수치가 높아 수술보류

미끄럼, 걸림 등 동일 면상의 추락/전도: W00-W19

▸ 부여번호: W01._____ · 4단위 번호부여(장소 분류): ._____

예) 아파트: .0 도로: .4 → 도로에서 미끄러짐: W01.4

임상검사 찾는 방법(CT, MRI, EKG 등)

- 입퇴원기록: 수술처치명
- 퇴원요약: 검사(laboratory, Lab)
- 경과기록: 객관적(objective, O)
- 의사지시기록
- 임상병리 검사: 검사지(Lab), 검사기록(flow sheet)
- 협의진단기록

표 4 • 척주 및 척수신경의 비교

척주(Vertebral column): 근골격계			척수신경(Spinal nerves): 신경계(31쌍)	
경(목)추(Cevical vertebrae)	C1-C7	7개	경(목)신경(Cervical nerves)	8쌍
흉(등)추(Thoracic vertebrae)	T1-T12	12개	흉(등)신경(Thoracic nerves)	12쌍
요(허리)추(Lumbar vertebrae)	L1-L5	5개	요(허리)신경(Lumbar nerves)	5쌍
천(엉치)추(Sacral vertebrae)	S1-S5	5개	천(엉치)신경(Sacral nerves)	5쌍
미(꼬리)추(Coccygeal vertebrae) 평균 3~5개(성인: 1개)			미(꼬리)신경(Coccygeal nerves)	1쌍

표 5 • 뇌와 척수의 구성: 백질과 회백질

뇌(brain)	척수(spinal cord)
· 안쪽: 백질(white matter)의 수질 · 표면/바깥쪽: 회백질(gray matter)의 피질	· 안쪽: 회백질의 피질 · 표면: 백질의 수질

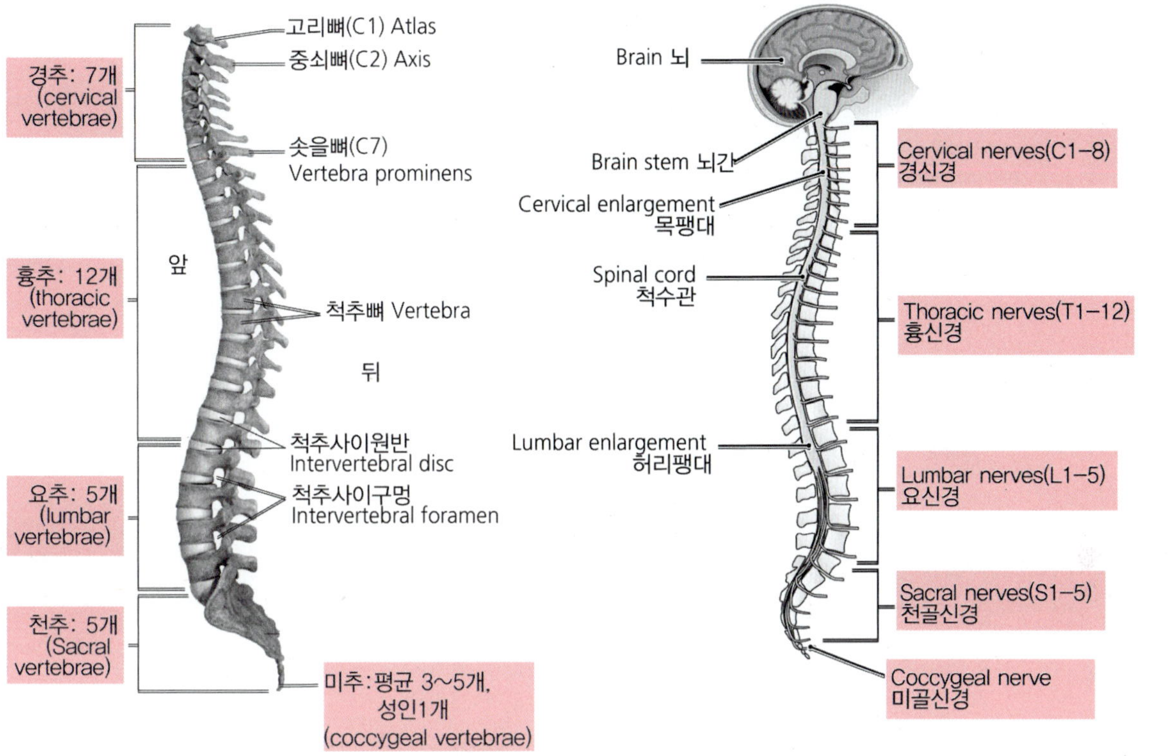

A. **척주**(vertebral column) B. **척수신경**(spinal nerve)

그림 1. 척주와 척수신경

중추신경계(Central nervous system; CNS)

↙ ↘

뇌(brain) + 척수(spinal cord) = 수막(뇌막, meninges)

말초신경계(Peripheral nervous system; PNS)

↙ ↓ ↘

<u>Cranial nerves 뇌신경(12쌍)</u>	<u>Spinal nerves 척수신경(31쌍)</u>	<u>Autonomic nerves 자율신경</u>
1. 후각신경	7. 안면(얼굴)신경	· 교감신경(Sympathetic nerves)
2. 시각신경	8. 내이(속귀)신경	· 부교감신경(Parasympathetic nerves)
3. 동안(눈돌림)신경: 눈운동	9. 설인(혀인두)신경	
4. 활차(도르래)신경: 눈운동	10. 미주신경: 목/내장	
5. 삼차신경(얼굴/혀/씹기)	11. 부신경: 목/등운동	
6. 외전(가돌림)신경: 눈운동	12. 설하(혀밑신경): 혀	

그림 2. 중추신경계와 말초신경계의 구분

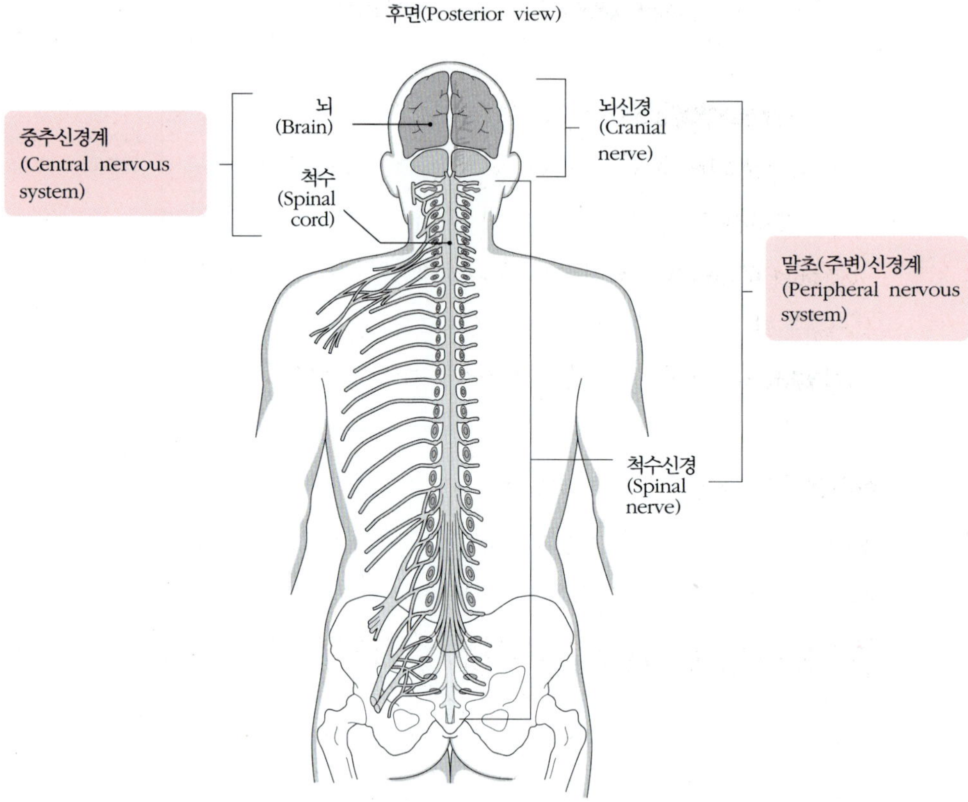

그림 3. 신경계의 분류

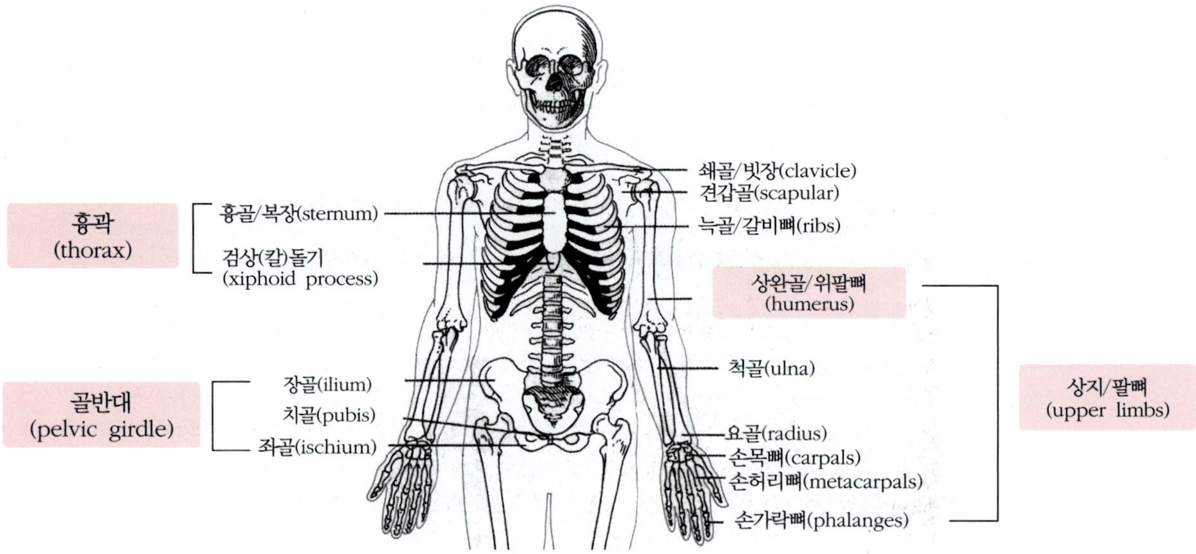

그림 4. 흉곽 및 상지의 뼈

차트 용어

- Alert 명료한(정신상태)
- Icteric=jaundice 황달(=hyperbilirubinemia)
- Extension 신전(펴기)
- Thumb 엄지손가락
- Flexion 굴곡(굽히기)
- Wrist 손목

약 어	원 어	
ABGA	Arterial blood gas analysis	동맥혈 가스 분석
CR $\bar{c}$ IF	Closed reduction and internal fixation	비관혈적 정복 및 내부고정술
EMG	Electromyogram	근전도 검사
Hct	Hematocrit	적혈구 용적
Hb, Hgb	Hemoglobin	헤모글로빈, 혈색소
H/S	Hartman's solution	하트만 용액(1 L =1,000cc)
MN	Midnight	자정(24시)
N-S	Non-specific = G-F = Free = Intact = WNL = full	특별한 소견 없음 = 정상
NSR	Normal sinus rhythm (heart)	정상 동방결절 리듬
OR $\bar{c}$ IF	Open reduction and internal fixation ‣ IF(내부고정술): screw(나사), pin(핀), wire(철사) 등	관혈적 정복 및 내부고정술
$\bar{q}$	Every	매
qid	Four times a day	하루에 4번
qod	Every other day	이틀에 한 번
ROM	Range-of-motion	운동범위
SSE	Soap solution enema	비눗물 관장
#	Number	횟수

표 6 • 뇌의 좌우 기능

좌측 뇌	우측 뇌
언변 좋음, 논리적, 분석적	공간감각 우세, 예술적, 감정에 약함

등록번호	122 22 66	성별 M
성명	오 합 격	
주민등록	800105－1234567	

입 퇴 원 기 록
Admission and Discharge Record

<table>
<tr><td colspan="4">주 소 :</td></tr>
<tr><td colspan="4">출신지 : 직 업 : 전 화 :</td></tr>
<tr><td colspan="4">연고자성명 : 황도진 관 계 주 소 : 전 화 :</td></tr>
<tr><td>입원 : 2017 년 5 월 15 일 과 병동 호</td><td></td><td colspan="2">20 년 월 일 과 병동 호</td></tr>
<tr><td>퇴원 : 2017 년 5 월 27 일 과 병동 호</td><td></td><td colspan="2">20 년 월 일 과 병동 호</td></tr>
<tr><td>재원일수 :</td><td></td><td colspan="2">20 년 월 일 과 병동 호</td></tr>
<tr><td colspan="3">최종진단명</td><td>분류번호</td></tr>
<tr><td colspan="3">주진단명 : Fx. distal humerus, Intercondyle Lt.</td><td></td></tr>
<tr><td colspan="3">(Intercondylar Fx.: comminuted Fx.)</td><td></td></tr>
<tr><td colspan="3">기타진단명 : High level of OT/PT</td><td></td></tr>
<tr><td colspan="3"></td><td></td></tr>
<tr><td colspan="3">수술 및 처치명</td><td></td></tr>
<tr><td colspan="3">수술명 : O/R & IF $\bar{c}$ 5 hole narrow DCP</td><td></td></tr>
<tr><td colspan="3">$\bar{c}$ 4 cortical screw</td><td></td></tr>
<tr><td colspan="3">$\bar{c}$ 1 cancellous screw (34mm)</td><td></td></tr>
<tr><td colspan="3">$\bar{c}$ 1 cortical screw (20mm)</td><td></td></tr>
<tr><td colspan="3">기타수술 및 주요검사</td><td></td></tr>
<tr><td colspan="3"></td><td></td></tr>
<tr><td colspan="4">치료결과 : 1. 완쾌 2. 경쾌 3. 호전안됨 4. 진단뿐 5. 가망없는 퇴원 6. 48시간내 사망 7. 48시간이후 사망</td></tr>
<tr><td colspan="4">퇴원형태 : 1. 퇴원지시후 2. 자의퇴원 3. 탈원 4. 전원</td></tr>
<tr><td colspan="4">병원감염 : 1. 수술후 2. 기타처치후 3. 비뇨기계 4. 호흡기계 5. 소화기계 6. 기타</td></tr>
<tr><td colspan="4">원사인 : 부검 : 예, 아니오</td></tr>
<tr><td colspan="4">계속적 진료 계획</td></tr>
<tr><td colspan="4">없음있음 (약속일 2017 년 월 일 시)</td></tr>
<tr><td colspan="2">담당 전공의 서명 : 이준심</td><td colspan="2">담당 전문의 서명 : 최동비</td></tr>
<tr><td colspan="2">의무기록 완성 : 2017 년 6 월 2 일</td><td colspan="2">의무기록사 서명 :</td></tr>
</table>

등록번호	122 22 66	성별 M
성명	오 합 격	
주민등록	800105 − 1234567	

퇴 원 요 약
Discharge Summary

Final Dx : Fx. distal humerus, Intercondyle Lt.

C.C : Lt. elbow pain

P.H : 상기 37세 남자환자는 2017년 5월 9일에 서울 은평구 보도에서 alcohol drunken state에서 slip down되어 인근 K병원에서 치료받음. elbow pain 지속되어 본원 OS OPD를 통하여 Adm. 함

Lab. X−ray Special study :

ESR/CRP 19.1/0.1
OT/PT 80/107

Clinical course of hospital

2017. 5. 15 : admission
2017. 5. 17~21 : Op risk 있어 수술연기하고, 환자외출하여 외래 consult 함.
2017. 5. 23 : operation
2017. 3. 27 : discharge

Tx.(operation) : O/R & IF $\bar{c}$ 5 hole narrow DCP
$\bar{c}$ 4 cortical screw
$\bar{c}$ 1 cancellous screw (34mm)
$\bar{c}$ 1 cortical screw (20mm)

Postop. Cx. : (−)

Resul t: improved

퇴원계획 : F/U at OPD (2017년 5월 31일)

전공의 : 이준심 수석전공의 : 탁희망 담당교수 : 주민음

등록번호	122 22 66	성별 M
성명	오 합 격	
주민등록	800105－1234567	

병 력 기 록
History

C.C : elbow pain

P.I : 1) Previous healthy
2) 2017년 5월 9일 Alcohol drunken state에서 slip down되어
서울 K병원에서 1차 치료를 받았음.
Imp) Fracture
3) 본 37세된 남자환자는 상기증상을 주소로 본원 OS OPD을 경유
하여 further evaluation 및 proper management 위해 내원함

PMHx. : Alcohol Hx. : 소주 2홉들이 1병/d x 2－3/wks x 20 yrs
Smoking Hx. : 1갑/d x 20 yrs
공무원 신체검사에서 간이 나쁘다는 얘기를 들음.
No known DM. pul tbc. hypertension

S/R : Lt. elbow pain (+) Fever/Chills (-)
No known DM, pul tbc, hypertension

S/R : Lt. elbow pain (+) Fever/chills (-)
Chest pain (-) Abd. pain (-)
A/N/V/D/C (-)

작성일 : 2017. 5. 15

Intern *Hong*

등록번호	122 22 66	성별	M
성명	오 합 격		
주민등록	800105－1234567		

신체검진기록
Physical Examination

V/S　T 36.5˚C　P : 82/min　R : 22/min

G/A　not so ill looking appearance
alert M/S

HEENT　normocephalus
not pale conjunctiva
not icteric sclera

Chest & Lung　symmetric expansion $\bar{c}$ retraction
CBS $\bar{s}$ ⓡ
No wheezing

Heart　RHB $\bar{s}$ ⓜ
No thrill
No heaving

Abd　Soft and flat
audible B.S
No tender point
L/S/K (－/－/－)

Back & Ext.　Lt. elbow area
ext. wound (－), tenderness (+)
swelling (+)　false motion (+)
crepitus (+)　false motion (+)
ROM elbow － flex, ext.: painful restriction
wrist － flex, ext: full
thumb － flex, ext: N-S
Motor － intact
Sensory － Free
Circulation － G-F

Imp) Fx. distal humerus intercondyle
Plan) Operation

Intern *Hong*

등록번호	122 22 66	성별 M
성명	오 합 격	
주민등록	800105-1234567	

경 과 기 록
Progress Notes

일 자	내 용	서 명
5.15	〈 Admission Note 〉	
	C.C : Lt. elbow pain	
	P.I : 본 37세된 남자환자는 상기 증상을 주소로 본원 OS OPD를 경유하여 further evaluation 및 proper management 위해 내원함.	
	2017년 5월 9일 Alcohol drunken state에서 도로에서 slip down되어 서울 K병원에 내원하였다.	
	Imp : Fx. distal humerus intercondyle	
	Plan: Operation	R1 *Lee*
5.16	〈 Preop. Evaluation 〉	
	1. Chest PA : WNL	
	2. EKG : NSR	
	3. CBC : WBC/Hb/Hct 6.130/15.0/44.6	
	4. ESR/CRP : 19/0.1 ↓	
	5. OT/PT : 5월 15일 80/107	
	5월 16일 63/94	
	* Abd U/S : diffuse liver disease (fatty liver)	
	6. S-electrolyte : 138/4.5/105/26	
	7. UA $\bar{c}$ micro : WNL	
	8. PT/PTT : 100 ↑/25.8	
5.17	high level of OT/PT로 Op. delay함.	
	5월 17일~21일까지 외출하기 원하여 외래에서 검사와 consult하게 함.	
	*내과(GI), 마취과 consult 보고, 수술할 예정임.	
		Lee

경 과 기 록

일 자	내 용	서 명
5.20	OT/PT 5월 15일 80/107 5월 16일 63/94 5월 18일 52/88	*Lee*
5.23	〈 Brief Op Note 〉 Surgon : 이민동 Assistans : 정순철/황도수/이준심 Anesthesia : GEA Preoperative diagnosis : Fx. distal Y-condyle humerus Lt. Postoperative diagnosis : Same as above Name of operation : O/R & IF $\bar{c}$ 5 hole narrow DCP $\bar{c}$ 4 cortical screw $\bar{c}$ 1 cancellous screw (34mm) $\bar{c}$ 1 cortical screw (20mm) Op findings : Hematoma and soft tissue were interposed between the facture fragments. Y-shaped comminuted fracture was noted in condyle. Elbow ROM 20-90 was found.	*Lee*
5.24	〈 POD #1 〉 OP wound : no oozing sign Lt. U/Ext : Motor, Sensory] intact Lt. long arm splint $\bar{c}$ elevation Hb/Hct 13.7/40.4 H/vac amount 110	*Lee*
5.26	〈 POD # 3 〉 S : No specific complaints O : 1) Op wound - clear 2) Lt. U/Ext: Motor, Sensory] intact Lt. long arm splint $\bar{c}$ elevation	*Lee*

경 과 기 록

일 자	내 용	서 명
5.26	3) Op wound closed observation	*Lee*
5.27	〈 Discharge note 〉 내과 외래로 간에 대한 Follow up 하도록 함. Rx Banan 2T Zeten 2T] #2 p.o bid x 7 days	*Lee*

등록번호	122 22 66	성별 M
성명	오 합 격	
주민등록	800105－1234567	

수술기록

Operation Record

날짜: 2017년 5월 23일 집도의: M.K. Choi
제 1 보조의: H.L. Nam 제 2 보조의: Q.M.Lee
참여간호사: Y. O. Yoon 순환간호사: H.Y.Lee

Preoperative diagnosis : Fx. distal Y－condyle humerus Lt.

Postoperative diagnosis : Same as above

Name of operation : OR & IF c̄ 5 hole narrow DCP
c̄ 4 hole cortical screw
c̄ 1 cancellous screw (34mm)
c̄ 1 cortical screw (20mm)

Operation type : Elective (*) Emergency ( )

Position of Pt. : Lt. lateral decubitus position

Skin preparation : 7.5% potadine soap (*) 75% alcohol ( ) 10% potadine (*)
Sterile drap (*) Others ( )

Op. findings : Hematoma and soft tissue were interposed between the fracture fragments. Y－shaped comminuted fracture was noted in condyle. Elbow ROM 20－90 was found.

Op. procedures :

Under the general endotracheal anesthesia, the patient was placed on the operating table in left lateral decubitus position and left upper extremity above the mayo. The with rubber tourniquet. A posterior skin incision was made beginning 5cm distal to the tip of the olecranon and extending proximally medial to the midline of the arm to 10 to 12cm above the olecranon tip. The skin and subcutaneous tissue were refl－ected to either side and then the olecranon, triceps tendon were exposed. The distal humeral area exposed by posterior Campbell approach then a tongue of the triceps aponeurosis were dissected and rased. The ulnar nerve was identified and gently retracted from its bed with a penrose drain. The triceps muscle were splitted in the midline and the tissue were reflected from the lower humerus by subperiosteal dissection. The condyle fracture site was exposed, and then the hematoma and soft tissue was removed by curett. The fractured site was exposed and manual reduction was done. Initally on the condylar area, 5 hole narrow DCP plate inserted & cortical screw was fixation on lateral side of fractured humerus after drilling, tapping, measu－ring depth.

Tissue of path : Yes, No Drains Sponge count correct? correct

Dictated/Written by H.L. Nam Surgeon's signature M.K. Choi

등록번호	122 22 66	성별 M
성명	오 합 격	
주민등록	800105－1234567	

협의진료기록
Consultation Record

의뢰사유 : For high OT/PT & anesthesia　　　마취과 민진도 선생님 귀하

본 37세 남자 환자는 Fx. distal humerus intercondyle (Lt.)로 입원 가료중입니다.
상기 소견에 대한 선생님의 고견을 선처 부탁드립니다.
감사합니다.

의뢰일 2017. 5. 16　　　의뢰의사 이주교/성동인

회 신 1 : 1. Problem: high OT/Pt (Body Wt. 83kg)
2. Dx.: distal humerus intercondyle Lt. Fx.
3. Op name:
4. Lab. OT/PT : 80/107 → 63/94
Hb/Hct : 15.0/44.6
PT/PTT : 100%/25.8
S－electro : 138/4.5/105/26
Viral marker : HBs Ag/Ab (－/+)
Abd. sono : fatty liver
EKG : NSR
5. G－I consult 해결된 후 (OT/PT normalized 된 후)
F/U consult 내주십시오.

회신일 : 2017. 5. 16　　　의뢰의사 이주교/성동인

의뢰사유 : F/U consult for operability
감사합니다.

회 신 2 : 아직 OT/PT 높은 상태입니다.
GI F/U 후에 연락주십시오.

회신일 : 2017. 5. 9　　　의뢰의사 이주교/성동인

회 신 3 : Rec) 1. Get permission for Anesthetics
2. Anesthetic plan: GEA
Premedication) Robinal 0.2mg IM
3. Intraop. postop. hepatic Cx. (hepatic failure, fulminant hepatitis) risk에 대해서 환자 및 보호자에게 충분히 설명하여 주십시오.

회신일 : 2017. 5. 22　　　의뢰의사 이주교/전수인

등록번호	122 22 66	성별 M
성명	오 합 격	
주민등록	800105－1234567	

협의진료기록
Consultation Record

의뢰사유: For high OT/PT & anesthesia　　　　GI 한승준 선생님 귀하

본 37세 남자 환자는 Fx. distal humerus intercondyle (Lt.)로 입원 가료중입니다.
상기 소견에 대한 선생님의 고견을 선처 부탁드립니다.
감사합니다.

의뢰일 2017. 5. 16　　　　의뢰의사 주기도/조인구

회 신 1: 〈 GI note 〉

Alcohol Hx: 소주 2홉, 1병/d x 2/wk. x 20yrs
HBS Ag/Ab (?/?)
: CK/LDH ↑와 함께 muscle origin으로 생각되는 AST 증가에 비추어
ALT의 증가는 상대적으로 많이 증가한 것으로 보여집니다.

회신일: 2017. 5. 16　　　　의뢰의사 신전파/장김치

의뢰사유: F/U consult for operability
감사합니다.

회 신 2 : SMA가 normalized된 후 수술하는 것이 좋겠습니다.
Rec) SMA F/U후 consult 해주십시오.

회신일: 2017. 5. 19　　　　의뢰의사 신전파/장김치

의뢰사유: F/U consult for operability

회 신 3 : Operation 시 hepatoxic event를 가급적 피해 주십시오.(마취약, bleeding에 의한 hypovolemic state, hypoxia etc.)
아직 Lab 자체는 증가되어 있으나 intra－ & postoperation SMA F/U하면서 (3일마다) close observation하여 주십시오.
감사합니다.

회신일: 2017. 5. 22　　　　의뢰의사 신전파/장김치

등록번호	122 22 66	성별 M
성명	오 합 격	
주민등록	800105 - 1234567	

협의진료기록
Consultation Record

의뢰사유: For 잇몸질환 — 마취과 윤주민 선생님 귀하

본 37세 남자 환자는 Fx. distal fumerus intercondyle(Lt.)로 입원 가료중입니다.
상기 소견에 대한 선생님의 고견을 선처 부탁드립니다.
감사합니다.

의뢰일: 2017. 5. 25 — 의뢰의사 고운도/오도용

회 신 3 : 〈 Periodontal Note 〉

Imp) Chronic periodontitis
일단 curative해서 치아 유지하기로 함.

Rec) CHX mounth gargle 250ml

회신일: 2017. 5. 25 — 의뢰의사 백찬호/전수형

등록번호	122 22 66	성별 M
성명	오 합 격	
주민등록	800105－1234567	

의사지시기록
Doctor's Orders

일 자	내 용	서 명
5.15	〈 Admission order 〉	
	1. T. diet	
	2. Chest PA	
	3. EKG	
	4. CBC $\bar{c}$ diff. count	
	ESR/CRP	
	5. SMA	
	6. PT/PTT	
	7. U/A $\bar{c}$ micro	
	8. S－electrolyte	
	9. HBs Ag/Ab	
	10. Both entire elbow AP & lat	
	11. Abd. u/s	
	12. Consult to GI	
	for high OT/PT & operability	
	13. consult to Anesthesia department	
	for high OT/PT & anesthesia	
	14. SMA $\bar{c}$ CK	
	LDH	*Lee*
5.17	15. 외출: 5월 17－20일까지 OS OPF F/U	
	16. SMA(5/18, 20)	
	17. OS, OPD F/U (5/20)	*Lee*
5.19	18. F/U consult to IM for operability	
	19. F/U consult to Anesthesia depat. for operability	
	20. SMA $\bar{c}$ CK (5/20)	
	LDH	*Lee*

의 사 지 시 기 록

일 자	내 용	서 명
5.21	21. F/U consult to Anesthesia dept.	
	22. F/U consult to IM OT/PT & for operability	
	23. SMA $\bar{c}$ CK ┐ 중복 LDH ┘ hold	*Lee*
5.22	〈 Preop. order 〉	
	24. NPO from M/N for OP	
	25. Get op permission	
	26. Get premedication from Anes. dept.	
	27. S−S enema	
	28. Px) H/S 1000cc IV	
	29. Px) Acopex 4.0 #2 IV bid 'AST' 'PM 10:00' 'on call'	
	30. prep) F/P/C 2pints 'AXM'	
	31. Send the Pt. to OR with X−ray & chart after full voiding	
	32. Premedication Robinal 0.1mg IM Dizepam 10mg P.O 'on call'	*Lee*
	〈 Postop. order 〉	
	33. NPO	
	34. Check V/S $\bar{q}$ 15 min × 4 ┐ $\bar{q}$ 30 min × 4 │ $\bar{q}$ 1 hr × 4 ┘ if V/S stabilized $\bar{q}$ 4h	
	35. Check Motor Sensory ┐ Circulation ┘ on Lt. u/exe.	*Lee*
5.23	36. Deep breathing & encourage cough	
	37. cold steaming	
	38. check H/V amount & frequent squeezing $\bar{q}$ 4hr	

의 사 지 시 기 록

일 자	내 용	서 명
5.23	39. stat 'CBC' 'S－electrolyte' 'ABG' 40. Px) Acopex 8.0 #4 sig IV qid 'AST' 41. Px) Tobra 240mg #2 sig IM bid 42. Px) Robaxin 2ⓥ #2 sig IV bid 43. Px) Esb 2 #2 sig IV bid 44. Px) Sendipen 3 #3 sig IM tid 45. Px) H/S 1000cc sig IV 46. Px) 5 D/S 1000cc sig IV 47. Px) 5 D/W 1000cc sig IV 48. Postop X－ray Lt. entire elbow AP & lat 49. CBC 50. DC # 43 # 44 # 45 51. Px) Lodine 6T ┐ MTC 6T │ #3 Sig PO tid Zestan 3T │ Cytotec 3T ┘	*Lee*
5.25	52. 치과 consult	*Lee*
5.27	53. Discharge 54. Px) Banan 2T ┐ #2 po bid x 7 days Zentan 2T ┘	*Lee*

〈오 합 격〉

★ 오합격 차트를 읽고 맞는 것에 O표 하시오.

1 **경과기록에 대한 설명으로 다르게 기재한 것은?**

① 술에 취한 상태에서 길에 미끄러져 팔을 다쳐 입원하였다.
② 복부 초음파 결과 정상이었다.
③ 환자는 5월 17-21일까지 병원 외래로 다녔다.
④ 'high level of OT/PT'로 수술을 연기하였다.
⑤ 왼쪽 상지의 감각은 정상이었다.

2 **진단명에 대한 분류번호로 맞는 것은?**

① S42.450, W01.9 ② S42.450, W01.4 ③ S42.491, W01.0
④ S42.451, W01.9 ⑤ S42.490, W01.4

3 **환자의 상태에 대한 설명으로 틀린 것은?**

① 외상과 눈의 공막에 황달도 없었다. ② 간이 좋지 않다는 지적을 받은 적이 있다.
③ 정신상태는 명료하였다. ④ 손목을 움직이는 데 통증과 제한이 있었다.
⑤ 심전도에 동방결절 리듬은 정상이었다.

4 **입원경로-수술-타과의뢰 건수가 맞게 연결된 것은?**

① OPD, 1, 3 ② ER, 1, 3 ③ OPD 1, 7
④ ER, 2, 7 ⑤ OPD, 2, 7

5 **수술 전 사항에 대한 내용과 다른 것은?**

① 수술동의서를 얻을 것
② 환자를 차트와 x-ray와 함께 수술실로 보낼 것
③ 근육주사용 하트만 용액 1L를 준비할 것
④ 비눗물 관장을 해줄 것
⑤ 밤 12시 이후부터 금식시킬 것

6 **기타진단명에 대한 분류번호는?**

① R71 ② R73.0 ③ R74.0
④ R76.8 ⑤ R73.9

7 **만일 환자가 퇴원 후 수술부위에 남아있던 핀을 제거하기 위해 입원하였다면 이때 부여할 수 있는 질병분류 번호는?**

① Z47.9 ② Z48.9 ③ Z47.88
④ Z47.0 ⑤ Z46.9

8 **처음 입원 시 수술받지 못하고 연기된 사실에 대한 분류번호로 맞는 것은?**

① Z53.0 ② Z53.9 ③ Z53.8
④ Z53.1 ⑤ Z53.2

9 **상기 환자의 골절 유형에 속하는 것은?**

① compound fracture
② infected fracture
③ simple fracture
④ puncture fracture
⑤ foreign body fracture

10 **입원기록지에는 누락된 것으로 추가로 부여할 수 있는 질병분류번호는?**

① K75.9
② K76.0
③ K76.9
④ K80.10
⑤ K80.51

02 뇌종양 Brain tumor

1.1 뇌종양(Brain tumor)

- ▶ 뇌조직과 수막의 비정상적 성장
- ▶ 뇌종양은 뇌부종(cerebral edema)과 수두증(hydrocephalus)의 원인이 될 수 있음
- ▶ 뇌척수액압력(CSF pressure) 상승 시 눈 뒤에 있는 시신경 가까이에 종창(swelling) 발생

표 1 • 뇌종양의 분류

원발성 종양	전이성 종양: 뇌(brain)로 전이
• 신경교종(glioma): 악성/장기(뇌, brain) – 성상세포종(astrocytoma) – 다형성 교모세포증(glioblastoma multiforme, GM) – 수아종(medulloblastoma) – 상의세포종(ependymoma) • 수막종(meningioma): 수막의 양성종양	• 전이성 종양(metastatic tumor): 10% • 원발성 → 뇌로 전이 – 원발성: 폐암, 유방암, 피부암(melanoma), 위장계 암

* 수막종증(meningiomatosis): D42.0, M9530/1(악성인지 양성인지 불분명)

1.2 치료

수 술

- ▶ 개두술 시행: 종양 절제한 후 흡인 또는 레이저를 사용하여 제거
- ▶ 수술 후 임상검사: CBC, 혈청전해질 농도 삼투성, PT, PTT 및 동맥가스분압측정
- ▶ 투약: 항경련제, 제산제, corticosteroids, 히스타민 수용제
- ▶ 무통제: 코데인
- ▶ 경한 통증 및 발열: acetaminophen
- ▶ 수술후 합병증: 뇌내압 상승, 출혈, 뇌척수액의 순환폐쇄

방사선요법 또는 화학요법 병행: 근치절제가 어려운 경우

약물요법

표 2 • 뇌종양의 분류

약 제	증 상
acetaminophen, 코데인	두통 해소
Dexamethasone	뇌부종 조절
Steroid(스테로이드)	수술 후 종창 제거
Phenytoin, pheriobarbital	경련 예방
Magnesium hydroxide(제산제)	스테로이드제제 복용, 스트레스 환자의 위자극 감소
Cimetidine, rantidine	위액분비물 감소, 스트레스성 궤양발생 감소
Prochlorperazine(진토제)	오심, 구토
Chemotherapy(화학요법)	종양세포의 증식 주기 저지(용량 분할 투여)

표 3 • 뇌의 기능

뇌의 부분	기 능
대뇌(Cerebrum)	사고, 추론, 운동 및 기억
소뇌(Cerebellum)	수의적(voluntary) 운동의 조절(균형, 자세유지)
시상(Thalamus)	신체감각(통증 등)의 연결장소
시상하부(Hypothalamus)	체온, 수면, 식욕, 정서 및 뇌하수체의 조절
교(Pons)	신경섬유로(nerve fiber tracts)의 연결
연수(Medulla oblongata)	심장, 혈관 및 호흡기계를 조절하는 센터

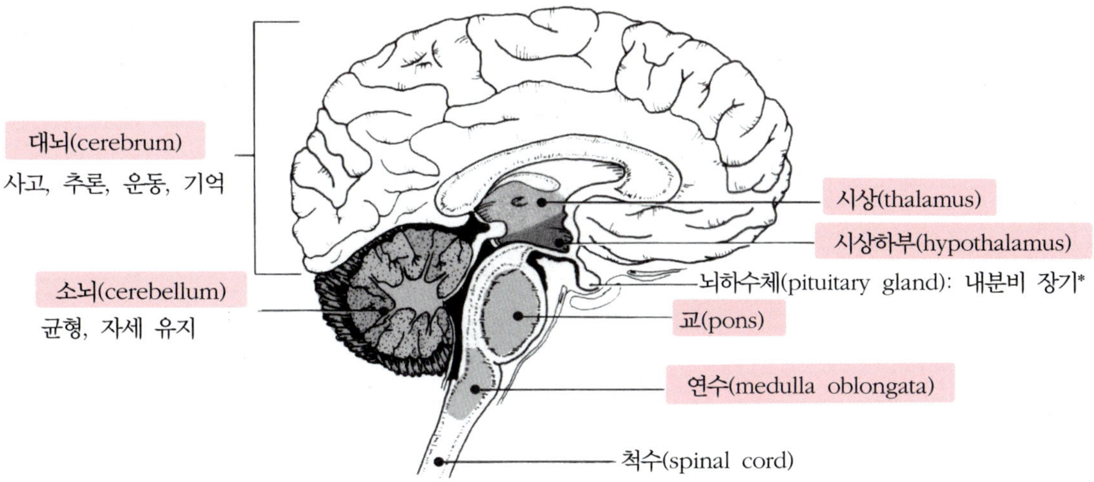

그림 1. 뇌(brain)의 구조와 기능

*내분비장기(9개): 뇌하수체, 송과체, 흉선, 갑상선, 부갑상선, 부신, 췌장, 고환, 난소

2.1 질병분류상 주의점

뇌종양(brain tumor)

▶ 원시성 신경외배엽 종양(primitive neuroectodermal tumor; PNET)

－M9473/3 뇌의 부위(악성 신생물) (C71.__)

수막종(meningioma): M9530/0

수막종증(meningiomatosis): M9530/1

▶ 조직병리보고서(Pathological report): 가장 확실한 진단명

중요 용어

▶ 포매(embedding): 조직학적 보고서
- 절편을 얇게 자른 후 그 절편의 원상 유지 위해 딱딱한 매체로 그 조직을 봉해 놓는 조작

▶ 신체의 면
- Sagittal plane(시상면): 신체 좌우 대칭 분리
- Frontal plane(전두면/이마면): 신체 앞·뒤 분리
- Transverse plane(횡단면): 신체 상·하부 분리

차트 용어

· Anaplastic	퇴행성	· Grayish	회색빛	· Rubbbery	고무같은
· Sagittal	시상	· Subgaleal space	모상하 공간	· Ventilator	인공호흡기

약 어	원 어	
ABGA	Arterial blood gas analysis	동맥혈가스분석
EEG	Electroencephalogram	뇌전도
EKG	Electrocardiogram	심전도
EOM	Extraocular movement	외안 운동
M/D/N	Moderate, development, nutrient	발육, 영양상태 적절
M/S	Mental status	정신상태
OT/PT	Oxaloacetic transaminase/pyruvic transaminase	간기능 효소검사
RHB	Regular heart beat	정상 심장박동
SPECT	Single photon emission computed tomography	단일 광전자 방출 전산화 단층촬영술
SSS	Superior sagittal sinus	상부 시상굴
VDRL	Venereal disease research laboratory (test for syphilis)	성병검사(매독검사)

등록번호	188 33 63	성별 F
성명	금 수 저	
주민등록	730107－1234567	

입 퇴 원 기 록
Admission and Discharge Record

<table>
<tr><td colspan="4">주 소 :</td></tr>
<tr><td colspan="4">출신지 :   직 업 :   전 화 :</td></tr>
<tr><td colspan="4">연고자성명 : 황우영   관 계 :   주 소 :   전 화 :</td></tr>
<tr><td>입원 : 2017년 8 월 30 일 과 병동 호</td><td rowspan="3">전과</td><td colspan="2">20 년 월 일 과 병동 호</td></tr>
<tr><td>퇴원 : 2017년 9 월 21 일 NS 과 병동 호</td><td colspan="2">20 년 월 일 과 병동 호</td></tr>
<tr><td>재원일수 :</td><td colspan="2">20 년 월 일 과 병동 호</td></tr>
<tr><td colspan="3">최종진단명</td><td>분 류 번 호</td></tr>
<tr><td colspan="3">주진단명 : Brain tumor</td><td></td></tr>
<tr><td colspan="3"></td><td></td></tr>
<tr><td colspan="3">기타진단명 :</td><td></td></tr>
<tr><td colspan="3"></td><td></td></tr>
<tr><td colspan="3">수술 및 처치명</td><td></td></tr>
<tr><td colspan="3">수술명 : Craniectomy $\bar{c}$ total removal of tumor</td><td></td></tr>
<tr><td colspan="3"></td><td></td></tr>
<tr><td colspan="3">기타수술 및 주요검사 : Brain MRI, Brain spect</td><td></td></tr>
<tr><td colspan="3">Cerebral angio</td><td></td></tr>
<tr><td colspan="3"></td><td></td></tr>
<tr><td colspan="3"></td><td></td></tr>
<tr><td colspan="4">치료결과 : 1. 완쾌 2. 경쾌 3. 호전안됨 4. 진단뿐 5. 가망없는 퇴원 6. 48시간내 사망 7. 48시간이후 사망</td></tr>
<tr><td colspan="4">퇴원형태 : 1. 퇴원지시후 2. 자의퇴원 3. 탈원 4. 전원</td></tr>
<tr><td colspan="4">병원감염 : 1. 수술후 2. 기타처치후 3. 비뇨기계 4. 호흡기계 5. 소화기계 6. 기타</td></tr>
<tr><td colspan="4">원사인 :   부검 : 예, 아니오</td></tr>
<tr><td colspan="4">계속적 진료 계획</td></tr>
<tr><td colspan="4">☐없음 ☑있음 (약속일 2017 년 2 월 1 일 시)</td></tr>
<tr><td>담당 전공의 서명 : 홍 철</td><td colspan="3">담당 전문의 서명: 성호주</td></tr>
<tr><td>의무기록 완성 : 2017 년 9 월 23 일</td><td colspan="3">의무기록사 서명 :</td></tr>
</table>

등록번호	188 33 63	성별 F
성명	금 수 저	
주민등록	730107－1234567	

퇴 원 요 약
Discharge Summary

Final Diagnosis : Meningiomatosis, Lt, parietal

C.C : Intermittent headache & nausea

onset : remote 7 years ago

recent 1 month ago

Brief history : 상기 44세 여자 환자는 7년 전부터 intermittent headache로 local에서 EEG 검사결과 뇌에 이상이 있다는 진단을 받고 치료한 적이 있다. 별 management 없이 지내던 중, 최근 1개월 전부터 Sx. aggravation되어 OPD를 경유하여 본 NS department에 admission하여 뇌종양으로 수술하였다.

Lab. X－ray Special : Brain CT

Brain MRI(postop): meningioma

Cerebral angiography(preop): meningioma

Pathology (OP) : meningiomatosis

Lt. parasagittal mass: meningioma

skull craniectomy: diffuse meningiomatous infiltrates

inter－trabecula space with full thickness involvement

퇴원 시 이상소견: OT/PT 288/130

Clinical course : 2017. 8. 30 : admission

2017. 9. 5 : operation

2017. 9. 21 : discharge

Tx.(operation) : Osteoplastic craniectomy and total removal of tumor

Postop. Cx : Cx (－)

Result : recovered

퇴원계획 : F/U at OPD (2017년 10월 4일)

Resident Sign: Hong

등록번호	188 33 63	성별 F
성명	금 수 저	
주민등록	730107－1234567	

경 과 기 록
Progress Notes

일 자	내 용	서 명
8.30	〈 Admission note 〉 C.C. Intermittent headache & nausea D : remote 7년 recent 1개월 전 본 44세 여자 환자는 local에서 뇌에 이상이 있다는 진단을 받고 치료 받은 적이 있다. 별 management 없이 지내던 중, 최근 1개월전부터 Sx. aggravation되어 OPD를 경유하여 본 NS department에 admission하였다. Brief history 7년 전부터 intermittent headache (+) local 의원에서 치료를 하였으며, 최근 4년간 Sx. 없다가 1년 전부터 vertex area skull mass palpated 되었다. 1달 전부터 Sx. recurred되어 OPD 경유 admission PHx : 7년 전 Appendectomy 1년 전 Hemorrhoidectomy ROS : Headache (+) － intermittent Nausea (+) Vomiting (－) Fever/chill (－/－)	*Hong*

경 과 기 록

일 자	내 용	서 명
8.30	P/Ex. : hard & protruding mass 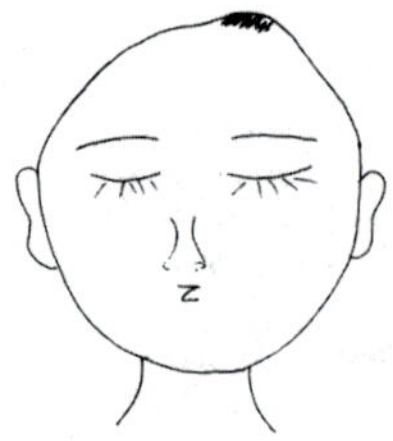 CBS $\bar{s}$ ⓡ RHB $\bar{s}$ ⓜ N/Ex : alert mental state isocoria $\bar{c}$ PLR (OU) Full EOM $\bar{c}$ nys CNF: intact cerebral function: intact cerebral function: intact Sensory: intact Motor: intact DTR: ++/++ Imp Brain tumor Lt. parietal R/O meningoma Plan Brain spect 4 vessel angiogram Brain CT $\bar{c}$ coronal OP : removal of tumor *Hong*	
8.31	cerebral angio : meningioma	*Hong*
9.1	foley removal 함	*Hong*

경 과 기 록

일 자	내 용	서 명
9.5	〈 OR note 〉 1. Preop Dx. : Lt. parasagittal meningioma 2. Postop Dx : Same as above 3. OP name : Craniectomy & tumor removal $\bar{c}$ Sinoplasty Duroplasty & Cranioplasty 4. Operator : K. J. Song M.D. 5. Assistants : A. Choi M.D/Hong 6. Op findings : 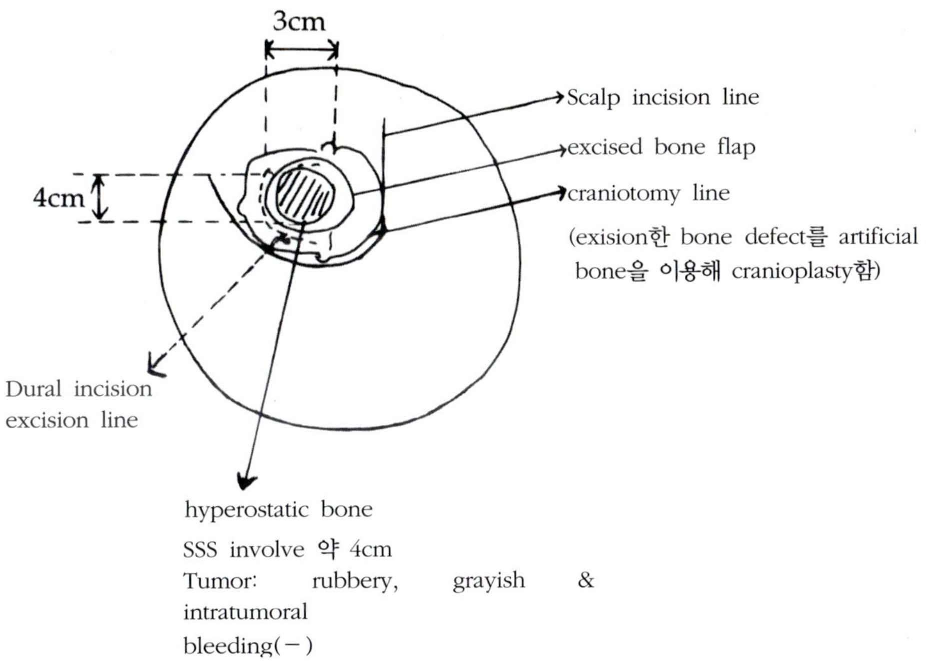	
9.5	1. Bone involve → remove 후 cranioplasty 함 2. dura에 붙은 tumor 함께 제거 후 dura repair 3. Forgatg catheter로 occlusion 시키고 tumor in SSS 모두 제거 후 lyodura로 SSS repair해 줌 4. Frozen Bx.: meningioma 5. tumor medial side의 sinus내 flow는 없었으나 medial wall과 flow는 유지되어 있어, lateral part만 resection 해내고, lyodura를 이용해서 sinoplasty해 줌 6. 8F Foley catheter $\bar{c}$ balloon을 이용하여 sinus flow를 차단	

경 과 기 록

일 자	내 용	서 명
9.5	〈 Immediate postop state 〉 1. Anesthesia로부터 full recovery는 되지 않은 상태 2. Pupil size & L/R : isocoric, prompt 3. Motor & sensory : painful stimuli에 all extremity weakness 소견 보이지 않음. 4. communication 가능함. 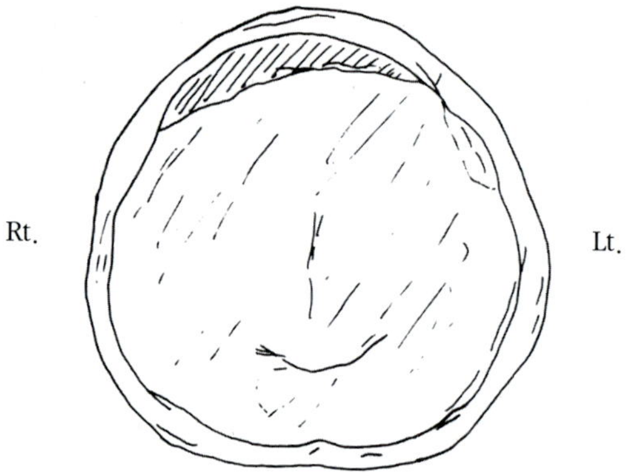 Immediate postop CT 1. Both frontal에 air density 2. Brain swelling은 심하지 않음 3. Op. site에 hemorrhagic density Plan) 1. Ventilator care 2. ICP control	*Hong*

경 과 기 록

일 자	내 용	서 명
9.8	〈 POD # 3 〉 1. V/S BP 120/80mmHg PR 70/min 2. N/Ex Alert mental state isocoric $\bar{c}$ PLR (OU) No facial weakness Motor ⎤ Sensory ⎦ grossly intact 3. Op wound : No problems	*Hong*

등록번호	188 33 63	성별 F
성명	금 수 저	
주민등록	730107－1234567	

협 의 진 료 기 록
Consultation Record

Request For Consultation To 소아과 한수국 선생님

for AVS angio & embolitation

본 44세 여환은 brain tumor(Parasagittal meningioma)로 입원 중입니다.
AVS angio & embolization에 관해 선생님의 고진선처를 부탁드립니다.
감사합니다.

2017. 8. 31 a.m.
Date Hour p.m

Prof. 한민부/홍철 M.D.
Signature of attending physician

Report of Consultation

Opinion and Recommendation

〈 Radiologic Report 〉

Chart & film review 하였습니다.
2017. 9. 1 오전 8: 30에 angio & embolization 실시할 예정입니다.

2017. 8. 31 a.m.
Date Hour p.m.

Prof. 한수국/홍철 R_1 M.D.
Signature of attending physician

등록번호	188 33 63	성별 F
성명	금 수 저	
주민등록	730107－1234567	

수 술 기 록
Operation Record

Surg. AP. H.J.Seong 1st Ass't M.B.Han 2nd Ass't ______ 3rd Ass't ______

Preoperative diagnosis : Parasagittal meningioma, Lt
Postoperative diagnosis : Same as above
Name of operation : Osteoplastic craniectomy, and tumor removal,
cranioplasty, duroplasty, sinoplasty
(Simpson grade I)

Procedures and Findings

Under general endotracheal anesthesia with N20, 02 and isoflurance, the patient was placed in supine position and head was flexed 30 degree. The entire scalp was prepared and drapped in usual aseptic manner. A Curvilinear scalp incision(U－shape like) was made left frontal, and subcutaneous tissue. pericranium denuded. Hyperostosised skull was seen at operation field. Four burr holes were made. (2 burr holes were made above SSS and 2 burr holes were made at tumor margin) and free bone flap obtained. After multiple dural tagging sutures. inverted U－shape dural incision was made and dural leaflets were reflected with holding sutures. Tumor and dura was excisioned en bloc. Superior sagittal sinus was invaded by tumor. Tumor consistency was rubbery, grayish and 3cm sized. Large draining vein was seen at the inferior portion of tumor(maybe Rolandic bein). After tumor resection, invaded SSS wall excisioned, and sinoplasty was done with Lyodura. Meticulous hemostasis was done with Surgicel, Aviten, Gelfoam. Excisioned dural defect was reconstructed duro－plasty with Lyodura watertightly. Bone defect was reconstructed with bone cement(methy methacrylate). Bone flap was approximated with wire suture. Hemovac inserted subgaleal space. Subcutaneous tissue and scalp closed layer by layer. During the procedure, patient to tolerated well.

Tissue to path. Yes No.   Drains (－)

Dictated/Written by M. B. Han   Surgeon's Signature H. J. Seong

등록번호	188 33 63	성별	F
성명	금 수 저		
주민등록	730107－1234567		

병 리 결 과 보 고 서
Pathological Record

처방명: Frozen biopsy　　처방의: 최용진　　주치의: 최용진

Gross Description :

Received fresh is a 2.3×2×1.2cm, rubbery pinkish white nodular mass, and a 3.5×3cm attached dura.

Frozen section diagnosis: Meningioma

Pathological diagnosis :

Intracranial mass, Removal: Meningiomatosis

Key word: Brain meningiomatosis

Result of staining : H－E (1)

date: 17. 08. 03

L. Y. Choi M.D.
Signature of Pathologist

등록번호 188 33 63　성별 F
성명 금 수 저
주민등록 730107 − 1234567

병 리 결 과 보 고 서
Pathological Record

처방명 : 작은 조직검사 (< 5 CM)　처방의 : 최용진　주치의 : 최용진
의뢰일 : 2017/09/06　병동 ID :
입역일 : 2017/09/20　진료과 :

Gross Description :

Received in formalin, specimen labelled as "이수석"

The specimen consists of two parts. The first one is several irregular fragments of grayish partly rubbery and partly friable tissue stated as superior sagittal sinus measuring about 3cc in volume. The second specimen is a round plate of hard bony tissue from scalp, measuring 6.5x6x2cm.

The outer surface shows ill definded elevation. On cut section. skull bone shows diffuse thickening with gritty surface.

Summary of sections: A1, 2: superior sagittal sinus.

B: decalcification

Pathological diagnosis

Skull, craniectomy :

Diffuse meningiomatous infiltrates in intertrabecular spaces with full thickness involvement.

Note: This meningioma does not show anaplastic change.

Keyword: Skull meningiomatosis

Result of staining

H − E (1)　MTB − 1
　MTB − 1

date : 2017. 09. 20

L. Y. Choi M.D.
Signature of Pathologist

등록번호	188 33 63	성별 F
성명	금 수 저	
주민등록	730107－1234567	

의 사 지 시 기 록
Doctor's Orders

일 자	내 용	서 명
8.30	〈 Admission order 〉	
	1. V/S $\bar{q}$ tid	
	2. BR	
	3. NRD	
	4. N/S 1 L IV	
	5. 20% Mannitol 400cc #4 IV qid ⓓ	
	6. Dexa 20mg #4 IV qid ⓓ	
	7. Zantac 2 Ⓐ # IV bid ⓓ	
	8. H_2 4 Ⓐ #4 IV qid ⓓ	
	9. CBC SMA PT/PTT	
	10. VDRL	
	11. EKG	
	12. Chest PA] "start"	
	13. U/A $\bar{c}$ ⓜ]	
	14. Brain CT $\bar{c}$ 예약	
	① axial & coronal view	
	② Bone setting	
	15. Brain SPECT 예약 (목 or 금)	
	as soon as possible	
	16. A－vessel Angio consult to Hong.M.D.	
	(for angio & embolization)	
	17. Bearse 3 Ⓣ]	
	Portal 6 Ⓒ] #3 p.o. tid ⓓ	
	Mgox 1.5g]	
	18. Pherytoin 600mg] #4 IV qid ⓓ × 2 day	
	N/S 40cc]	
	19. 18) 후에 Hydantoin 300mg] # p.o. tid ⓓ	
	Normo 3Ⓣ]	

〈금 수 저〉

★ 금수저 차트를 읽고 맞는 것에 O표 하시오.

1 주진단명에 대한 분류번호로 맞는 것은?

① D32.0, M9530/0 ② C70.0, M9530/3 ③ D42.0, M9530/1
④ C70.0 M9530/0 ⑤ D42.0, M9530/3

2 환자에 대한 내용으로 맞게 분류한 것은?

① 간헐적인 두통과 구토를 주소로 내원하였다.
② 개인의원에서 MRI 결과 뇌종양으로 진단받았다.
③ 8개의 폴리카테터와 balloon을 이용하여 굴 흐름을 차단하였다.
④ 수막종에 퇴행성 변화가 보였다.
⑤ 한달 전부터 두개골 정수리 부분에 궤양이 촉진되었다.

3 동결절편 결과 나타난 진단명으로 맞는 것은?

① D33.2 ② D32.0 ③ C79.30
④ C79.4 ⑤ C79.31

4 환자의 병력에 대한 내용으로 다르게 기재한 것은?

① OT/PT 수준이 높은 상태로 퇴원하였다. ② 퇴원 후 외래에서 치료받기로 계획하였다.
③ 수술 직후 ventilator care를 받았다. ④ 뇌혈관조영술은 수술 후에 시행하였다.
⑤ 7년 전 충수돌기절제술을 하였다.

5 주진단에 대한 주수술명의 분류번호로 맞는 것은?

① 01.6 ② 01.53 ③ 01.24
④ 01.59 ⑤ 01.31

6 OT/PT에 대한 의미로 맞는 것은?

① 정상수치보다 낮을 때 간기능이 좋지 않음을 의미한다.
② 혈청효소검사로 혈청내의 효소의 수준을 나타낸다.
③ 바륨을 입으로 삼킨 후 식도, 위 및 작은창자를 x-ray로 촬영한다.
④ 염료를 피부를 통해 간으로 바늘을 넣어 주입하고 담관을 x-ray로 촬영한다.
⑤ 뇌척수액압력 상승 시 시신경 가까이에 종창이 발생한다.

7 과거력상 입원 전에 받은 수술명에 대한 분류번호로 맞는 것은?

① 49.46 ② 01.24 ③ 01.59
④ 02.06 ⑤ 49.59

8 의무기록의 기재내용 중 ventilator의 의미로 맞는 것은?

① 환기 ② 인공호흡기 ③ 혈액순환기
④ 공기청정기 ⑤ 환풍기

9 **수술 내용으로 맞게 기재한 것은?**

① U자 모양의 곡선 머리덮개 절개를 왼쪽 두정골(마루뼈)에서 시행했다.
② 상부 시상굴에 종양을 제거 후 lyodura로 수복했다.
③ Hemovac은 모상위 공간에 삽입했다.
④ 종양은 돌같고, 회색빛으로 약 3cm 크기였다.
⑤ 기관내 전신마취하에 복와위로 눕혀 있었다.

10 **입원기간 동안 시행했던 검사가 아닌 것은?**

① EEG ② MRI ③ VDRL
④ CT ⑤ Chest PA

03 손가락 심지굴근의 열상

Laceration of (finger) flexor digitorum profundus

그림 1 • 마취기록지

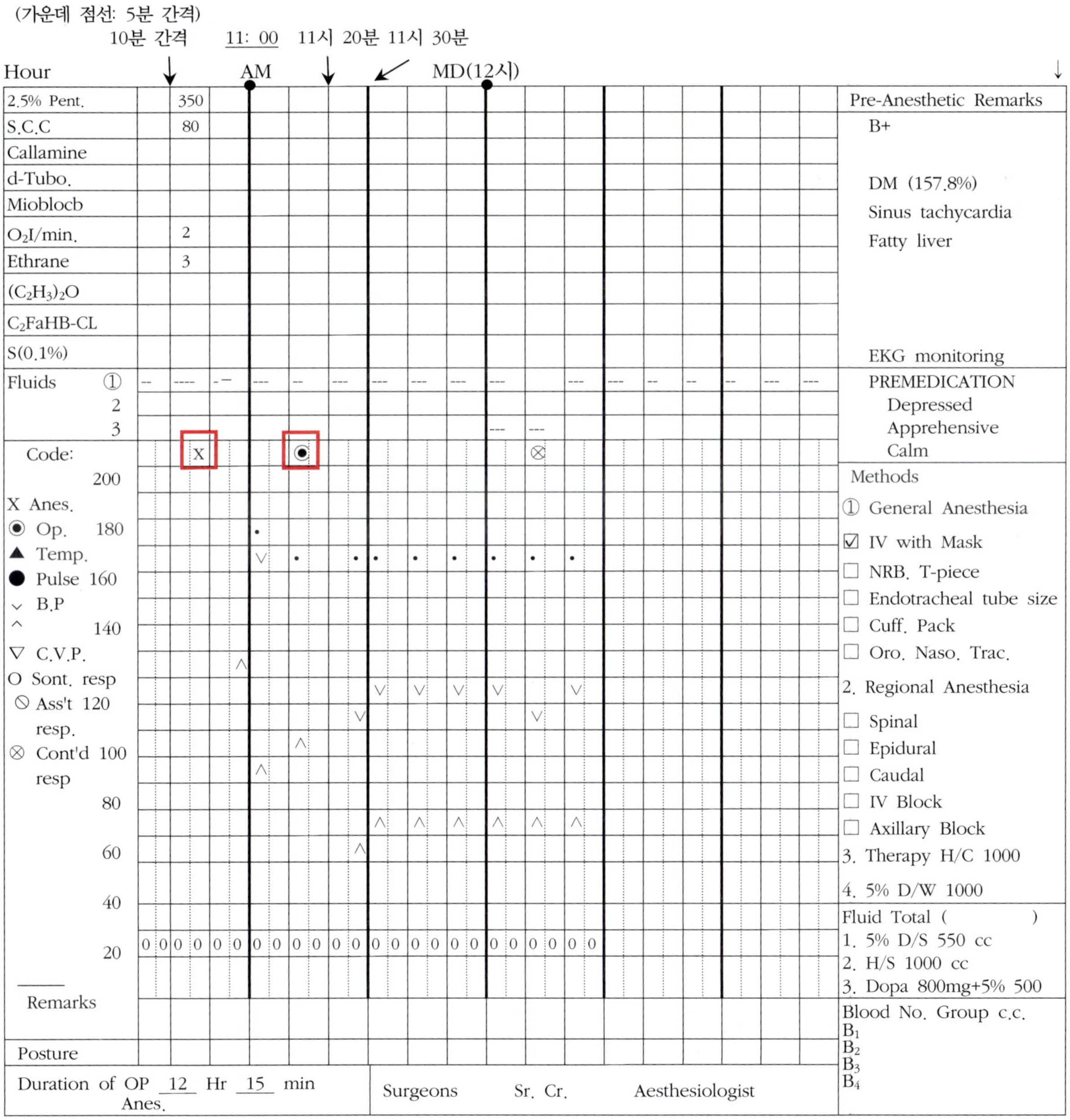

(가운데 점선: 5분 간격)
10분 간격 11: 00 11시 20분 11시 30분
AM MD(12시)

Hour	
2.5% Pent.	350
S.C.C	80
Callamine	
d-Tubo.	
Mioblocb	
O_2l/min.	2
Ethrane	3
$(C_2H_3)_2O$	
C_2FaHB-CL	
S(0.1%)	
Fluids ① 2 3	

Code:
X Anes.
⊙ Op.
▲ Temp.
● Pulse
⌄ B.P
^
∇ C.V.P.
O Sont. resp
⊘ Ass't resp.
⊗ Cont'd resp

200, 180, 160, 140, 120, 100, 80, 60, 40, 20

0 0 0 0 0 0 0 0 0 0 0 0 0 0 0 0 0 0 0 0 0 0 0 0 0 0

Remarks

Posture

Duration of OP 12 Hr 15 min
Anes.

Surgeons Sr. Cr. Aesthesiologist

Pre-Anesthetic Remarks
B+
DM (157.8%)
Sinus tachycardia
Fatty liver
EKG monitoring

PREMEDICATION
Depressed
Apprehensive
Calm

Methods
① General Anesthesia
☑ IV with Mask
☐ NRB. T-piece
☐ Endotracheal tube size
☐ Cuff. Pack
☐ Oro. Naso. Trac.
2. Regional Anesthesia
☐ Spinal
☐ Epidural
☐ Caudal
☐ IV Block
☐ Axillary Block
3. Therapy H/C 1000
4. 5% D/W 1000

Fluid Total ( )
1. 5% D/S 550 cc
2. H/S 1000 cc
3. Dopa 800mg+5% 500

Blood No. Group c.c.
B_1
B_2
B_3
B_4

1.1 마취기록지 해독 방법

마취기록지 시간 표시

□ 10분간격 - 10분씩 계산
| 30분간격 - □과 □ 사이의 가운데 굵은 선
⋮ 5분간격 - □ 한 칸 중 가운데 점선

- 오전 11시~MD(12:00)까지: □ 6개(10분씩 계산)
- 마취 시작 시간 X: 오전 10시 45분
- 수술 시작 시간 ◉: 오전 11시 15분
- 마취 종료 시간 ⊗: 오후 12시 15분

〈그림 1〉

1.2 마취 종류

전신마취(General anesthesia): Endo, Intro 내(內)

- Endotracheal(기관내), Endobroncheal(기관지내), IV(정맥내), IM(근육내)
- Inhalation[흡입, open drop(개방점적식)], Rectal(직장)

부분마취(Regional anesthesia)

- Spinal(척수), Epidural(경막외), Nerve block(신경차단)

국소마취(Local anesthesia)

- 회복실기록지가 없음
- 수술기록지에서 국소마취제 확인하여 기록

표 1 • 마취기록지(Anesthesiology Record)의 기호

기 호	의 미	
◉	start of operation	수술시작
X	start of anesthesia	마취시작
⊗	end of anesthesia	마취종료
∨	systolic blood pressure	수축기 혈압
∧	diastolic blood pressure	이완기 혈압
O	respirations	호흡
●	pulse rate	맥박률
△	temperature	체온

*혈압(BP): 120/80(정상) → 120: 수축기 혈압, 80: 이완기 혈압

2.1 체위의 종류

앙와위(Supine position=dorsal position, 배측위)

- 수술대에 등을 대고 똑바로 눕는 체위
- 복부, 골반, 흉곽, 하지수술

복와위(Prone position) ↔ 앙와위(supine position)

- 수술대에 대고 엎드리는 체위
- 척추수술

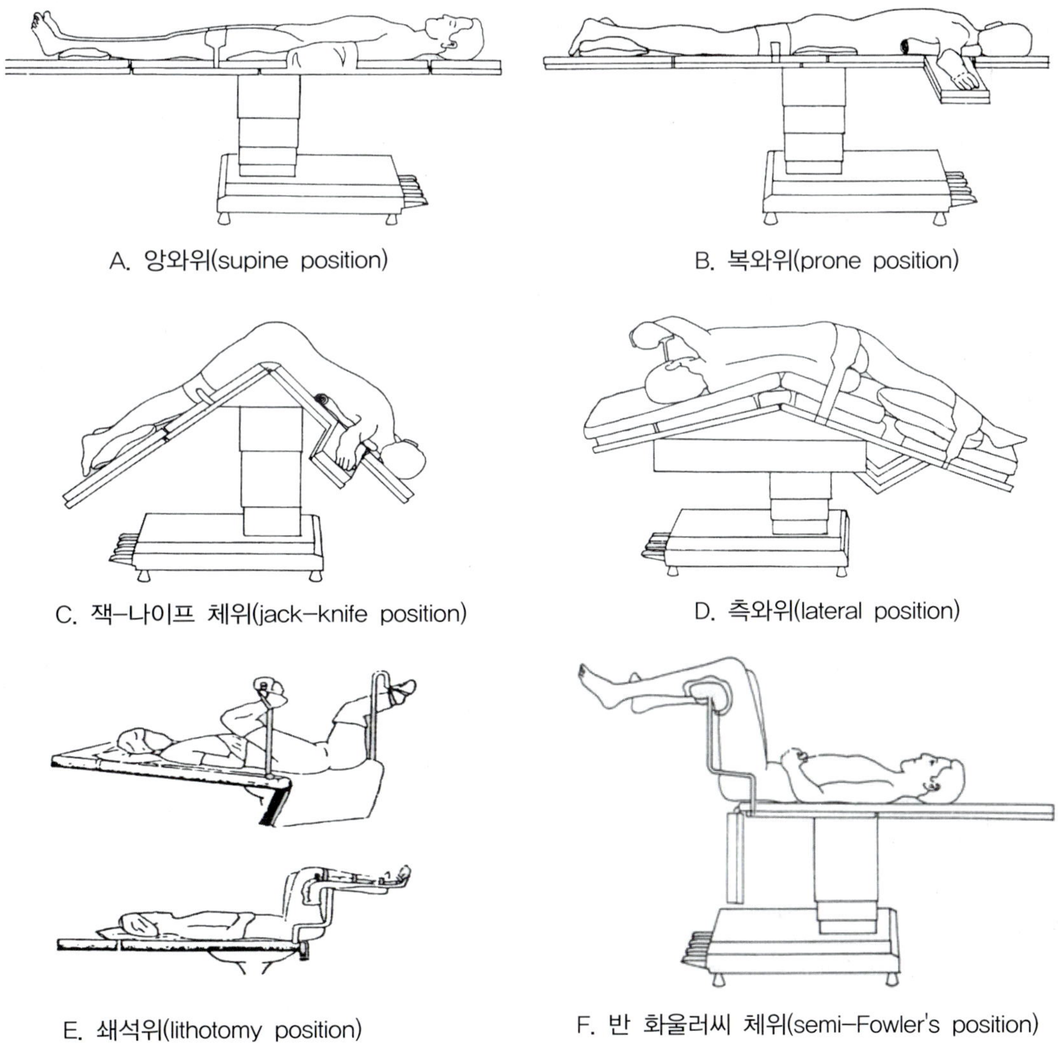

그림 2. 체위(position)의 종류

쇄석위(Lithotomy position)

- 배위(dosal position)에서 무릎을 구부려 다리를 발걸이(stirrup)에 올리는 체위
- 방광경 검사, 회음부, 항문수술

반 화울러씨 체위(Semi-Fowler's position, S-F position)

- 배위(dorsal position)에서 무릎을 25°~30°로 올린 체위
- 갑상선 절제술

측와위(Lateral position)

- 우측 또는 좌측 어느 한 부분이 아래로 가는 체위
- 식도, 콩팥, 폐, 둔부수술

잭-나이프 체위(Jack-knife position)

- 복와위(prone position)에서 수술대 상부의 꺾어진 곳에 둔부가 오도록 하는 체위
- 치핵절제술, 미골수술, 구불결장경검사(sigmoidoscopy)

2.2 봉합사

- 봉합사는 혈관을 결찰하여 지혈효과
- 손상받은 조직이 치유될 때까지 조직 지지

표 2 • 봉합사의 분류

흡수성 봉합사(Absorbable suture)	비흡수성 봉합사(Non absorbable suture)
• **특징**: 치유과정에서 조직에 의해 녹아 흡수 • **크기**: 9-0(0이 9개) ~No.5 – 번호가 크면 실 굵어짐 – [0]이 많아지면 실 가늘어짐 예) NO.1 〈 NO.2, 0000 〈 00 • **종류**: – plain catgut – chromic catgut – dexon – vinyl	• **특징**: 상처 치유과정 중에 흡수되지 않음 • **종류 및 크기** – silk: 크기/1호~7호, 번호가 클수록 실 굵어짐 – nylon or dafilon: 피부봉합 – dacron polyester fiber: 크기/9-0~No.5 – polyprophylene: 크기/9-0~No.5 – cotton – stainless steel

2.3 수술 시 구성팀

의사팀

▶ Surgeon(수술집도의): 실제 수술 시행

▶ 1st Ass't(First Assistant): 제1수술보조의사

– 수술부위 확보, 혈액 흡인, 수술부위에서 떨어진 조각 제거

▶ 2nd Ass't(Second Assistant): 제2수술보조의사

– 1st Ass't와 동일

간호사팀

▶ 소독간호사(scrub nurse)

– 수술복장, 외과적 손소독, 소독가운 및 소독장갑 착용

– 수술기구 및 물품 제공, 거즈세기(sponge count) 등 물품 수 확인

▶ 순환간호사(circulating nurse)

– 수술실 복장, 물품 및 기구 제공, sponge count

– 수술 시 모든 장비의 작동 점검

3.1 질병분류

손상외인(V01–Y98): KCD–7(3권)

예) · 추락(fall) → 미끄러짐(slipping) → W01.__ + 장소분류

· 사고(accident) → 운수(transport) → 충돌(collision) → 승객 V43.___

· 재난(misadventure) → 실패(failure) → 수술(surgery) → Y62.__: T81. + Y62.

파열(rupture) = 열상(laceration) = 외상성(traumatic) → 손상(injury)

3.2 차트의 기재방식

SOAP 형식: 경과기록, 퇴원요약, 협의진료기록

① S(Subjective information): 주관적인 정보 = CC

– CC(chief complain): 환자 또는 가족이 호소하는 것

예) abdominal pain(복부 통증), headache(두통)

② O(Objective information): 객관적인 정보 = 임상검사

- 임상검사, 신체조사결과

  예) U/S(초음파), CT, B.P.(혈압)

③ A(Assessment): 평가 = 진단명

- 주관적 및 객관적 정보를 토대로 진단명, 의사 판단

④ P(Plan): 계획

- 향후 진단 및 치료 계획

진단명의 분류번호 찾는 방법

- 퇴원요약지의 최종진단명
- 병리조직기록지의 진단명
- 수술기록지(postop. dx 수술 후 진단명)
- 경과기록지의 O(objective, 객관적) 또는 A(assessment, 평가)의 진단명
- 협의진단기록지의 imp, R/O 진단명(타기록지의 imp, R/O은 번호 부여 안함)
- 입퇴원기록지의 최종진단명
- 임상병리기록지(감염, 빈혈, 간염, 매독 등)

3.3 상반된 용어

- 신전(펼치기, extension): 사지를 펴는 것
- 굴곡(굽히기, flexion): 굽힘(bending)

약 어	원 어	
A/N/V/D	Anorexia, nausea, vomiting, diarrhea	식욕부진, 오심, 구토, 설사
Ass't	Assistant	보조의사
BPB	Brachial plexus block	상완 신경총 마취
BR	Bed rest	안정
FDP	Flexor digitorum profundus	심지굴근(깊은 손가락 굽힘근)
FDS	Flexor digitorum superficialis	천지굴근(얕은 손가락 굽힘근)
GA	General anesthesia	전신마취
G-F	Grossly free = N-S = WNL = intact	육안으로 정상
HBs Ag	Hepatitis B surface antigen	B형 간염 표면 항원
HCV	Hepatitis C virus	C형 간염 바이러스
HD	Hospital day	재원일수
LFT	Liver function test	간기능검사
PR	Pulse rate	맥박
PSVT	Paroxysmal supraventricular tachycardia	발작성 심실상 빈맥
VSD	Ventricular septal defect	심실중격결손

등록번호	111 22 33	성별 M
성명	이 대 길	
주민등록	801101－1234567	

입 퇴 원 기 록
Admission and Discharge Record

주 소 :			
출신지 :	직 업 :	전 화 :	
연고자성명 :	관 계 :	주 소 :	전 화 :
입원 : 2017년 9 월 9 일 과 병동 호		20 년 월 일 과 병동 호	
퇴원 : 2017년 월 일 과 병동 호		20 년 월 일 과 병동 호	
재원일수 :		20 년 월 일 과 병동 호	

최종진단명	분 류 번 호
주진단명 : Rt. 2nd finger FDP complete laceration	
Rt 3, 4, 5th finger FDP, FDS	
기타진단명 : complete laceration	
Rt 2nd finger digital N. laceration	
(ulnar side)	
수술 및 처치명	
수술명 : Rt. 2nd finger FDP tenorrhaphy	
Rt. 2nd finger digital N. neurorrhaphy	
Rt. 3,4th finger FDP, FDS tenorrhaphy	
Rt. 4th finger FDP tenorrhaphy	
기타수술(처치) 및 주요검사 :	

치료결과 : 1. 완쾌 2. 경쾌 3. 호전안됨 4. 진단뿐 5. 가망없는 퇴원 6. 48시간내 사망 7. 48시간이후 사망	
퇴원형태 : 1. 퇴원지시후 2. 자의퇴원 3. 탈원 4. 전원	
병원감염 : 1. 수술후 2. 기타처치후 3. 비뇨기계 4. 호흡기계 5. 소화기계 6. 기타	
원사인 :	부검 : 예, 아니오
계속적 진료 계획	
없음있음 (약속일 20 년 월 일 시)	
담당 전공의 서명 : 정복교	담당 전문의 서명 : 이수박
의무기록 완성 : 2017 년 10 월 20 일	의무기록사 서명 :

등록번호	111 22 33	성별 M
성명	이 대 길	
주민등록	801101 - 1234567	

응 급 기 록
Emergency Record

주 소	서울시 강남구 대치동 218			전 화	423-2830	직 업	회사원
동행인	황 윤 보	성별/연령	F/38	전 화	423-2830	환자와의 관계	남 편
내원수단	□ 도 보 □ 구급차 □ 경찰차 기 타						
내원경위	식구들과 음식 준비하던 중 넘어지면서 식칼에 Rt hand 부딪치면서 Rt 2nd, 3rd, 4th, 5th finger deep laceration되어 업고 내원함						
내원시교육	□ 접수안내 □ 침상낙상방지 □ 도난방지, 소지품관리 □ 보호자수 제한						
응급처치후 처리	입원 (PS)과 ( ) 호 □외래의뢰 □귀가 □자퇴 □타병원 □사망 □기타						

활력 증후		혈압mmHg	맥박/분	호흡/분	체온/℃	의식수준		체중	Kg
시간		130/80	94/min	22/min	36°4	기 타			
시간		/							

작성자 RN 양 탁 순

주증상:	의뢰과	전공의 의뢰시간	진찰시간	서 명
	1 과			
기왕력 : □고혈압 □당뇨병 □심장질환 □결핵 □수술력	2 과			
알러지 및 예방주사 : □특수알레르기 □주사약부작용 □파상풍예방주사	3 과			
병 력 :	4 과			

C/C: Rt hand (palm)

deep laceration 2nd & 5th

onset: 9/8 10:00(PM)

P/I by knife

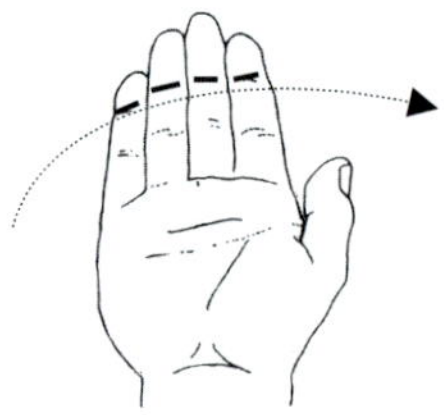

Rt hand (palm)

imp) multiple laceration

Rt hand 2~5th

1nt 김

〈 PS ER Note 〉

C/C) Rt hand bleeding

onset: 10:00 PM 9.8

vector: knife

P/I) 음식 준비 중 넘어지면서 칼에 찔려 L/C을 통해 transfer 정

응 급 실 기 록

PE) 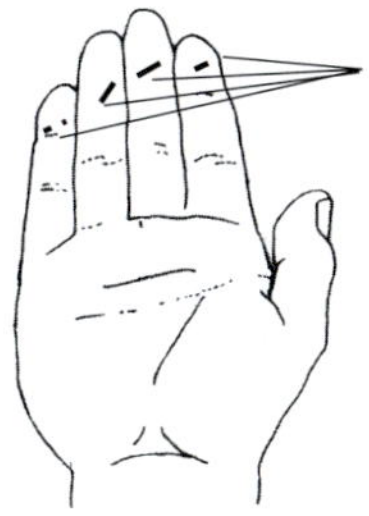

motor: 2, 3, 4, 5th finger flexion
sensory: 2, 4th finger
ulnar side weakness
circulation: intact

Imp) Rt 2, 3, 4, 5th finger deep laceration

Plan) Adm.

Rx) 1) NPO

2) Meicelin 1.0g IV (AST)
Akocin 150mg IM

3) CBC $\bar{c}$ plt é BUN/cr s-glucose
UA PT PTT Blood typing & X-Match

4) Prep/ WB 3ⓟ

5) Chest PA Lat $\bar{c}$ Reading (st)
EKG (p)

6) 5% D/W 1L ⎫ IV (20gtt)
Nacl 600mmEg ⎭

7) Rt (hand Ap & oblique (st)

정

등록번호	111 22 33	성별	M
성명	이 대 길		
주민등록	801101 − 1234567		

퇴 원 요 약
Discharge Summary

Date of Admission	2017. 9. 9
Date of Discharge	2017. 9. 23

\# 1. Rt. 2nd finger FDP complete lac.
2. Rt. 3, 4, 5th finger FDP. FDS complete lac.
3. Rt. 2nd finger digital N lac. (ulnar side)

P.I : 집에서 넘어지면서 칼을 손으로 짚어 다쳐서 L/C 거쳐
본원에 옴 (ER)

P.H : DM, Fatty liver로 12년 본원 내과 입원 및 F/U 해오다
최근에는 가끔 약국에서 약 복용해 옴

Lab. ABGA : 7.389-36.5-127.9-21.8-22.9-98.6
CBC : 16.3-46-7.200-15만
Bun/cr : 5/0.8
E : 135-4.0-106-217
SGOT/PT : 80/54 Glucose : 217
VDRL : negative HBsAg/Ab (−/−)

\# 1. Rt. 2nd finger FDP tenorrhaphy.
2. Rt. 2nd finger digital N. neurorrhaphy (ulnar side)
3. Rt. 3, 5th finger FDP, FDS tenorrhaphy
4. Rt. 4th finger FDP tenorrhaphy

OPD F/U
Dynamic splint

옥

등록번호	111 22 33	성별 M
성명	이 대 길	
주민등록	801101 - 1234567	

병 력 기 록
History

CC) Rt hand bleeding

onset : N : 00 PM 9.8

vector : knife

PI) 음식준비 중 헛디뎌 넘어지면서 칼을 손으로 짚어 C/C가 develop
→ L/C을 거쳐 본원 권유 받아 내원

PHx) DM (+)
Arrythmia (+)
Fatty liver (+)
로 '12 본원 내과 Adm. & F/U 해오다 최근은 intermittent drug store medication 중임

Tb (-) HBP (-) present medication (-)
Op. Hx (+) : 20yrs 전 appendectomy

SHx)

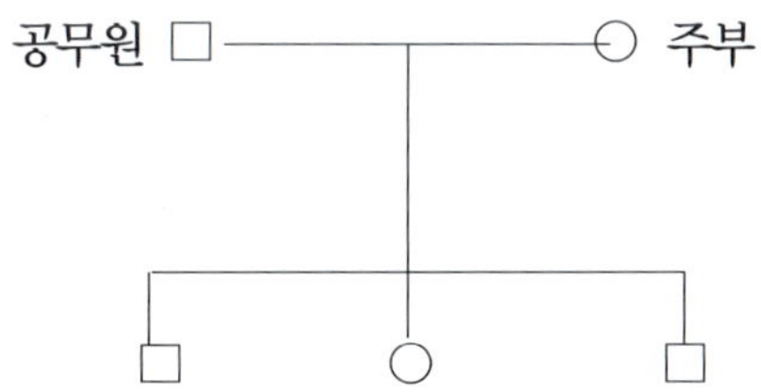

FHx): 아들이 VSD가 있어 Dacron으로 patch repair하였으나 수술로 인한 pleura 손상이 있어 hemothorax 발생하여 thoracotomy 받았음
부인은 IUP 35wks에 입원하여 분만하였으며 이때 선재성 당뇨병이 있었음

ROS): fever (-) chilling (-) A/N/V/D/C (-/-/-/-/-)
cough (-) sputum (-) rhinorrhea (-)
nasal obst (-) sorethroat (-)

양

병 력 기 록

PEx) G/A Acutely ill looking app.
alert

HEENT slightly icteric
non anemic

Chest : RHB $\bar{s}$ ⓜ
CBS $\bar{s}$ ⓡ symm expansion

Abd : soft flat

Ext : G－F
no pitting

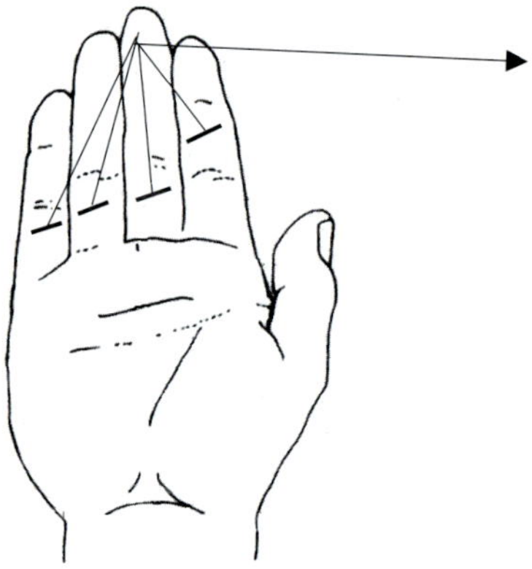

deep lac.
2nd finger
FDP rupture
ulnar side sensory weakness
3rd finger: FDP, FDS rupture
4th finger: FDP, FDS rupture
ulnar side sensory weakness
5th finger: FDP, FDS rupture
circulation: intact

Imp) Rt 2, 3, 4, 5th finger deep laceration
plan) Exploration

양

등록번호	111 22 33	성별 M
성명	이 대 길	
주민등록	801101 − 1234567	

경 과 기 록
Progress Notes

일 자	내 용	서 명
'17.9.8	〈 Admission Note 〉 생 략	
'17.9.9	〈 Brief op. note 〉 · 10: 30 AM 9.9 BPB 시도하였으나 fail함 · 환자 과거력상 Arrythmia, DM, alcoholic fatty liver, smoking: 2−3 pack/day for 20yrs 마취과 Dr에게 설명하였으며 general anesthesia 시도 하겠다함 11: 00 AM 경 실시 → fail 함 환자 respiration 없는 상태에서 mask ambu. bagging 시도 → 원활한 respiration 안됨. 2−3회 정도의 intubation 재시도하였으나 fail → upper & lower lip cyanotic change 보였으며 PR 〉200 있은 후 50정도로 down됨. 마취과 의사 2−3회 cardiac massage 실시 하였으며 PS 주치의가 2−3회 cardiac massage 실시 → 곧 바로 회복됨 CS Resident 연락 후 방문함. · self 살아 나면서 cyanotic change는 사라지고 환자 의식 돌아옴 · 계속 BP 90−100/90 PR 〉170으로 check되어 수술하지 못한 채 회복실로 옮김. · 회복실에서도 계속 PR〉170 check되었으며 내과 주치의에게 연락 후 EKG & ABGA 실시 후 내과 의국 방문 · 내과주치의가 EKG & ABGA 결과본 후 verapamil 5mg IV slowly order냄 · Verapmil inj 후에도 PR 160−170 계속 유지 · 내과 주치의가 회복실 방문 후 cardiac massage 시행 → PR 90 정도로 down됨 → ICU 가는 것이 어떻겠느냐고 문의하였으나 V/S stable 하신 후 general ward로 올라가서 attack 있을 때 EKG 다시 찍고 내과 연락 하라고 함 · General ward로 올라옴. BP 110/70 PR 95	

경 과 기 록

일 자	내 용	서 명
	〈 Immediate Post Op. Note 〉 S : No specific complain O : V/S BP 110/70 PR 95 dyspnea (-) palpitation (-) cyanotic change (-) A : stable state P : EKG monitoring 안되므로 if Sx attack시 EKG check하기로 함. (bed side prep EKG)	
9.12	〈 Brief Op. Note 〉 1. Op. date: '17. 9. 12 2. Operator: prof. 이수박 3. Assistant: 홍희주, 양주구, 정복교 4. Pre. op dx: Rt 2, 3, 4, 5th finger deep lac. Post op : #1. Rt 2nd finger FDP complete lac. 2. Rt 3, 4, 5th finger FDP, FDS complete laceration 3. Rt 2nd finger digital N(ulnar side) laceration 5. Op. name: #1. Rt 2nd finger FDP tenorrhaphy 2. Rt 3rd 5th finger FDP FDS tenorrhaphy 3. Rt 4th finger FDP tenorrhaphy 4. Rt 2nd finger digital N. neurorrhaphy(ulnar side) 6. Procedure: See OR	홍
9.13	S : Rt hand pain O : V/S stable smoking 계속 금지시켰으나(담배도 압수함) smoking하심(in 병실) flap color: pinknish oozing (-) marginal bleeding (+) dehiscence (-) hematoma (-) A : post op. stable P : observation DM diet smoking control	정

경 과 기 록

일 자	내 용	서 명
9.15	S : No specific complain O : V/S stable 계속 smoking 하심 보호자와 환자에게 다시 설명함 pinknish oozing (−) marginal bleeding (±) dehiscence hematoma (−) A : post op stable P : DM diet dynamic splint apply smoking control	정
9.17 #5	S : Rt hand pain O : dynamic splint로 PT하고 있음 Rt 2, 4, 5th finger ulnar side sensory weakness A : post op stable P : observation dynamic splint 유지	정
9.19 #7	S : Rt hand pain O : dynamic splint RT 잘하고 있음 oozing (−) hematoma (−) dehiscence (−) A : post op. stable P : dynamic splint	정
9.21 #9	S : Rt 3rd finger pain O : dynamic splint PT 잘하고 있음 mild swelling hematoma (−) blood clot (+) dehiscence (−) A : post op stable P : Rt hand PT	황

등록번호	111 22 33	성별	M
성명	이 대 길		
주민등록	801101 - 1234567		

협의진료기록
Consultation Record

Request For Consultation To 마취과 박종민 선생님

Summary of Present Finding

상기 환자는 Rt 2, 3, 4, 5th finger tendon rupture 후 9/9 BPB→ GA하에서 op 실시하려 하였으나 PSVT attack있어 fail한 환자입니다.
과거력상 PSVT Hypertriglycemia, DM, fatty liver 있어 본원 내과에 '17 10월까지 F/U 해오던 환자입니다. 9/12 op. 예정으로 내과적으로는 op. risk는 없을 것이라고 하십니다. 귀과적 evaluation & Anes. & op. 여부에 대한 선생님의 고견을 부탁드립니다. 감사합니다.

2017. 09. 11 — 김도대/정보교 M.D.

Date Hour — Signature of Attending Physician

Report of Consultation

Opinion and Recommendation

High Op. Risk

Rec) Brachial plexus block

Premed) Atrophine 0.5mg ┐
Nubain 10mg ┘ IM

2017. 9. 13 — Prof. 박종민 M.D.

Date Hour — Signature of Attending Physician

등록번호	111 22 33 성별 M
성명	이 대 길
주민등록	801101－1234567

협의진료기록
Consultation Record

Request For Consultation To 내과 장준화 선생님

Summary of Present Findings

상기 환자는 '17. 9. 8 Rt 2, 3, 4, 5th finger tendon rupture로 17. 9. 12 tenorrhaphy 시행한 환자로 12년에 PSVT, hypertriglycemia, DM으로 본원에 입원한 Hx 있으며 그 이후 OPD F/U 하다 intermittent 하게 Drug store medication 하였습니다.
환자 fatty liver에 대한 F/U 원하고 있습니다.
귀과적인 Evaluation 및 Treatment 부탁드립니다.
감사합니다.

2017. 09. 16 Prof. 이주교/성동인 M.D.
Date Hour Signature of Attending Physician

Report of Consultation

Opinion and Recommendation

Dx : Rt 2, 3, 4, 5th finger tendon rupture (9/8/17)
S/P Tenorrhaphy (9/12/17) in our hospital
Problem : Known fatty liver
PHx : arrythmia, DM (DMC) hypertriglycemia (Bezalip 400mg bid) : 12년 8월
SHx : alcohol (+) － 소주 1병 맥주 2－3병/ 1－2day for 20yrs.
smoking (+) － 2－3 pack/day for 20yrs
Lab : CBC : 13.9 － 41 － 5700 PLT : 11만
LFT (8월 17년) OT/PT 64/63 r－GT : 129

2017. 9. 18 장준화/박찬구 M.D.
Date Hour Signature of Attending Physician

협 의 진 료 기 록

(17. 10. 1) GOT/PT 18/10 δ-GT : 73

(17. 9. 11) GOT/PT 80/54 13 : 1 T : 0.8

(17. 9. 10) GOT/PT 56/60

HBs Ag/Ab (−/−)

Abd U/S (17. 7) : prominent fully infiltration of liver mild splenomegaly

Imp) Increased SGOT/GPT

Rec) ① HBC Ab

② Anti: HCV Ab

③ if possible, Do Abd U/S

④ fatty liver F/U

등록번호	111 22 33	성별 M
성명	이 대 길	
주민등록	801101－1234567	

방사선 소견서
X－Ray Report

☑ Ambulatory
☐ Portable
☐ Emergency
☐ New ☑ Old

☐ X－ray
☐ C－T
☑ U－S
☐ Others

판독일자: 17/09/11

진 료 과		병 실	03215	판독의사	이 x x

Part & Type OF Examination
Abd U/S

History & Clinical Findings OT/PT 56/60

Findings
2017－09－21

Abdominal ultrasonogram :

Hepatic parenchymal echoes are diffusely and moderately increased.
The wall echoes of portal veins and diaphragmatic echoes are decreased.
Liver is otherwise normal in size and contour with no focal lesion,
no dilated duct and no abnormal vasculatures.
Extrahepatic bile duct and MPV are not dilated.
Gallbladder is normal with no intraluminal pathology.
Pancreas is intact.
Both kidneys are not remarkable.
Splenic size is enlarged (11.7cm in size).
No intraperitoneal free fluid is seen.
No enlarged lymph nodes are noted in intra－and retroperitoneum.

Imp. : As compared with the previous sonogram taken on July－19－17
1. Persistent finding of moderate degree of fatty infiltration of liver with no remarkable interval change
2. slightly more enlarged mild splenomegaly
otehwise unremarkable

지구민 / 손창주

Acr Codes : 43－541.76 44－542.76 44－543.76

등록번호	111 22 33	성별	M
성명	이 대 길		
주민등록	801101 - 1234567		

마 취 기 록 지

Anesthesia Record

Anes. No.______ Phys. Stat. □, **1,②,3, 4, 5**

Wt. **78Kg** Ht **180cm** Hb______

Preop. Dx **Finger deep laceration Rt. 2, 3, 4, 5** Op. Prop. **Exploration**

Post. Dx **SAA** Op. perf. **none**

Premedication **A/S 0.5mg** Nubain **8mg**

Hour 11: 00 AM ∨ MD ∨ Total(mg)

2.5% Pent.	350	
S.C.C	80	
Callamine		
d-Tubo.		
Mioblocb		
O_2l/min.	2	
Ethrane	3	
$(C_2H_3)_2O$		
C_2FaHB-CL		
S(0.1%)		×
Fluids ①		-- -- -- --- - --- --- --- --- X--- ⊗ --- --- -- -- -- --- ---
2		
3		-- --

Code:
X Anes.
◉ Op.
▲ Temp.
● Pulse
⌄⌃ B.P
▽ C.V.P.
O Sont. resp
⦸ Ass't resp.
⊗ Cont'd resp

Scale: 200, 180, 160, 140, 120, 100, 80, 60, 40, 20

Remarks

0 0 0 0 0 0 0 0 0 0 0 0 0 0 0 0 0 0 0 0 0 0 0 0

Posture

Duration of OP 12 Hr 15 min

Anes.

Surgeons Sr. Cr. Aesthesiologist

Pre-Anesthetic Remarks

B+

DM (157.8%)

Sinus tachycardia

Fatty liver

EKG monitoring

PREMEDICATION

Depressed

Apprehensive

Calm

Methods

① General Anesthesia

☑ IV with Mask

☐ NRB. T-piece

☐ Endotracheal tube

☐ Cuff. Pack

☐ Oro. Naso. Trac.

2. Regional Anesthesia

☐ Spinal

☐ Epidural

☐ Caudal

☐ IV Block

☐ Axillary Block

3. Therapy H/C 1000

4. 5% D/W 1000

Fluid Total ( )

1. 5% D/S 550 cc
2. H/S 1000 cc
3. Dopa 800mg + 5% 500

Blood No. Group c.c.

B_1

B_2

B_3

B_4

등록번호	111 22 33	성별 M
성명	이 대 길	
주민등록	801101 − 1234567	

마 취 기 록 지

Anesthesia Record

Anes. No.______________ Phys. Stat. □, 1,②,3, 4, 5

Wt. **78Kg** Ht **180cm** Hb__________

Preop. Dx **Finger deep laceration Rt. 2, 3, 4, 5** Op. Prop. **Exploration**

Post. Dx **SAA** Op. perf. **none**

Premedication **A/S 0.5mg** Nubain **10mg**

Hour ∨ MD ∨ 1:00 PM ∨ 2:00 PM ∨ ∨ Total(mg)

2.5% Pent.																			
S.C.C																			
Callamine																			
d-Tubo.				2	21														
Mioblocb																			
O_2l/min.																			
Ethrane																			
$(C_2H_3)_2O$																			
C_2FaHB-CL																			
S(0.1%)																			
Fluids ①	--	--	-‒	---	②-	---	---	---	---	---	④-	---	---	--	--	--	---	---	
2																			
3								③	--	--									

Code: X Anes. ◉ Op. ▲ Temp. ● Pulse ∨ B.P ∧ ▽ C.V.P. O Sont. resp ⃠ Ass't resp. ⊗ Cont'd resp

Scale: 200, 180, 160, 140, 120, 100, 80, 60, 40, 20

Remarks

Posture

Duration of OP 12 Hr 15 min

Anes.

Surgeons Sr. Cr. Anesthesiologist

Pre-Anesthetic Remarks
- B+
- DM(+)
- PSVT
- Alcholic fatty liver
- OT/PT(80/54)
- EKG monitoring

PREMEDICATION
- Depressed
- Apprehensive
- Calm

Methods
- □ General Anesthesia
- ☑ IV with Mask
- □ NRB. T-piece
- □ Endotracheal tube
- □ Cuff. Pack
- □ Oro. Naso. Trac.
- ② Regional Anesthesia
- □ Spinal
- □ Epidural
- □ Caudal
- □ IV Block
- □ Axillary Block
- □ *BPB*

3. Therapy H/C 1000
4. 5% D/W 1000

Fluid Total ( )
1. 5% D/S 550 cc
2. H/S 1000 cc
3. Dopa 800mg + 5% 500

Blood No. Group c.c.
- B_1
- B_2
- B_3
- B_4

등록번호	111 22 33	성별 M
성명	이 대 길	
주민등록	801101－1234567	

수 술 기 록
Operation Record

날짜: 2017년 9월 12일 집도의: S.P. Lee M.D
제 1 보조의: H.J. Hong M.D. 제 2 보조의: P.K.Jung M.D.
참여간호사 순환간호사

Preoperative diagnosis : #1 FDP rupture 2nd finger (complete)
2. FDP, FDS rupture, Rt 3,4,5th finger (complete)
3. Digital n, rupture, Rt 2nd finger (ulnar side)

Postoperative diagnosis : S/A

Name of operation : #1. Tenorrhaphy FDP, Rt 2, 4th finger
FDP, FDS, Rt 3, 5th finger
2. Neurorrhaphy Rt 2nd finger (ulnar side)

Findings and Procedures :

1) The patient was placed on the operating table in supine position under general anesthesia via orotracheal intubation
2) The operating field was cleansed and the draping was done as the usual manner.
3) Pneumatic tourniquet was applied at 250 mmHg.
4) After confirmation of the FDP 2nd finger, FDS, FDP 3,4,5th finger and ulnar side digital nerve were ruptured.
5) Tenorrhaphy of FDP Rt 2, 4th fingers and FDP, FDS 3, 4th fingers was done by Modifed Kessler's mtd and continuous running suture with 4-0 mersilk, 6-0 prolene.
6) Neurorrhaphy of ulnar side digital nerve, Rt 2nd finger was done with 10-0 nylon.
7) Skin was repaired with 6-0 prolene.
8) Wet bulky dressing was done.
9) The pt was sent to R.R. without any specific problem.

Tissue of path: Yes, (No) Drains ⊖
Dictated / Written by H. J. Hong Surgeon's signature S. P. Lee

등록번호	111 22 33	성별 M
성명	이 대 길	
주민등록	801101－1234567	

당뇨병 관리기록
Diabetes Management Record

Date / Medication							9/9
Body Wt.							80Kg
Diet (Cal)							NPO
Medications							
Insulin (U)							
Injection site							
Blood sugar 7 am 11 am 4 pm 9 pm							157 09 181 118
Acetone							
Hypoglycemia							
Date / Medication	**9/10**	**9/11**	**9/12**	**9/13**	**9/14**	**9/15**	**9/16**
Body Wt.							
Diet (cal)	GD	GD	NPO	1800cal DGD 4	1900cal DGD #4	1900cal GDO#4	1900cal DGD#4
Medications							
Insulin (u)							
Injection site							
Blood sugar 7 am 11 am 4 pm 9 pm	161 372 193 200	166 274 152 189	166 못함 87(6pm) 248	169 123 227 163	153 198 188 267	157 103 X(부재) 187	171 224 154 204
Acetone							
Hypoglycemia							

〈이 대 길〉

★ 이대길 문제를 읽고 맞는 것에 O표 하시오.

1 환자의 손상외인에 대한 분류번호가 맞는 것은?

① W18.0 ② W19.0 ③ W17.8
④ Y01.0 ⑤ Y02.8

2 의무기록지 중 FDP의 정식용어(full term)로 옳은 것은?

① fibrin degradation product ② flexor digitorum profundus
③ flexor digitorum phenomenon ④ flexor digitorum proximalis
⑤ fibrin digitorum profundus

3 진단명의 분류번호가 맞게 조립된 것은?

㉠ S61.0	㉡ S61.7	㉢ S63.4	㉣ S64.9	㉤ S64.0	㉥ S66.18
㉦ S66.60	㉧ E14.79	㉨ K76.0	㉩ I47.1	㉪ I49.9	

① ㉠－㉢－㉣－㉥－㉨－㉪ ② ㉠－㉤－㉦－㉧－㉨－㉩
③ ㉡－㉤－㉦－㉧－㉨－㉪ ④ ㉡－㉣－㉥－㉧－㉨－㉩
⑤ ㉡－㉢－㉣－㉥－㉩－㉪

4 소화기 내과 협의 진단 시 내린 권고 사항이 아닌 것은?

① 복부 초음파 검사 ② C형 간염항체 ③ 간기능 검사
④ B형 간염중심 항체검사 ⑤ 지방간 follow-up

5 의무기록 내용과 다르게 설명된 것은?

① 손가락 혈관순환에 이상이 있다. ② 비장(지라)종대가 있고 비장의 크기가 11.7cm이다.
③ 충수돌기 절제술을 전에 받았다. ④ 처음 마취시간은 오전 10시 45분이다.
⑤ 처음 수술시간은 오후 12시 5분이다.

6 환자의 부인에 대한 병력을 분류한다면?

① O47.9 ② E14.79 ③ O24.4
④ O24.3 ⑤ E11.79

7 수술분류번호가 맞게 되어 있는 것은?

① 83.64 ② 83.99 ③ 04.79
④ 82.45 ⑤ 04.43

8 HD #5째 되는 날 섭취 칼로리는?

① 1900 cal ② 1800 cal ③ 1700 cal
④ 1600 cal ⑤ 1900 cal

9 **아들에 대한 병력은 수술시점에서 분류한 번호가 맞게 조립된 것은?**

① S27.11, Q21.09, 35.53, 34.09
② Q21.09, S27.10, 35.72
③ T81.2, J94.2, 35.53, 34.09
④ T82.5, Z87.7, J94.2, 35.53, 34.09
⑤ S27.11, J94.2, 35.53, 34.09

10 **마취과에서 권고한 마취와 그 후 실제 시행한 마취방법은?**

① BPB, BPB
② BPB, GA
③ GA, GA
④ GA, BPB
⑤ RA, RA

04 팔로4징후 및 동맥관개존증
Tetralogy of Fallot & patent ductus arteriosus

1.1 선천성 심질환(Congenital heart disease)

팔로4징후(Tetralogy of Fallot; TOF)

- 4가지(tetra) 결함을 포함하는 선천성 기형
- 선천성 심장질환 중 증상이 가장 심함
- 곤봉상손가락(clubbing finger), 호흡곤란(dyspnea), 청색증(cyanosis), 실신(syncope), 웅크리고 앉는 특징적 자세 등이 나타남.

팔로4징후(TOF)의 선천성 기형: 대동맥 + 폐동맥

- 대동맥 우측편재(Shift of the aorta to the right)
- 심실중격결손(Ventricular septal defect; VSD)
- 폐동맥협착(Pulmonary artery stenosis; PS)
- 우심실 비대(Hypertrophy of the right ventricle; RVH)

청색증(Cyanosis)

- 혈액의 산소량이 부족하여 생긴 피부 및 점막의 변색
- 어린이가 팔로사징인 경우 청색증이 심하여 "푸른 아기(blue baby)"라고 함

동맥관개존증(개방, Patent ductus arteriosus; PDA): 대동맥+폐동맥

- 개존(patent): 열려 있음
- 정상적으로 생후 6개월 이내 닫혀져야 하는 대동맥(aorta)과 폐동맥(pulmonary artery)사이의 동맥관(ductus arteriosus)이 열려 있음
- 자궁내 풍진(rubella, German measles) 감염, 미숙아 유아호흡곤란증후군과 관련
- 치료는 동맥관을 닫는 수술

중격결손(Septal defects)

- 심방 또는 심실사이의 중격(septum)에 작은 구멍이 있음

- 인공심폐기(heart-lung machine)에 혈액순환 유지
- 치료는 수술
  - 심방중격결손(Atrial septal defect; ASD)
  - 심실중격결손(Ventricular septal defect; VSD)
    - 출산 시 발생하는 VSD는 스스로 닫힘

1.2 혈관(Blood vessels)

심장 및 혈관 용어

- **동맥**(artery): 큰 혈관으로 산소가 많은 혈액을 심장에서 온몸으로 운반
- **소동맥**(arteriole): 동맥보다 작은 동맥
- **모세혈관**(capillaries)
  - 가장 작은 혈관
  - 동맥과 소동맥으로부터 인체세포로 산소와 영양분이 풍부한 혈액 운반
- **정맥**(vein): 인체조직으로부터 심장으로 산소가 부족한 피를 운반하는 혈관
- **소정맥**(venule): 정맥보다 작은 정맥

울혈성 심부전(심장기능상실, Congestive heart failure)

- 심장이 적절한 양의 혈액을 펌프할 수 없음
- 혈액이 동맥으로 나가지 않고 정맥을 통하여 심장으로 들어오게 됨
  - **폐부종**(pulmonary edema): 폐의 미세한 공기낭(sac)으로 모세혈관의 액이 새어 나옴

관상동맥질환(Coronary artery disease)

- 심장을 둘러싸고 있는 동맥의 질환
- 관상동맥은 대동맥으로부터 바로 분지하는 두 개의 큰 혈관으로 심장에 산소 공급
- 관상동맥질환은 보통 atheroscLerois(죽상경화증)의 결과
  - 관상동맥의 내면에 지방화합물이 축적

죽상동맥경화증의 2가지 위험

① **혈전성 폐쇄**(thrombotic occlusion)

- 동맥의 거친 내면이 관상동맥 혈액을 비정상적으로 응고(clotting)시킴

② **허혈(ischemia): 혈액의 흐름이 감소**

- 괴사(necrosis): 완전히 막혀 심근의 괴사
- 색(infarction): 죽은 심근(myocardium) 조직의 부분

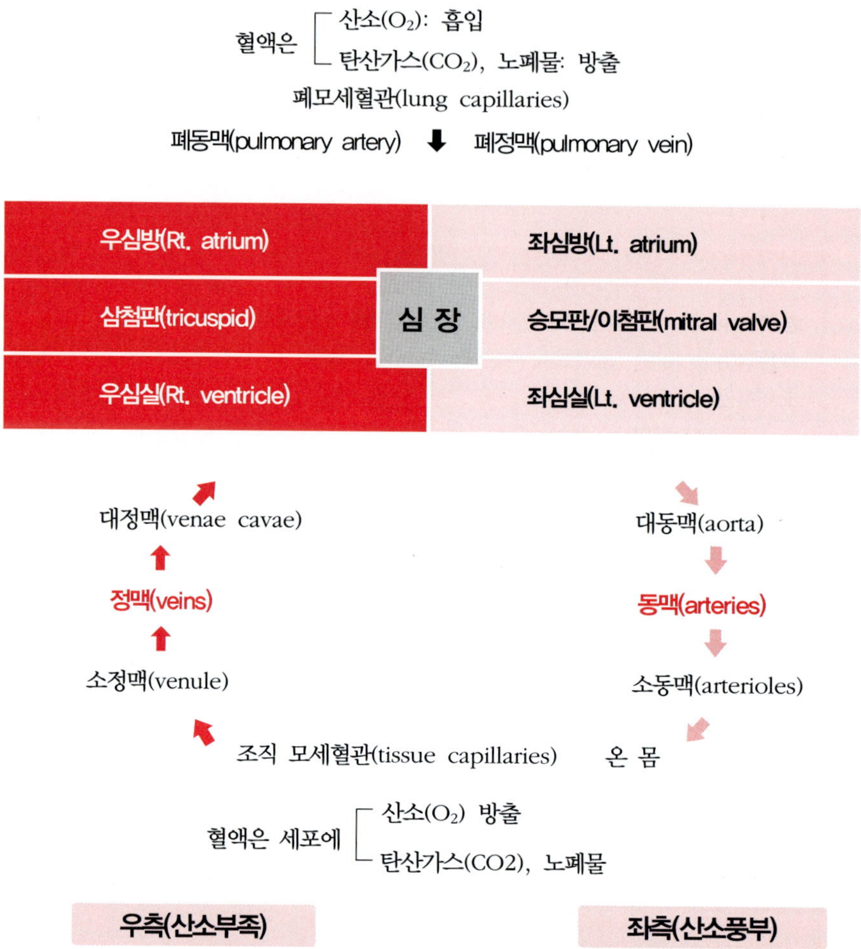

그림 1. 혈류의 순환(Circuit of blood flow)

- ▸ 좌심방, 좌심실 ⇨ 산소화(oxygenated)
- ▸ 우심방, 우심실 ➡ 산소 부족(oxygen-poor)

심근경색증(Myocardial infarction; MI): 심장발작(heart attack)

- ▸ 관상동맥이 동맥경화증이나 혈전으로 인해 내강이 막혀 심장에 혈액공급이 되지 않아 심근조직(myocardium)이 파괴되는 과정

협심증(Angina pectoris): 가슴의 통증

- 심근의 산소요구량이 증가함으로써 가슴에 갑작스런 통증이 나타나는 증후
- 통증이 어깨에서 왼쪽팔로 진행
- 설하제(nitroglycerine)를 혀 아래 투여함으로써 통증이 사라짐
- 베타-차단제(Beta-blocker): nadolo(Corgard)와 atenolo(Tenormin) 칼슘통로 봉쇄약물(Calcium channel blocker)

1.3 부정맥(Arrhythmia): 비정상적 심장의 리듬

심방실차단(Heart block, atrioventricular block)

- 동방결절(Sinoatrial node; SA node):
  - 심장의 박동이 처음 발생하는 위치
  - pacemaker를 삽입하는 부위
- 동방결절(SA node)을 통하여 히스속(bundle of His)으로 흥분의 전도가 부적절
- 동방결절의 손상은 방실결절(AV node)을 활성화하는 힘을 약화시켜 흥분파가 심실에 도달하지 못하게 함
- 심박동조절기(cardiac pacemaker)의 삽입수술(implantation)로 심차단을 교정하여 정상 리듬으로 되돌림
  - **부분심장차단(partial heart block)**: 일시적으로 부전(failure)이 발생하면 심장은 규칙적 간격에서 한 리듬의 한 박동을 놓치게 됨.
  - **완전심장차단(complete heart block)**: 흥분파가 동방결절(SA node)로부터 방실결절(AV node)로 도달하지 못하면 심실은 심방보다 천천히 수축
    → 심방실 차단(A-V blocker): Ⅰ도(I44.0), Ⅱ도(I44.1), Ⅲ도(I44.2)

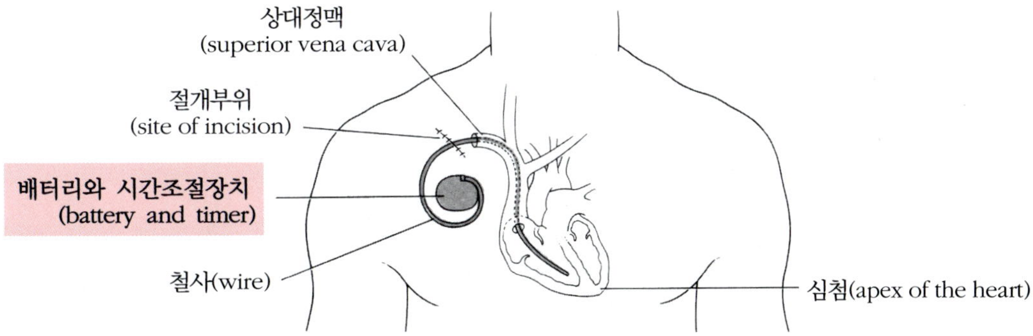

그림 2. 영구적인 심박동조절기

2.1 임상 처치

초음파검사(Ultrasound tests)

① **도플러 심초음파계(Doppler ultrasound flowmeter)**

- 혈관 외에 음파에 초점을 두어 적혈구의 반향음으로 혈류를 측정
- 협착부분에 혈류 속도가 증가
- 팔, 목, 다리의 동맥과 정맥에 혈관폐색이 있는지 조사

② **초음파 심음향도(Echocardiography; ECHO)**

- 고음파(초음파)의 파동을 가슴에 전달하여 심장의 판막, 심실, 심방, 심장표면으로부터 되돌아오는 반향음을 전기적으로 구성하여 기록
- 심장의 구조와 움직임을 볼 수 있음

혈관조영술(Angiography)

▸ 염료(dye)를 혈중 또는 심장, 심실로 주입하고 심장과 가슴의 큰 혈관에 x-ray 촬영

심장 자기공명영상(Cardiac MRI; Magnetic resonance imaging)

▸ 자기파(magnetic wave)를 심장에 보내 영상을 만듦
▸ 수술 전에 선천성 심장질환, 심장종양, 큰 혈관병소에 관한 자세한 정보를 얻는 데 사용

2.2 기타 처치검사(Other procedure)

심장카테터법, 심도관법(Cardiac catheterization)

▸ 가늘고 유연한 도관(catheter)을 정맥 또는 동맥으로 밀어 넣고 심장에 이르게 함
▸ 혈류의 압력과 흐름의 양상 찾는 데 사용

심전도검사(Electrocardiography; EKG, ECG)

▸ 심장을 통한 전기의 흐름을 기록하는 과정

홀터감시(Holter monitoring)

▸ 새로운 완벽한 심전계(심장의 전류를 측정하는 기구, electrocardiograph)
▸ 24시간 동안 심장의 arrhythm(부정맥)을 관찰할 수 있음

피부경유내강경유심장동맥성형술(Percutaneous transluminal coronary angiography; PTCA): 풍선 카테터 확장술(Balloon catheter dilation)

- 끝에 풍선(balloon)이 달려 있는 카테터를 대퇴동맥(thigh)을 통하여 삽입
- 이 관은 대동맥을 지나 관상동맥까지 갈 수 있음
- 삽입 후 밸룬을 조심스럽게 부풀리면 동맥내 지방축적물이 플라크가 눌리게 됨
- 혈관통과가 좋아짐

차트 용어

· Coarse	거친	· Cynosis	청색증	· Flat	평평한
· Extubation	발관(삽입관 제거)	· Hemipalsy	편마비	· Poliomyelitis	소아마비/회백수염

약 어	원 어	
ASD	Atrial septal defect	심방중격결손
A-V	Atrioventricular	방실의(A-V block 방실차단)
BCG	Bacille Calmette Guerin Vaccine	BCG 생백신
CICU	Cardiac intensive care unit	심장수술 중환자실
CO_2	Carbon dioxide	이산화탄소
D/C	Discontinue	중지
DPT	Diphtheria, pertussis, tetanus (vaccine)	디프테리아, 백일해, 파상풍(백신)
e′	Electrolyte	전해질
Echo	Echocardiography	초음파 심장촬영술
HR	Heart rate	심장박동률
NCP	Normocephaly	정상두부
NFD	Normal forcep delivery	정상 겸자분만
NSVD	Normal spontaneous vaginal delivery	정상 자연질분만
O_2	Oxygen	산소
PDA	Patent ductus arteriosus	동맥관 개존증(개방)
PMHx	Past medical history	과거력
p.r.	Per rectum	직장을 통해
RCA	Right coronary artery	우관상동맥
RV	Right ventricle	우심실
S/P	Status post	상태 후
TOF	Tetralogy of Fallot	팔로사징
TS	Thoracic surgery	흉부외과
TSICU	Thoracic surgery intensive care unit	흉부외과 중환자실
VSD	Ventricular septal defects	심실중격결손

등록번호	188 55 77	성별	M
성명	황 금 빛		
주민등록	160105-1234567		

입 퇴 원 기 록
Admission and Discharge Record

<table>
<tr><td colspan="3">주 소 :</td></tr>
<tr><td colspan="3">출신지 :   직 업 :   전 화 :</td></tr>
<tr><td colspan="3">연고자성명 : 유용린   관 계 :   주 소 :   전 화 :</td></tr>
<tr><td>입원 : 20 년 월 일 과 병동 호</td><td rowspan="3">전과</td><td>2016 년 12월 17일 TS 과 병동 호</td></tr>
<tr><td>퇴원 : 20 년 월 일 과 병동 호</td><td>2016 년 12월 31일 PED과 병동 호</td></tr>
<tr><td>재원일수:</td><td>2016 년 월 일 과 병동 호</td></tr>
</table>

최종진단명	분 류 번 호
주진단명 : Tetralogy of Fallot	
기타진단명 : Patent ductus arteriosus	
Atrial septal defect	
Postop. artrioventricular block	
수술 및 처치명	
수술명 : Total correction of tetralogy of Fallot	
Ligation of patent ductus arteriosus	
Repair of atrial septal defect	
기타수술 및 주요검사 : Pacemaker implantation	

<table>
<tr><td colspan="2">치료결과 : 1. 완쾌 2. 경쾌 3. 호전안됨 4. 진단뿐 5. 가망없는 퇴원 6. 48시간내 사망 7. 48시간이후 사망</td></tr>
<tr><td colspan="2">퇴원형태 : 1. 퇴원지시후 2. 자의퇴원 3. 탈원 4. 전원</td></tr>
<tr><td colspan="2">병원감염 : 1. 수술후 2. 기타처치후 3. 비뇨기계 4. 호흡기계 5. 소화기계 6. 기타</td></tr>
<tr><td colspan="2">원사인 :   부검 : 예, 아니오</td></tr>
<tr><td colspan="2">계속적 진료 계획</td></tr>
<tr><td colspan="2">☐없음 ☑있음 (약속일 2017 년 1 월 21 일 시)</td></tr>
<tr><td>담당 전공의 서명 : 한명민</td><td>담당 전문의 서명 : 홍후영</td></tr>
<tr><td>의무기록 완성 : 2017 년 1 월 18 일</td><td>의무기록사 서명 : 김우희</td></tr>
</table>

등록번호	188 55 77	성별 M
성명	황 금 빛	
주민등록	160105－1234567	

퇴 원 요 약
Discharge Summary

Final dx : TOF
AV block (HR 60－80/m)
2nd degree of AV block of wenckebach type
Repair of ASD with prosthesis, open

C.C : Cynosis

P.I : '16. 2. NFD
'16. 4. 서울 명진병원에서 TOF로 진단받고
6. 정밀검사 위해 서울 S대학병원에 입원(4일간) 하였음
'16. 12. 3. 본원 흉부외과 외래에서 검사 후 심장수술받기 위해 입원함

PMHx : Tbc/DM/HT (－/－/－) Op history (－)

Op. & procedure : TOF total correction (98/12/20)

Tx. : Post op. AV block 있어 Holter 등으로 W/U하고 Pacemaker implantation 하여 HR 60－100 가량 유지함. Alupent 5mg P.O. Tid. medication함.

Discharge & Medication

Alupent 5mg
CSV 5mg
ADT 5mg
p.o. tid x 5일

F/U : '16. 1. 18. OPD

Han

등록번호	188 55 77	성별	M
성명	황 금 빛		
주민등록	160105－1234567		

경 과 기 록
Progress Notes

일 자	내 용	서 명
'16/12/13	〈 Admission Note 〉	

C.C Cyanosis

P.I 본 10개월된 남아는 서울 명진병원에서 임신 36주만에 태어나 10일간 인큐베이터에 있었으며, 선천성 심장질환으로 진단받은 후 사회사업과의 도움으로 서울 S대학병원 소아과에 입원하여 Cardiac US, Angio, MRI 검사하여 TOF로 진단받고 수술을 받기 위해 기다려 왔음

‘16. 2. 23 NFD
‘16. 4. 20 서울 명진병원에서 TOF로 진단받고 수술 권유받음.
6. 정밀검사 위해 서울 S대학병원에 입원(4일간)하였음.
‘16. 12. 13 본 병원 흉부외과 외래에서 검사 후 심장수술 받기 위해 소아과로 입원함.

PMHx Tbc/DM/HT (－/－/－) OP history (－)
약물부작용, 알레르기 없음.
임신 36주, 2.6kg로 태어나 10일간 인큐베이터에 있었음.
타병원에서 Anemia로 철분제제 투여해 옴.
Developmental problems: 뒤집기

S/R General: lip cyanosis at severe crying
Respiratory: cough (+)
Hematopoietic: anemia (서울 S대학병원부터 철분제 먹어 왔음)
Neurological: asymmetry at crying (face)

Physical Exam

Skin	cyanosis at lip & nail
Head	NCP $\bar{s}$ scar
Face	anormaly: Rt. hemifacial palsy
Lung	sym exp $\bar{s}$ retraction
Heart	pansystolic murmur Gr.II.
Abdomen	soft & flat

경 과 기 록

일 자	내 용	서 명
12/13	Initial problem list #1 pansystolic ⓜ, known TOF #2 facial palsy A : R/O TOF R/O cbr. thrombosis P : Brain CT Cardic cath, Echo Operation: TOF correction	*Han*
12/17	〈 Transfer out note 〉 TOF 수술받을 환자입니다. Echo : large VSD, Overriding of aorta. PS. hypoplastic PA. Left PDA. bifurcation of aortic arch 보이는 환자입니다. general condition 좋은 상태입니다. 수고하십시오.	*Han*
12/17	〈 TS transfer in note 〉 Problem : #1 TOF BHx : 1) known congenital heart disease (TOF) since birth. 2) '16. 6. 20 서울 S대학병원에서 Cardiac catheterization 시행 TOF(hypoplastic PA PAI 100mm^2/m^2 combined PS hypoplastic inf. septum Rt arch Lt. PDA divided desc arch) 3) OP 위해 본원 소아과로 입원 – 흉부외과로 전과됨 PHx : B/H herniorrhaphy S/R : cyanosis (+) P/E : Pansystolic ⓜ Ass.) TOF Plan) Total correction	*Yoo*
12/20	〈 Op note 〉 Operator : Y.H.Hong Assist : L.U.Kim / I.Y.Park / R.Y.Yoo Preop. Dx : TOF Postop. Dx : same Op name : TOF total correction VSD closure transannular patch pulmonary valvotomy ASD primary closure Left PDA ligation	*Park*

경 과 기 록

<table>
<tr><th>일 자</th><th>내 용</th><th>서 명</th></tr>
<tr><td>12/24</td><td>〈 간호일지 〉 CVICU
1) Total correction하고 오면서 ventilator care함.
→ Endotracheal tube Extubation.
2) O_2 5 L/min via O_2 hood 중임.
3) chest−tube (Rt. pleura, Mediastinum) removed
4) Lt. lung에 plural effusion 있어 Lasix, Aldactone으로 management
→ 현재 effusion 많이 빠져서 호전양상임.
5) secretion 많아서 nasotracheal suction 함.
6) Dopa(1:1) 1.5u/ns로 2.9㎍/Kg/IV로 infusion 중임.

BUN/Cr 8.0/0.3
혈압 77/50 맥박 139 호흡 43 체온 35.8℃
CBC 15.4 − 4.05 − 11.7 − 35 − 238
e′ 138 − 3.9 − 101</td><td>Nr. Choi</td></tr>
<tr><td>12/26</td><td>〈 POD #6 〉
S : fever (−) oral feeding moderate
O : HR 120 BP 80/50
Wound OK
Lab) WBC 11,700 Hb. 10.6 e′137−4.4−97
CRP 0.99
EKG : complete A−V block
A : 2nd degree A−V block
P : kupral D/C
tebutaline 0.5mg p.o. tid.
Pacemaker implantation</td><td>Park</td></tr>
<tr><td>12/29</td><td>〈 Transfer Out Note 〉
S : HR 90 → 75 last night
BP 75/39 − UVI pacing rate 130 restarted.
playing well
oral intake moderate

Problem #1 S/P Total correction of TOF
#2 complete AV block
Opinions
Postop. AV block가 있어 pacing 중 입니다. pacing하지 않으면 심박동이 70까지 떨어지므로 당분간 pacing하고 후에 Holter와 PO Mx에 대한 문의는 주의경 선생님 order를 따르시기 바랍니다.</td><td></td></tr>
</table>

경 과 기 록

일 자	내 용	서 명
12/31	〈 Transfer in note 〉 Problems #1 S/P Total correction ·VSD closure ·Transannular patch ·pulmonary valvotomy ·ASD primary closure S/P Lt. PDA ligation #2 Complete AV block Opinions #1 TOF로 total correction후 POD #11인 환자로 HR 120－140 → pacemaker apply한 후 130/min BP 70/40 Wt. gain (－) sweatting (+) U/O 150－250 cc/day (다소 적은 듯함) Lab) 12. 26 WBC 11700 Hb 10.6 e′ 137－44－97 CRP 0.99	R1 *Han*
12/31	〈 POD #11 〉 12. 27. Postop. Echo 결과 1) No residural VSD 2) Good contractility. No pericardial effusion dysrhythm 3) Mild residural PS (Supra valvular) Moderate to mild ≃ 2.6 m/sec 4) R/O secondary coronary to RV fistula Suspected minimal RCA dilatation (2.8－2.9mmPMX) 5) Suprasternal & subcostal view는 관찰못함. #2. Postop. bradycardia 생겨(ward 온후). pacemaker 130/min으로 setting 현재 pacemaker off하면 HR : 70정도 내려가 계속 사용중임. Holter monitoring하려 (12/30)했으나 bradycardia때문에 1월 4일로 연기함.	R1 *Han*

경 과 기 록

일 자	내 용	서 명
'17/1/1	〈 POD #12 〉 S Irritable O fever (−) V/S stable Urine output 120cc ↓↓ sweatting (++) EKG monitoring : 130회 pacing 중임 (self x). poor food intake B.S. : coarse Constipation (+) → Dulcolax 1/4 supp. PR A AV block Constipation Coarse breathing sound P Lung care (T−suction freq.) Dulcolax PR 삽입 EKG monitoring	R1 *Han*
1/14	〈 Discharge 〉 Tx. : Postop. AV block 있어 Holter 등으로 W/U하고, pacemaker implantation하여 HR 60−100 가량 유지함. Alupent 5mg p.o. Tid. medication함. F/U : 1. 18. 홍후영 OPD에서 F/U 할 계획임.	R1 *Han*

등록번호	188 55 77	성별	M
성명	황 금 빛		
주민등록	160105 - 1234567		

영상의학결과보고서

Cardiac Report

시행일 : 2016. 12. 17	시행의 :	진료과 :
검사자 :	처방의 :	병동 :

임상소견

No clinical information

Heart MRI

Sequence: T1WI, axial, oblique sagittal, both oblique coronal.
Cine MRI of left PDA in oblique coronal plane.
Cine MRI of aortic arch in sagittal plane.

Right aortic arch level에 두 개의 lumen(7mm와 6mm 직경)으로 aortic arch가 나뉘는 rare anomaly로써 persistent 4th aortic arch로 생각되며 left PDA(2mm in diameter)가 left innominate artery에서 기시하여 left pulmonary artery에 insertion하는 것이 관찰되며 oblique coronal plane과 cine MRI상에서 내부에 flow가 관찰됨(echo 소견과 일치) 약 8mm의 VSD가 perimembraneous to outlet septum에 관찰되며 약 3mm size의 ASD가 secundum type으로 관찰됨. Pulmonic valve의 annulus는 약 1cm로 측정됨.

결 론

TOF with right aortic arch.
Persistent 4th aortic arch.
Left PDA arising from left innominate artery.
Perimembraneous VSD with outlet extension.
Pulmonary arterial index는 241.7 (distal right pulmonary artery 6mm, distal left pulmonary artery 9mm)

판독의사 : 양주응

등록번호	188 55 77	성별	M
성명	황 금 빛		
주민등록	160105－1234567		

영상의학(심장계)결과보고서

Echocardiographic Report

등록번호 : 188 55 77 　검 사 명 : 소아 Echocardiogram 　환자성명 : 홍상순
검 사 일 : '16. 12. 27 　진료과/병동 : 　성명/나이 : M/10개월 　시행의 : 정동우

Tape No : P17－1524 　BSA : 　m^2 　WT : 8.4kg 　HT : 70cm

Measurements

AOD __14.2_mm LVDd __22.3__mm SV __8.5__m L LAD __23.5__mm

LVDs __16.9_mm CO __6.11__ 1/min LA/AO __1.65__ LVEDV __16.8__ ml

EF __51__% RVD __13.8__ mm LVESV __8.3__m L %FS __24__ %

IVST __6.5__ mm EPSS _____mm PWT ____5.8____mm

PG (　) max_______(mm/Hg) mVCF ______ circ/sec

Peak Velocity (　) _____(m/s) mVA 2DE ____ cm^2

PG (　) max_______(mm/Hg) Dopp _______ cm^2

Peak Velocity (　) ______(m/s)

PG (　) max _______(mm/Hg)

Peak Velocity (　) ______(m/s)

Mitral Valve: AMVL Exursion ________________ mm

AMVL E－F slope ________________ mm/sec

2－D

Situs________ Atrio－vent conn___________________ Vent－Arter conn________

RA_________ LA_______________ Atrial septum _________

RV_________ LV_______________ Ventricular septum_______

TV________mm MV_____________mm Wall motion__________

PV________mm AoV_____________mm

PA_________ Aorta_____________ Aortic Arch__________

SVC_________ IVC___________________________ Pulm. Vein____________________

Coronary arteries (R)_______________ (L)______________

Comments

S/P TOF. bifurcated Ao arch PDA developmental delay
→ Total correction ('16. 12. 20)

1) no residual VSD
2) good contractility no pericardial effusion, dysarrhythmia
3) mild residual PS(supravalvar), moderate to mild PR(velocity 1.7～1.8m/sec)
≃ 2.6m/sec
4) R/O secondary coronary to RV fistula
Suspected minimal RCA dilatation (2.8～2.9mm at prox. RCA)
5) Suprasternal & subcostal view는 관찰못함

M.D. 조주만

등록번호	188 55 77	성별 M
성명	황 금 빛	
주민등록	160105-1234567	

홀 터 보 고 서
Holter Report

Referred by :	Indications : 745.2	Date : 02-Jan-17
from :	Medications : Other Drugs	Hook-up date : 05-Jan-17
		Time : 15 : 55 : 00
		Duration : 24 : 00 : 57

ORS complexes

3 Ventricular ectopics which represent 〈 1% of total ORS complexes

3 Supraventricular ectopics which represent 〈 1% of total ORS complexes

Paced ORS complexes which represent 〈 % of total ORS complexes

Ventricular Ectopy	Supraventricular Ectopy
3 Isolated	3 Isolated
O Bigeminal Cycles	O Couplets
O Couplets	O Runs
O Runs	O Beats in Runs
O Beats in Runs	O Beats Longest at O BPM at
O Beats Longest at O BPM at	O Beats Fastest at O BPM at
O Beats Fastest at O BPM at	

Heart Rates

56	MIN at 01:38:40	06-Jan-17	S-T Levels Channel
71	AVG		mm at
128	MAX at 08:07:48	06-Jan-17	Longest RR at

Interpretation:

Predominant rhythm was sinus rhythm.

There were episodes of 2nd degree A-V block of wenckebach type with varying degree of conduction.

Intermittently episodes of A-V block with 2:1 conduction were noted.

Three isolated vpcs and three aberrant conduction (wide ORS) were noted.

CONC.) 2nd degree of A-V block of wenckebach type (including 2 : 1 block)

Rare isolated vpcs

Sign : 윤희민

등록번호	188 55 77	성별 M
성명	황 금 빛	
주민등록	160105－1234567	

간 호 기 록
Nurses Record

진단명 : TOF

분만정보 : NFD by 의사에 의함 분만, 출생체중 2.6kg

부모학력 및 직업 : 아버지 대졸, 회사원

입원동기

4월 20일 서울 명진병원에서 TOF 진단받음.
6월 18일 정밀검사 위해 입원 (3－4일)
12월 13일 외래 진찰받고 당일 입원함 (수술, 정밀검사 위해)

예방접종 DPT(+) Hepatitis(+) Poliomyelitis (+) BCG (+)

8개월된 남아로 TOF 진단하에 12월 13일에 입원
facial hemipalsy 있어 brain CT(12/14), ECG,
2－D+ Doppler Echocardiogram(12/14)
Heart MRI (12/17)
12/20 Op. 후 TSICU로 전송감.

Brain CT : normal
ECG : normal
2－D+ Echo : TOF, Large PM, VSD,
Overriding of Aorta
Combined PS, Lt. PDA minimal flow

간호사 임웅순

〈황 금 빛〉

★ 황금빛 차트를 읽고 맞는 것에 O표 하시오.

1 환자 출생 시 신생아 분류번호는?

① O60.2　② P07.31　③ P07.14　④ P07.20　⑤ P07.30

2 환자의 병력을 설명한 것 중 틀린 것은?

① 입원 전 빈혈로 철분제제를 복용했다　② 환아는 출생 후 10일 동안 인큐베이터에 있었다.
③ 처음 선천성 심장병은 2016년 4월이었다.　④ 출생 시 정상분만, 몸무게는 정상 이하였다.
⑤ 뒤집기에 대한 발달상의 문제가 있었다.

3 환아의 진단명에 맞는 분류번호가 맞는 것은?

① Q21.09　② Q25.5　③ Q21.19　④ Q25.3　⑤ Q21.8

4 선천성 심장질환으로서 팔로사징의 기형에 속하지 않는 것은?

① 폐동맥 협착　② 심실중격결손　③ 대동맥 좌측편재
④ 우심실 비대　⑤ 대동맥 우방전위

5 AV block의 분류번호가 맞게 짝지어진 것은?

① I44.1, I97.1　② I44.1, I97.8　③ I44.2, I97.9
④ I44.3, I97.1　⑤ I44.3, I97.8

6 의무기록의 내용과 동일한 것은?

① 변비가 있어 Dulcolax $\frac{1}{4}$을 직장을 통해 삽입했다.
② 장티푸스, 파상풍, 간염, 백일해, BCG의 예방접종을 했다.
③ 볼과 손톱에 청색증이 있었다.　④ 오른쪽 반측안면에 마비와 머리에는 반흔이 있었다.
⑤ 복부는 단단하면서 평편하였다.

7 환아의 수술 또는 처치분류번호가 아닌 것은?

① 39.64　② 35.51　③ 35.81　④ 35.99　⑤ 38.85

8 경과기록의 설명으로 틀린 것은?

① 수술 후 2일째에 기관내관을 제거했다.　② 입원 시 청색증이 있었다.
③ 심방실차단은 수술 후 6일째에 시작되었다.　④ 수술 후 심장계 중환자실에 있었다.
⑤ 수술 후 12일째 거친 숨소리가 있었다.

9 소아과와 중환자실의 재원일수가 맞게 짝지어진 것은?

① 소아과 18일, 중환자실 4일　② 소아과 7일, 중환자실 7일
③ 소아과 18일, 중환자실 7일　④ 소아과 16일, 중환자실 14일
⑤ 소아과 16일, 중환자실 7일

10 입원경로가 맞는 것은?

① 타병원에서 수술을 받고 외래로 입원하였다.　② 외래를 통해 흉부외과로 입원하였다.
③ 소아과로 입원하여 흉부외과로 퇴원하였다.　④ 소아과로 입원하여 소아과로 퇴원하였다.
⑤ 흉부외과로 입원하여 흉부외과로 퇴원하였다.

05 화상 흉터 수축 후
Post burn scar contracture

1.1 화상(Burns)

- 화상의 정도: 전체 체표면적에 대한 화상을 입은 면적의 비율
- 측정방법: "Rule of nine" 사용
- 전체를 100%로 하여 화상부위의 피부표면 용적을 예상
  - 머리와 목: 9%
  - 앞몸통: 18%, 뒤몸통: 18%
  - 상지: 각각 9%, 하지: 각각 18% → 사지만 총 54%
  - 회음부: 1%

1.2 질병분류상 주의점

표 1 • 화상 및 부식(Burns and corrosions)

분 류	화 상	부 식
•First-degree burns(1도 화상) 홍반(erythema), 지각과민	________.1	________.5
•Second-degree burns(2도 화상) 수포(blisters), 표피손실(epidermal loss)	________.2	________.6
•Third-degree burns(3도 화상) 조직의 심부괴사(necrosis), 전층 피부 손실	________.3	________.7
· 신체표면의 10% 미만	T31.0	T32.0
· 신체표면의 10～19%	T31.1	T32.1
· 신체표면의 20～29%	T31.2	T32.2
· 신체표면의 30～39%	T31.3	T32.3
:	:	:

① **화상 부위의 정도(degree) 및 신체표면**

Burn of trunk, second degree, 60% of body surface involved
: 체간 면적 60%의 2도 화상 T21.2, T31.6

② **동일한 부위에서 화상의 정도가 다를 경우 높은 정도로 분류**

Burn of chest wall, 2nd degree: 흉벽 2도 화상

Burn of buttock, 3rd degree: 둔부(볼기) 3도 화상 T21.3

③ **화상이나 부식을 입은 신체부위가 다르면 각각 분류**

Burn of wrist, third degree: 손목 3도 화상

Burn of calf, second degree: 종아리 2도 화상 T23.36, T24.22

④ **부식 부위의 정도**

Corrosion of first degree of palm: 손바닥의 1도 부식 T23.54

표 2 • 중독 및 부작용(Poisoning and adverse effect)

약물 및 화학물질표 KCD-7(3권)		
• 제19장	T36.______ - T65.______	: 약물, 약제 및 생물학적 물질의 의한 중독
• 사고(Accident)	X40.______ - X49.______	
• 의도적 자해(suicide, 자살)	X60.______ - X84.______	: self-harm
• 의도불명확	Y10.______ - Y34.______	
• 치료상 부작용	Y40.______ - Y59.______	: 약물의 부작용

[참고] . ______는 장소표시: KCD-7(1권) 발생장소 번호 pp. 967-970 찾음

▸ Toxic effect of thallium, suicidal attempt in the mountain T60.4, X68.8
: 산에서 자살하려고 탈륨먹고 중독되어 옴

▸ Dermatitis due to properly applied antifungal antibiotics L27.0, Y40.7
: 처방대로 바른 항진균성 항생제로 인한 피부염

외과·내과적 처치로 인해 발생한 합병증(T80–T88)

▸ **처치의 합병증**
- 처치에 의한 출혈, 혈종(hematoma), 쇼크, 우발적 천자 및 열상
- 수술부위의 파괴, 감염(infection), 남겨진 이물, 혈관성 합병증

▸ **기계적 합병증**
- 인공삽입물에 의한 고장, 전위, 누출, 위치이상, 기계적 폐쇄, 천공, 돌출상태

▸ **합병증 제외**
- 척수천자로부터 누출된 뇌척수액
- 결장조루술 후 기능불량
- 심장수술에 의한 기능적 심장장애
- 위 수술 후, 요추궁 절제후 및 수술 후 맹관 증후군

▶ Postoperative wound infection T81.4, Y62.0
: 수술 후 상처의 감염

[참고] 수술 또는 처치후 합병증 + 손상외인 → 일반 임상과 : T____ + Y_____
산과: O____ + Y_____

차트 용어

- Amputation 절단
- Debridement 좌멸괴사조직제거술
- Buttock 둔부(볼기)
- Scar 흉터(반흔)
- Contracture 수축
- Palm 손바닥

약 어	원 어	
GEA	General endotracheal anesthesia	기관내 전신마취
	− IV, IM, Endotracheal anesthesia	− 정맥내, 근육내, 기관내 마취법
	− rectal, open drop anesthesia	− 직장, 개방점적식 마취법
IM	Intramuscular	근육내
IVP	Intravenous pyelogram	정맥내 신우조영도
KUB	Kidney, ureter and bladder	신장, 요관 및 방광의 X-ray 검사
LLQ	Left lower quadrant	좌하복부(왼쪽 아랫배 부위)
LOM	Limitation of movement	운동 제한
SR	System review	신체각계조사(병력)
= ROS	Review of system	
STSG	Split thickness skin graft	중간층 식피 이식술

등록번호	220 11 33	성별 M
성명	최 은 인	
주민등록	731020 - 1234567	

입 퇴 원 기 록

Admission and Discharge Record

<table>
<tr><td colspan="4">주 소 : 서울시 강남구 논현동</td></tr>
<tr><td colspan="2">출신지 : 서울시 강남구 논현동</td><td>직 업 :</td><td>전 화 :</td></tr>
<tr><td>연고자성명 : 민수석</td><td>관 계 :</td><td>주 소 :</td><td>전 화 :</td></tr>
<tr><td colspan="2">입원 : 20 년 월 일 과 병동 호</td><td rowspan="3">전과</td><td>2017 년 월 일 과 병동 호</td></tr>
<tr><td colspan="2">퇴원 : 20 년 월 일 과 병동 호</td><td>2017 년 월 일 과 병동 호</td></tr>
<tr><td colspan="2">재원일수 :</td><td>2017 년 월 일 과 병동 호</td></tr>
<tr><td colspan="3">최종진단명</td><td></td></tr>
<tr><td colspan="3">주진단명 : Post burn scar contracture on Lt. hand, palm</td><td></td></tr>
<tr><td colspan="3"></td><td></td></tr>
<tr><td colspan="3"></td><td></td></tr>
<tr><td colspan="3">기타진단명 :</td><td></td></tr>
<tr><td colspan="3"></td><td></td></tr>
<tr><td colspan="3"></td><td></td></tr>
<tr><td colspan="3">수술 및 처치명</td><td></td></tr>
<tr><td colspan="3">수술명 : Debridement</td><td></td></tr>
<tr><td colspan="3">Release by partial excision of scar contracture</td><td></td></tr>
<tr><td colspan="3">and split thickness skin graft</td><td></td></tr>
<tr><td colspan="3">기타수술 및 주요검사 : Colostomy wound: delayed closure</td><td></td></tr>
<tr><td colspan="3">(secondary suture)</td><td></td></tr>
<tr><td colspan="3"></td><td></td></tr>
<tr><td colspan="3"></td><td></td></tr>
<tr><td colspan="4">치료결과 : 1. 완쾌 2. 경쾌 3. 호전안됨 4. 진단뿐 5. 가망없는 퇴원 6. 48시간내 사망 7. 48시간이후 사망</td></tr>
<tr><td colspan="4">퇴원형태 : 1. 퇴원지시후 2. 자의퇴원 3. 탈원 4. 전원</td></tr>
<tr><td colspan="4">병원감염 : 1. 수술후 2. 기타처치후 3. 비뇨기계 4. 호흡기계 5. 소화기계 6. 기타</td></tr>
<tr><td colspan="3">원사인 :</td><td>부검 : 예, 아니오</td></tr>
<tr><td colspan="4">계속적 진료 계획</td></tr>
<tr><td colspan="4">없음 (있음) (약속일 2017년 3월 6일) 종양내과 외래에서 항암제치료 시작할 예정임</td></tr>
<tr><td colspan="2">담당 전공의 서명 : 이한길</td><td colspan="2">담당 전문의 서명 : 강지편</td></tr>
<tr><td colspan="2">의무기록 완성: 2017년 월 일</td><td colspan="2">의무기록사 서명 : 정수오</td></tr>
</table>

등록번호	220 11 33	성별 M
성명	최 은 인	
주민등록	731020－1234567	

퇴 원 요 약

Discharge Summary

1. Final Dx : Post burn scar contracture on Lt hand, palm

2. C.C. : Post burn scar contracture on Lt hand.
   (due to previous burn, 2016. 12. 28)

3. KUB : R/O Renal stone
   U/A : RBC 40－50, hematuria

4. Procedures : Debridement
   Release by partial excision of scar contracture
   and split thickness skin graft

5. OPD care for further evaluation

6. Discharge medication: CBO oint 2 tubes

Signature of Doctor 정한길

등록번호	220 11 33	성별 M
성명	최 은 인	
주민등록	731020－1234567	

병 력 기 록
History

1. C.C : Post burn scar contracture on Lt. hand, palm

2. Personal history : N－C

3. S.H : N－C

4. Past history : 2016년 12월 4일 자살하려고 집에서 가스통을 폭발시켜 CO poisoning 상태에서 both hand, wrist에 괴사를 동반한 약 12%의 화상을 입고 본 병원에 입원하여 Rt. wrist amputation, Lt 2－5th finger amputation 후 2월 28일 퇴원하였음

5. F.H : father : gastric ca.
(8 years ago, total gastrectomy, no recurrence)
daughter : ankyloglossia

6. P. I: Lt. hand palm contracture에 대한 operation을 권유받고 외래를 통하여 입원함

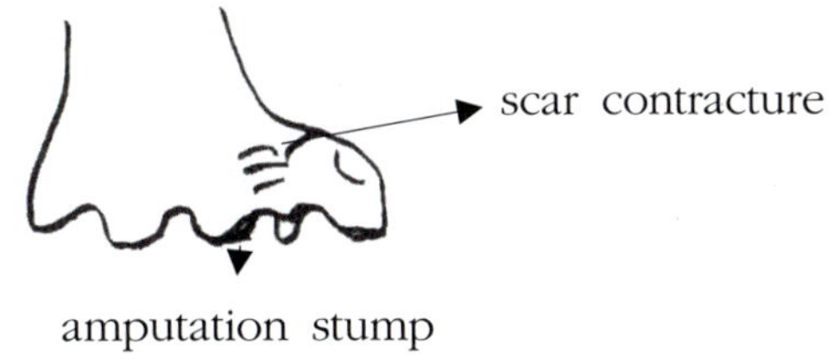

〈Lt. hand〉

7. S/R : vomiting (－) dyspnea (+) nausea (－)
constipation (－) abdominal pain (+)
LOM on left hand － web space (+)

Dr's sign 김국홍

등록번호	220 11 33	성별 M
성명	최 은 인	
주민등록	731020 - 1234567	

신 체 기 록
Physical Examination

키(Height):　체중(Weight):　체온(T):　맥박(P):　호흡(R):　혈압(B.P.):

G/A: Relatively well looking appearance
M/S: alert
HEENT : not anemic conjunctiva
　　not icteric sclera
Chest: CBS $\bar{s}$ ⓡ
　　RHB $\bar{s}$ ⓜ
Abdomen: Soft
　　not tenderness
　　normoactive B.S.
Extremity:

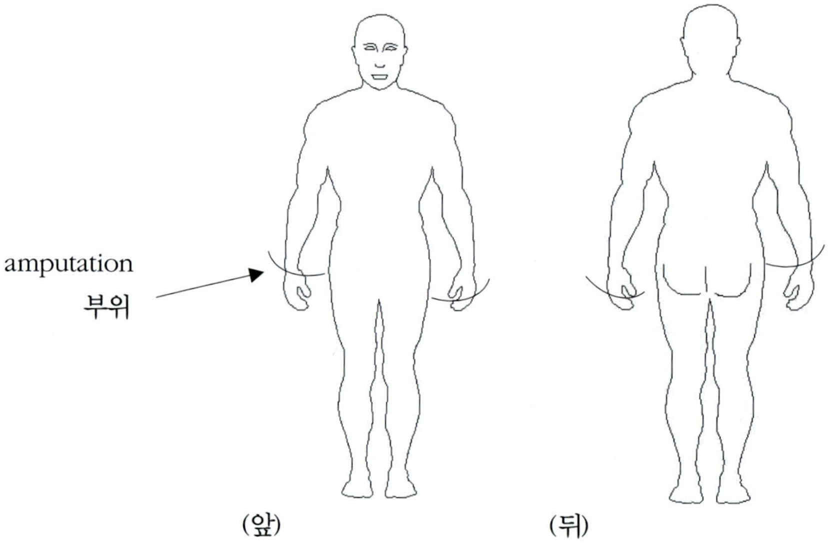

Dr's sign 김국홍

등록번호	220 11 33	성별 M
성명	최 은 인	
주민등록	731020－1234567	

경 과 기 록
Progress Notes

〈 Admission Note 〉

12.4 The 44 years old male patient was admitted to the PS via OPD because of post burn scar contracture on Lt. hand, palm.

* Old chart review

2016년 12월 4일 가스폭발에 의한 화상으로 입원하여 2017년 2월 28일까지 GS에서 치료받음. OS로 transfer되어

1. 2017. 1. 1 : both finger disarticulation
2. 2017. 1. 10 : Rt wrist amputation
3. 2017. 2. 11 : Rt wrist amputation revision의 3회에 걸친 수술 후 퇴원

PS OPD에서 Lt hand contracture에 대한 skin graft 권유받고 오늘 외래를 통하여 입원

Imp) Post burn scar contracture on Lt. hand, palm

Plan) Release by partial excision of burn scar & STSG

이한길

12.5 Operation Record

1. Op. name : Debridement
   Release by partial excision of scar STSG
2. Pre. op. diagnosis : Post burn scar contracture on Lt. hand
3. Post op. diagnosis : ditto.
4. Operator : Prof. J. M. Lee
5. Assistant : R_2 U.H. Seo
   Int. O.W. Choi
6. Anesthesia : G/E/A

이한길

12.8 POD #3

hematuria (+)

Uro. consult 이한길

12.10 POD #5

Good condition 이한길

12.12 Discharged 이한길

등록번호	220 11 33	성별 M
성명	최 은 인	
주민등록	731020 - 1234567	

협의진료기록
Consultation Record

Request For Consultation To

Summary of Present Findings To Dr. 비뇨기과 양동주 과장님

Physician of Department

두 번째 입원으로 지난번 입원 시 오른쪽의 손목과 왼쪽 2-5번째 손가락의 절단술을 시행한 후 퇴원하였습니다. 퇴원 후에도 계속 abdominal pain이 있으면서 가끔씩 hematuria 소견을 보였다고 합니다. 이번 입원 후 3일 전에 scar에 대한 release 후 STSG 시행하였는 바, 오늘 다시 hematuria 소견을 보여 상담 드리오니 고진선처 바랍니다. 감사합니다.

2016. 12. 6 a.m.
Date Hour p.m.

Prof. 유상지/이한길 M.D.
Signature of Attending Physician

Report of Consultation

Opinion and Recommendation

〈 Urology Reply 〉

1. C/C : hematuria
   turbid urine
   frequency (+)
   chillness (+)
   nausea (+)
   LLQ pain for 3days
2. Lab : U/A (RBC 40 - 50)
   K.U.B : suspicious stone density at Lt. renal area
3. Imp : R/O renal stone
4. Rec. : IVP
5. Inj. : Pethidine 50mg IM

2016. 12. 7 a.m.
Date Hour p.m.

Prof. 양동주 M.D.
Signature of Attending Physician

등록번호	220 11 33 성별 M
성명	최 은 인
주민등록	731020－1234567

(수술) 검사 마취 **신 청 서**

병　명: 왼쪽 손 및 손바닥 화상 수축 후
수술/검사명 : STSG
주치의사 : 이 한 길

본인은 본인(또는 상기 환자)에게 행하여질 수술, 검사 및 이에 수반되는 마취의 필요성과 그 내용, 의학상 일반적으로 예상되는 합병증과 후유증에 대하여 금일(이 한길)의사로부터 자세한 설명을 들었으며, 본 수술, 검사로써 불가항력적이거나 일반적으로 야기될 수도 있는 합병증 또는 후유증, 환자의 특이체질로 인한 우발사고가 있다는 것을 충분히 이해하면서 귀 병원에 상기 수술 또는 검사를 실시하여 줄 것을 본 서면으로 요청하며, 이에 따른 일반적인 후유증이나 합병증에 대하여 민·형사상의 제소 또는 이의를 제기하지 않을 것을 자필 서명, 날인으로 서약합니다.

* 기 왕 력	:	☑ 없음	☐ 있음
* 특 이 체 질	:	☐ 알레르기	☐ 당뇨병
		☐ 고혈압	☐ 출혈소인
		☐ 심장병	☐ 약으로 인한 사고
		☐ 마취사고	☐ 기타 ________

2016. 12. 4　10시 30분 오전
오후

상기환자 또는 대리인 박 두 위　인 *Park*
주　소: 서울시 서대문구 남가좌동 234－51
증　인: 홍주황　인 *Hong*
주　소: 환자와 동일

* 본 신청서는 본인의 서명이나 날인으로 유효하나 미성년자 또는 본인이 서명하기 어려운 신체적, 정신적 지장이 있을 때는 보호자 또는 가까운 가족이 대리서명 또는 날인해야 한다.

귀 하

등록번호	220 11 33	성별	M
성명	최 은 인		
주민등록	731020 – 1234567		

수 술 기 록

Operation Record

날짜 : 2016년 12월 5일　　　집도의 : J. M. Lee
제 1 보조의 : U. H. Seo M.D.　　　제 2 보조의 : O.W. Choi M.D.
참여간호사 :　　　순환간호사

Preoperative diagnosis : Post burn scar contracture on Lt. hand, palm

Postoperative diagnosis : SAA

Name of operation : Release by partial excision and STSG

Findings :

The scar contracture with motion limitation on Lt hand, palm was noted.
There was some discharge on folded area on scar tissue.
Dermatome: Brown electric dermatome
Donor site: Lt. buttock

Procedures :

Under the general endotracheal anesthesia, the patient was placed in the supine position and the Lt. arm extended. The operation site was prepared and draped as the usual manner. The rotating rubber tourniquet was applied on Lt. arm for reducing oozing. The incision line was designed as the drawing and the skin incision was made and deepened into the subcutaneous tissue. The scar tissue was removed and the medium thickness skin was obtained from Lt. buttock and covered the defect of recipient site of Lt. palm. The compressive dressing was applied. The patient was tolerated whole the procedures and sent to the recovery room in good conditions.

Tissue to path. ________　　　Drains ________

Dictated/Written by U. H. Seo. M.D.　　　Surgeon's Signature J. M. Lee M.D.

〈최 은 인〉

★ 최은인 차트를 보고 맞는 답에 O표 하시오.

1 첫 번째 입원 당시의 화상에 대한 진단분류번호가 맞게 분류된 것은?

① T30.0, T31.01 ② T29.3, T31.10 ③ T22.0, T23.39, T31.19
④ T23.37, T31.11 ⑤ T22.0, T31.21

2 첫 번째 입원 시 3번 수술을 시행하였는데 수술분류번호가 맞게 조립된 것은?

ㄱ. 84.01 ㄴ. 84.02 ㄷ. 84.04 ㄹ. 84.06
ㅁ. 86.61 ㅂ. 86.99 ㅅ. 84.3 ㅇ. 86.04

① ㄱ－ㄷ－ㅅ ② ㄱ－ㄹ－ㅂ ③ ㄷ－ㅁ－ㅅ
④ ㄷ－ㅂ－ㅇ ⑤ ㅁ－ㅅ－ㅇ

3 수술 후 3일째 되는 날 혈뇨로 인하여 비뇨기과에 협의진단을 하였다. 그 내용과 다른 것은?

① 정맥내 신우촬영법(콩팥깔대기 조영술)을 촬영하도록 권유하였다.
② 신장, 요도 및 방광촬영을 통해 신장결석이 의심되는 소견이 나왔다.
③ 소변보는 빈도수가 증가하였다.
④ 3일 동안 왼쪽 아랫배의 통증이 있었다.
⑤ 오한과 오심이 있었다.

4 이번 입원기간 중에 실시한 수술명을 분류한 것 중 옳은 것은?

① 86.61 ② 86.65 ③ 86.3
④ 86.4 ⑤ 86.67

5 이번에 성형외과에 재입원하게 된 주요 원인 및 주진단 분류번호는?

① 손바닥 흉터에 대한 피부이식술, L90.5 ② 손등 흉터에 대한 피부이식술, T90.5
③ 손바닥 흉터에 대한 피부이식술, T90.9 ④ 손등 흉터에 대한 피부이식술, L94.9
⑤ 손바닥 흉터에 대한 피부이식술, T94.9

6 가족력을 읽고 그 내용과 분류번호가 맞게 짝지어진 것은?

ㄱ. 아버지가 8년 전에 위암수술을 받고 완치되었다.
ㄴ. 딸이 설유착증이다. ㄷ. 딸이 구개열이다.
ㄹ. Z85.9 ㅁ. Z80.0 ㅂ. C16.99 ㅅ. Q38.1

① ㄱ－ㄷ－ㅁ－ㅅ ② ㄱ－ㄴ－ㄱ－ㅅ ③ ㄱ－ㄴ－ㅁ－ㅅ
④ ㄱ－ㄷ－ㅂ－ㅅ ⑤ ㄱ－ㄴ－ㅂ－ㅅ

7 이번 성형외과에 입원하게 된 것은 지난번 입원 후유증으로 인한 것이다. 이것의 분류번호는?

① T23.39 ② T29.3 ③ L90.5
④ T95.2 ⑤ T95.1

8 과거력상 나타난 가스폭발에 대한 분류번호가 맞는 것은?

① T58, X47.0 ② T97, Y87.0 ③ T58, Y17.0
④ T97, Y87.2 ⑤ T58, X67.0

9 환자가 피부를 절제하고 이식한 부위는?

① 상지 ② 하지 ③ 가슴
④ 대퇴부(넙다리부) ⑤ 둔부(볼기)

10 만약 피부이식 부위에 거부반응이 생겨 3개월 후 다시 입원하였다면 이에 대한 합병증분류번호는?

① T81.8 ② T86.8 ③ T86.9
④ T81.3 ⑤ T85.8

06 측두부위의 경막상 혈종
Epidural hematoma of temporal area

1.1 혈종(Hematoma)

- 기관, 공간 혹은 조직에서 보통 혈병으로 된 혈액이 국소적으로 집합된 것
- 혈관벽의 파손이 원인

경막상 혈종(Epidural hematoma)

- 경막 위에 혈액 축적

경막하 혈종(Subdural hematoma)

① **정의**: 경막하강에 혈액 축적

② **분류**: ▸ 중증형, 급성형: 뇌의 파상과 지주막의 열상으로 혈액과 뇌척수액의 양쪽이 강내에 들어가 뇌의 직접적인 손상과 경막하 압박이 부가
▸ 만성형: 교상정맥의 파열 결과로 혈액만이 경막하강내에 삼출

③ **원인**: 보통 두부의 폐쇄성 외상

④ **증상**: ▸ 삼출은 점차 진행하고 외상 후 수주 내에 두통, 진행성 혼미, 편측마비가 옴
▸ 천막허니아의 징후인 동공의 산대가 나타남

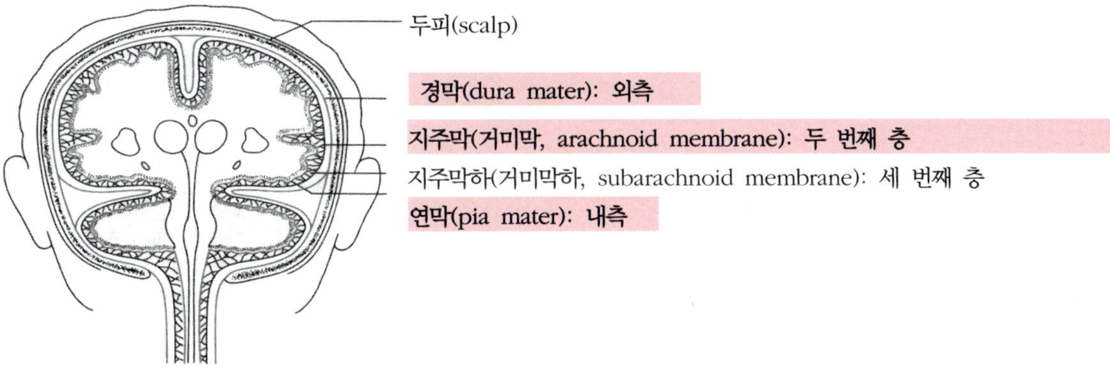

그림 1. 수막(meninges)의 층: 뇌+척수=중추신경계

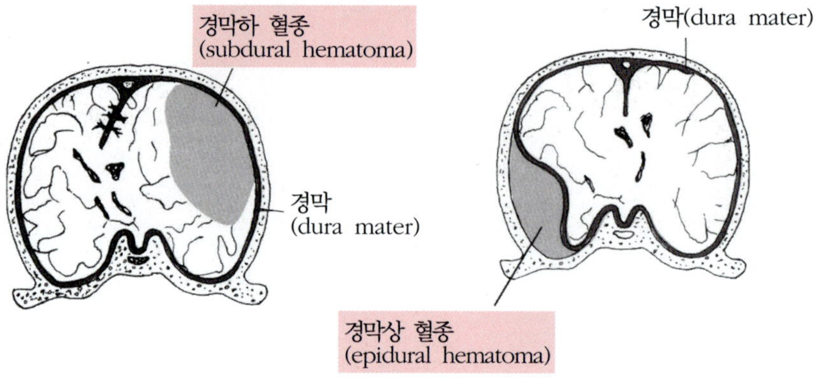

그림 2. 경막하 및 경막상 혈종

1.2 혈관 장애(Vascular disorders)

뇌혈관 사고(Cerebrovascular accident; CVA)

- 뇌졸중(stroke), 중풍, 뇌경색(cerebral infarction)
- 대뇌 혈액공급의 장애
- 뇌 안에 국소부분의 허혈(ishemia)의 결과

뇌졸중의 3가지 유형

① **혈전성(thrombotic)** : 뇌로 가는 동맥의 혈액응고(thrombus)가 혈관폐색(occulusion) 초래

– 항응고제 치료, 동맥내막절제술(endoarterectomy: 동맥내면의 죽상경화성 플라크 절제)

– 일과성 허혈발작(transient ischemic attacks; TIAs)

: 전체적 폐색 이전에 혈관이 순차적으로 막히는 증상

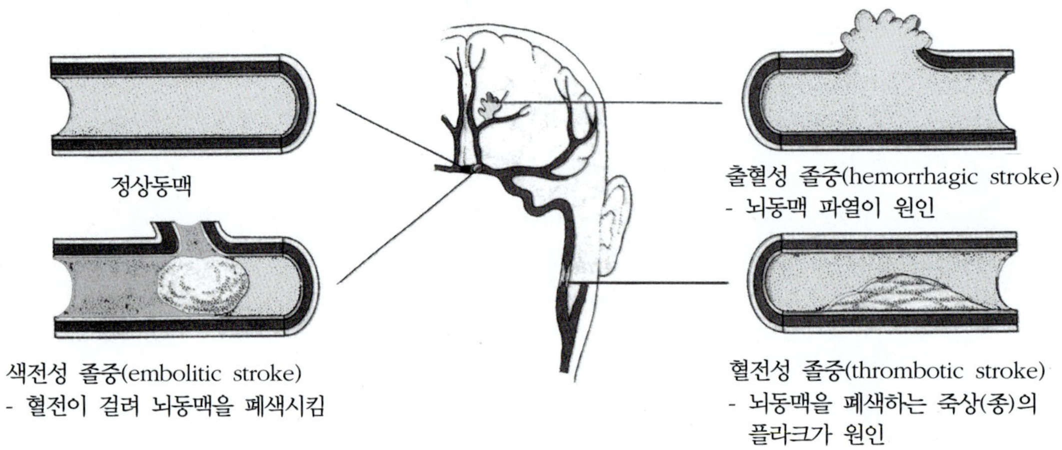

그림 3. 뇌졸중(stroke)의 유형

② **색전성(embolic)**: 색전(embolus)이 대뇌동맥을 떠돌다 작은 혈관에서 막힘

③ **출혈성(hemorrhagic)**: 대뇌동맥으로부터 혈액의 방출

뇌졸중의 위험요인(risk factors)

▸ 고혈압, 당뇨병, 심질환, 흡연, 비만, 약물남용(코카인), 콜레스테롤치 상승

2.1 두개내 출혈(Intracranial hemorrhage)

경막상출혈(Extradural hemorrhage; EDH)

① **정의**

- 중뇌막 동맥(middle meningeal artery)으로부터의 출혈
- 급성으로 진행되어 지혈을 하지 않으면 생명 잃음
- 두부의 손상 → 무의식 → 의식의 명료기(lucid interval) → 혼수(coma)

경막하출혈(Subdural hemorrhage; SDH)

① **정의**: 경막과 지주막(거미막) 사이 공간에 출혈(정맥에서의 출혈이 많음)

② **발생**: 경막상 출혈보다 빈번

③ **원인**: 전두엽 또는 후두엽 부분의 손상

거미막하 출혈(Subarachnoid hemorrhage; SAH)

① **정의**: 지주막과 연막 사이의 출혈

② **원인**

- 뇌기저부의 지주막하에 동맥의 동맥류 파열
- 두개골의 골절에 의해 뇌막의 표면 파열
- 고혈압(가장 중요)

2.2 외상성 장애(Traumatic disorders)

표 1• 뇌좌상과 뇌진탕의 비교

뇌좌상(Cerebral contusion)	뇌진탕(Cerebral concussion)
• 머리의 직접적인 외상으로 뇌조직의 타박상 • 신경학적 결손이 24시간 이상 지속 • 두개골 골절과 연관 – 경막하혈종(subdural hematoma) 및 경막상혈종 (epidural hematoma) 발생 – 영구적인 뇌손상 또는 간질 초래	• 손상(injury) 후 일시적인 의식상실 • 대개 24시간 이내 회복 • 뇌조직의 구조적 손상의 증거는 없음 • 심한 뇌진탕은 혼수(coma) 상태 발생 가능

3.1 정위적 뇌수술(Stereotaxic neurosurgery)

- 입체정위고정기(stereotaxic instrument)를 이용하여 두개골 고정
- 3차원적으로 측정하여 뇌수술 표적의 위치를 정함
- 전기소작(electrocautery), 한랭발생(cryogenic)의 기구 또는 레이저를 가진 probe를 뇌 속으로 넣어 뇌수술 시행
- 최근의 gamma knife(고에너지 방사선)가 달린 정위방사선수술(stereotaxic radiosurgery)
  - 깊고, 접근 어려운 두개강내 뇌종양과 비정상적인 혈관응어리를 외과적 절개없이 치료

3.2 신경과 영역의 질환

편두통(Migraine)

- 머리의 한쪽에 주로 발생
- 쿡쿡 쑤시며 메스꺼움이 동반되는 두통

표 2 • 두개골 및 안면골의 비교

두개골(머리뼈, Cranial bones)	안면골(얼굴뼈, Facial bones)
• 전두골(이마뼈, Frontal bone) • 두정골(마루뼈, Parietal bone) • 측두골(관자뼈, Temporal bone) ► 악관절(Temporomandibular joint, TMJ) - 측두골과 하악골 연결 ► 유양돌기(꼭지돌기, Mastoid process) • 후두골(뒤통수뼈, Occipital bone) • 접형골(나비뼈, Sphenoid bone) • 사골(벌집뼈, (Ethmoid bone)	• 비골(코뼈, Nasal bones) • 누골(Lacrimal bone) • 상악골(위턱뼈, Maxillary bone) • 하악골(아래턱뼈, Mandibular bone) • 관골(광대뼈, Zygomatic bone) • 서골(Vomer)

* □: 두개골의 동(굴) sinus of skull

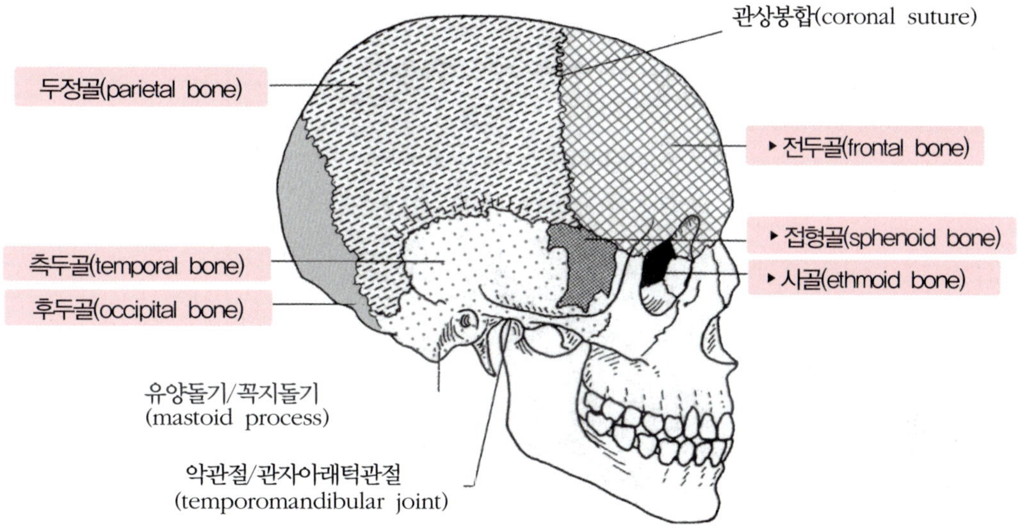

그림 4. 두개골/머리뼈(Cranial bones): 측면

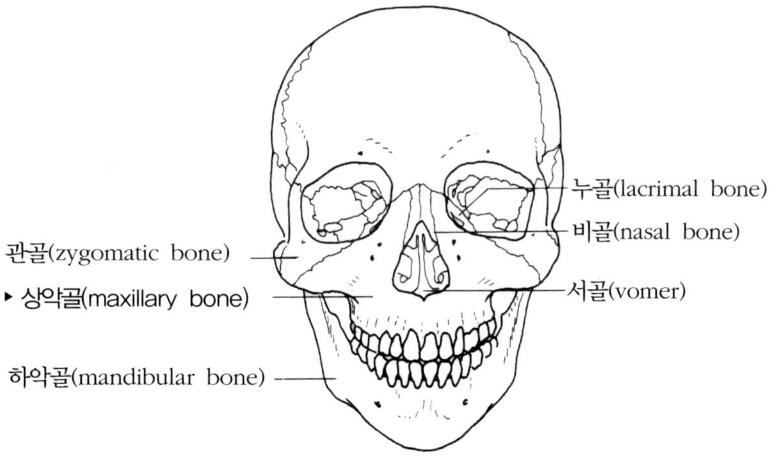

그림 5. 안면골/얼굴뼈(Facial bones)

3.3 수술분류번호 비교

- 진단명: Brain tumor(뇌종양)
- 수술명: Craniectomy and total removal of tumor(머리뼈절제술 및 종양제거) 01.59

- 진단명: Epidural hematoma, Rt, temporal area(오른쪽 측두부 경막위 혈종)
- 수술명: Osteoplastic craniotomy and hematoma removal(뼈형성 개두술 및 혈종제거) 01.24

차트 용어

· Compression	압박	· Drowsy	졸음	· Fibula	비골(종아리뼈)	· Motor	운동신경
· Sluggish	느릿느릿 움직임	· Stiffness	경직	· Thigh	대퇴(넙다리뼈)=femur	· Tibia	경골(정강뼈)
· Iisocoria	동공등대, 두 눈의 동공 크기 동일 ↔ anisocoria 동공 크기 다름						

약 어	원 어	
ABR	Absolute bed rest	절대 안정
AJ	Ankle jerk	발목반사
BJ	Biceps jerk	이두근반사
CBS	Clear breathing sound	깨끗한 호흡음
DTR	Deep tendon reflex	심부건반사
EDH	Epidural hemorrhage	경막외 출혈
EOM	Extraocular movements	외안구 운동
EVD	External ventricular drainage	외심실 배액
FTP	frontotemporo-parietal craniectomy	전두측두-두정 두개절제술
GCS	Glasgow Coma Scale	글라스고우 무의식 척도 점수화
	‣ $E_2M_3V_2$ Eye(1-4), Motor(1-6), Verbal response(1-5) 눈, 운동, 언어 점수화 → 점수 낮을수록 깊은 혼수상태	
GEA	General endotracheal anesthesia	기관내 전신마취
HS	Hartman's solution	하르트만 용액(1 L =1,000cc)
ICH	Intracerebral hemorrhage	두개내 출혈
KJ	Knee jerk(neurologic examination)	슬개(무릎) 반사(신경학적 검사)
LOC	Loss of consciousness	의식상실
LRT	Lower respiratory tract	하호흡기
N/V	Nausea and vomiting	오심 및 구토
OU	Both eyes(Latin: oculus uterque)	양쪽 눈
	[OU(oculus dexter): 오른쪽 눈, OS(oculus sinister): 왼쪽 눈]	
PC	Packed cell	농축세포
PLR	Prompt light reflex	눈이 신속하게 반응
ROM	Range of motion	운동범위
ROS	Review of system	신체각계조사
SDH	Subdural hematoma	경막하 혈종
TIAs	Transient ischemic attacks	일과성 허혈발작
TJ	Triceps jerk(neurologic examination)	삼두근반사(신경학적 검사)
TMJ	Temporomandibular joint	악관절(관자뼈아래턱 관절)
T-P	Temporoparietal bone	측두 두정골(관자마루뼈)

등록번호	220 13 55	성별 M
성명	유 기 적	
주민등록	640205－1234567	

입 퇴 원 기 록
Admission and Discharge Record

주 소 :	보 험 : 산재보험		
출신지 :	직 업 :	전 화 :	
연고자성명 : 변주연	관 계 :	주 소 :	전 화 :

	전과	
입원 : 2017년 4 월 20 일 NS 과 병동 호		20 년 월 일 과 병동 호
퇴원 : 2017년 5 월 29 일 과 병동 호		20 년 월 일 과 병동 호
재원일수 :		20 년 월 일 과 병동 호

최종진단명	분 류 번 호
주진단명 : Epidural hematoma, Rt. temporal area	
기타진단명 : Scalp contusion, Rt. FTP	
Basal skull Fx. on ant. cranial fossa	
Subdural hematoma, Lt, FTP	
ICH, Lt. T－P	
수술 및 처치명	
수술명 : Osteoplastic craniotomy (Lt. FTP) and	
hematoma removal	
기타수술 및 주요검사 : Stereotactic aspiration $\bar{c}$	
closed drainage	

치료결과 : 1. 완쾌 2. 경쾌 3. 호전안됨 4. 진단뿐 5. 가망없는 퇴원 6. 48시간내 사망 7. 48시간이후 사망	
퇴원형태 : 1. 퇴원지시후 2. 자의퇴원 3. 탈원 4. 전원	
병원감염 : 1. 수술후 2. 기타처치후 3. 비뇨기계 4. 호흡기계 5. 소화기계 6. 기타	
원사인 :	부검 : 예, 아니오
계속적 진료 계획	
없음·있음 (약속일 2017 년 6 월 7 일 시)	
담당 전공의 서명 : 한 요 한	담당 전문의 서명 : 이주역
의무기록 완성 : 20 년 월 일	의무기록사 서명 :

등록번호	220 13 55	성별 M
성명	유 기 적	
주민등록	640205－1234567	

퇴 원 요 약
Discharge Summary

Final Dx : Basal skull Fx. on ant. cranial fossa
Epidural hematoma Rt. temporal area
Scalp contusion Rt, FTP
Subdural hematoma Lt, FTP
ICH Lt, T－P

C.C : Deep drowsy mental state

P. I : 상기 53세 남자는 17년 4월 20일 오전 11시에 건축 작업현장에서 4m 높이에서 추락하는 사고로 local에서 응급치료를 받은 뒤 곧 본원 ER로 긴급 후송되어 NS에서 응급수술을 받음

Lab. & X－ray Findings :

ESR/CRP 19/0.1
OT/PT 80/107

Clinical course :

17. 4. 20. : admission
17. 4. 20 : operation
17. 5. 29 : discharge

Tx :

1. Osteoplastic craniotomy Lt. FTP and hematoma removal
2. Stereotactic aspiration $\bar{c}$ closed drainage

Postop Cx : negative
Result : improved
Plan : F/U at OPD (2017. 6. 7)

Han

등록번호	220 13 55	성별 M
성명	유 기 적	
주민등록	640205－1234567	

병 력 기 록
History

C.C : Drowsy m/s

T : '17. 4. 20
P : 인천의 안세시멘트 공사장
V : 4m 높이 건물에서 falling down injury

ROS(S/R) : LOC (+)
neck/back pain (－/－)
N/V (+/+)
headache(+)

P/Ex

G/A : acute ill looking appearance
deep drowsy mental state
HEENT : scalp swelling & tender on RT. FTP area
Neck : supple
Chest & Lung : symmetric expansion $\bar{s}$ retraction
CBS $\bar{s}$ ⓡ
Heart : RHB $\bar{s}$ ⓜ
Abd : Soft and flat
Back & Ext. : No grossly abnormality
N/Ex : Deep drowsy mental state
isocoria $\bar{c}$ sluggish LR (OU)
EOM : full range of motion
Motor / Sensory ─ intact
DTR's Bj (++/++) Kj (++/++)
Tj (++/++) Aj (++/++)
Ankle clonus : (－/－)
Babinski's Sy : (↓/↓)

Imp) Sull Fx.
Cbr. contusion
Scalp contusion Rt. FTP
Ac's EDH Rt. T
Ac's SDH Lt. FTP
T－ICH Lt. T

17. 4. 20 Signature Hong

등록번호	220 13 55	성별 M
성명	유 기 적	
주민등록	640205－1234567	

경 과 기 록
Progress Notes

일 자	내 용	서 명
4.20	〈 Admission Note 〉 P.I : 상기 53세 남자는 17년 4월 20일 오전 11시에 건축 작업현장에서 4m 높이에서 추락하는 사고로 인천 믿음병원에서 응급치료를 받은 뒤 곧 본원 ER로 긴급후송되어 NS에서 응급수술을 받음 PHx : T － 15. 3. 8 11AM P － 인천 안세시멘트회사 V － 2m falling down injury → 1。 care at 인천 믿음병원 LOC (+) headache (－) N/V (+/+) dizziness (－) nasal/ear bleeding (+: both/－) neck stiffness (+) No known pul tbc, DM, HiBP Hx P/Ex V/S BP 180/120 mmHg PR 96/min RR/22/min BT 38℃ G/A acute ill looking appearance M/N M/D HEENT scalp swelling & tender on Rt. FTP area not pale conjunctiva not icteric sclera Both nasal bleeding Neck supple Chest & Lung : symmetric expansion $\bar{c}$ retraction CBS $\bar{s}$ ⓡ Heart : RHB $\bar{s}$ ⓜ Abd : Soft and flat Back & Ext. : No grossly abnormality N/Ex : Deep drowsy mental state Isocoria $\bar{c}$ sluggish LR(OU) No facial weakness EOM: full range of motion	Han

경 과 기 록

일 자	내 용	서 명
4.20	Motor / Sensory] grossly intact DTR's Bj (++/++) Kj(++/++) Tj (++/++) Aj(++/++) Ankle clonus: (−/−) Babinski's Sy: (↓/↓) GCS 3 / 3 / 5] 11 Imp) 1. Cbr. contusion 2. Scalp contusion Rt, FTP 3. Basal Skull Fx. anterocranial fossa clinically 4. Ac's EDH Rt. T 5. Ac's SDH Lt. FTP 6. D−T ICH on Lt. T−P	*Han*

〈Brain CT〉

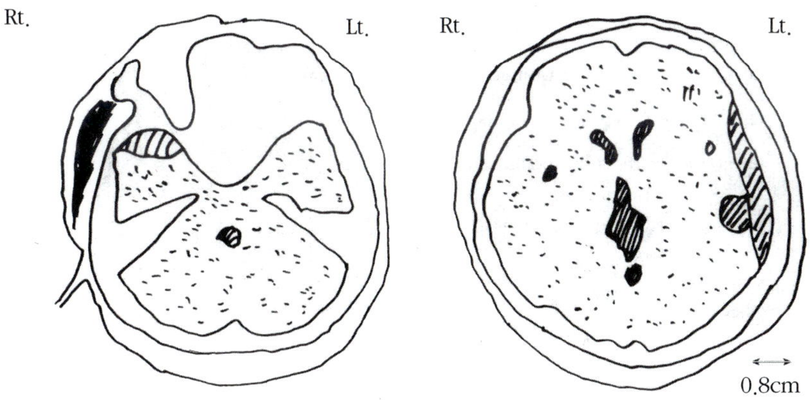

일 자	내 용	서 명
4.20	〈 Brief Op Note 〉 Surgeon : 김의주 Assistants : 이주역/한요한 Anesthesia : GEA Preoperative diagnosis : Ac's subdural hematoma, Lt. FTP T−ICH on Lt. T−P Ac's epidural hematoma on Rt. temporal base Postoperative diagnosis : Same as above Name of operation : Osteoplastic craniotomy Lt, F−T−P removal of hematoma	*Han*

경 과 기 록

일 자	내 용	서 명

4.20 〈 Immediate Postop Evaluation 〉

1. V/S BP 130/80 RR 60/min
2. N/Ex Stuporous mental state
   Rt. anisocoric $\bar{c}$ P.L.R (O.U)
   No facial weakness
   Motor / Sensory] grossly intact
3. Post-op brain CT scan

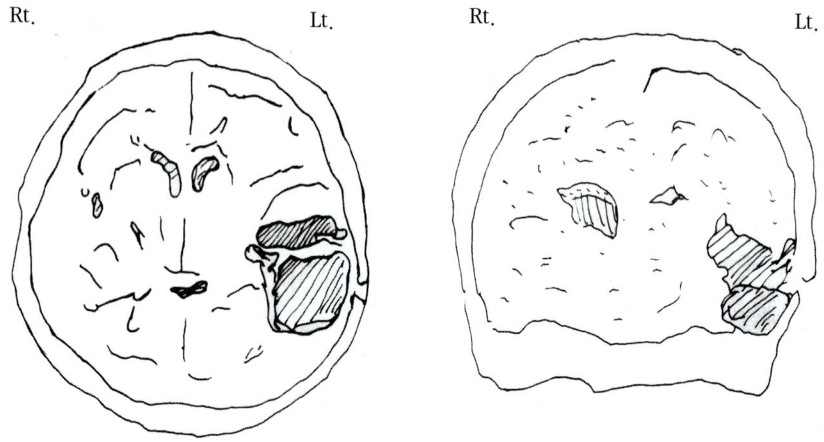

4. Plan : Stereotactic aspiration $\bar{c}$ closed drainage

Han

4.20 〈 Stereotactic aspiration with closed drainage 〉

Under the local anesthesia with 2% lidocaine, the patient was prepared & drapped as usual manner. A linear scalp incision was made on Lt. temporal area with No.15 blade, using previous wound & Burr hole site. The dura mater was punctured with sharp needle.

Under the stereotactic frame fixation, the proximal portion of catheters were inserted the catheter into the hematoma 3.0cm from skull inner table & removed the guider. The darkish hematoma was gush out through the catheter tube and the distal portion of catheter was connected with 3 way connecter. The incised scalp was sutured with 2-0 nylon & the catheter was fixed to the scalp. The cobb tube & EVD was connected. The patient under the procedure is well tolerated.

Han

경 과 기 록

일 자	내 용	서 명
4.21	〈 POD #1 〉 1) V/S BP 130/80 mmHg PR 68/min 2) N/Ex Deep drowsy mental state isocoric $\bar{c}$ P.L.R (O.U) No facial weakness Motor / Sensory] grossly intact 3) H/V 300cc drain Stereotactic tube 30cc drain 4) Plan ① Extubation 시행 ABGA: PH－PO_2－PCO_2 : 7.4－41－131 ② Gen post－op care ③ Transfusion: Hb/Hct 9.9/29.4	*Han*
4.23	〈 POD #3 〉 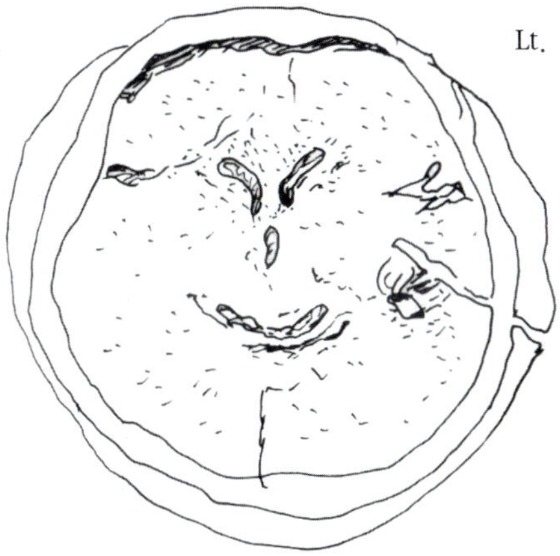 Nearly total evacuating state of DT－ICM on Lt. T－P Marked scalp swelling Stereotactic tube: 10cc drain N/Ex : Drowsy mental state isocoric $\bar{c}$ P.L.R (O.U) EOM: full range of motion No facial weakness Motor Sensory Plan : Stereotactic tube remove Scalp wound care General conservative care	*Han*

일 자	내 용	서 명
4.27	〈 POD #7 〉 Sl. drwosy mental state $\bar{c}$ confusion isocoric $\bar{c}$ P.L.R (O.U) No facial weakness Motor ⎤ grossly intact Sensory ⎦ Plan 1. F/U Brain CT 2. ABR 3. Conservative management	
5.7	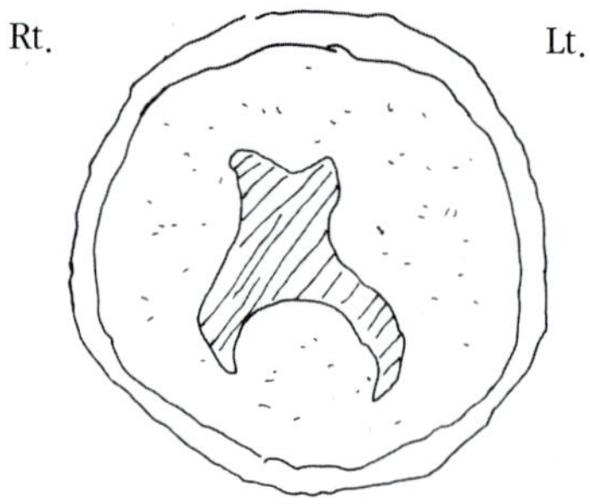 DT−ICH(Lt. TP) much relieved	*Han*
5.21	〈 POD #31 〉 Sl. drowsy mental state $\bar{c}$ confusion isocoric $\bar{c}$ P.L.R (O.U) No facial weakness Motor ⎤ grossly intact Sensory ⎦ Plan 1. F/U Brain MRI 2. Conservative management	R1 *Han*
5.29	〈 POD #38 〉 Sl. drowsy mental state $\bar{c}$ confusion isocoric $\bar{c}$ P.L.R (O.U) No facial weakness Motor Sensory Plan 1. Discharge 2. NS OPD F/U	R1 *Han*

등록번호	220 13 55	성별 M
성명	유 기 적	
주민등록	640205 − 1234567	

수 술 기 록

Operation Record

날짜: 2017년 4월 20일 집도의: M.J. Kim
제 1 보조의: J. H. Lee 제 2 보조의: Y.H.Han
참여간호사: 순환간호사 :

Preoperative diagnosis : Subdural hematoma, Lt. FTP
T − ICH on Lt. T − P
Epidural hematoma on Rt. temporal base
Postoperative diagnosis : Same as above
Name of operation : Osteoplastic craniotomy Lt. F − T − P
removal of hematoma

Findings & Procedures :

Under the general endotracheal anesthesia with ONO and isoflurane, the patient was placed on the supine position turning head to right side. The entire scalp was drapped and prepared as usual manner. The scalp incision was made on left FTP area question mark shaped. The scalp bleeding was controlled by application of multiple Dandy application and scalp was reflected inferiorly. The bone was drilled and burr holes were made on left FTP area. The bone flap was made by sawing and fracture on the base. The exposed dura was tense and it was incised X − shaped.

The blood clot was removed and the bleeding from bridging vein was noted. The bipolar coagulator was used for cauterization and gelfoam was applied. The remainded temporal lobe was severely contused and there showed multiple bleeding goci so temporal lobe was sucked and bleeding was controlled. Finaly contused brain was removed partially and remainded temporal lobe showed normal brain configuration.

So resected base was coated surgicel anf gelfoam. The copious irrigation with saline and there was no bleeding or oozing. So dura was closed. The dura was tented on craniotomy margin. The H/vac was inserted and the muscle layer and skin layer sutured. The patient tolerated well above procedure and sent to CT room.

Dictated by : J. H. Lee Surgeon's signature : M. J. Kim

등록번호	220 13 55	성별	M
성명	유 기 적		
주민등록	640205 - 1234567		

협의진료기록

Consultation Record

Request For Consultation To 피부과 최동찬 선생님

진단명 및 의뢰사유 :

Transportation of pt.
Ambulatory of pt.
Please examine this patient with special reference of for skin lesion on Rt. back & thigh

본 53세 남자 환자는 EDH, SDH로 의심하에 입원 가료중입니다. 상기분야에 대한 선생님의 고진선처 부탁드립니다.

2017. 05. 03

Date Hour

이주홍 / 김민주

Signature of Attending Physician

Report of Consultation

Imp: Generalized skin eruption due to drugs
R/O: Acute urticaria
D: since: 2days

Skin finding: well-dermocated, round-shaaped, erythematous patches on the trunk.
R) ESP-oint 20 gm(tid)

2017. 5. 3

최동찬 M.D

등록번호	220 13 55	성별 M
성명	유 기 적	
주민등록	640205－1234567	

협의진료기록

Consultation Record

Request For Consultation To 정형외과 여대세 선생님

진단명 및 의뢰사유

Transportation of pt.

Ambulatory of pt.

Please examine this patient with special reference of for swelling $\bar{c}$ tenderness on the Rt knee

본 53세 남자 환자는 EDH, SDH로 의심하에 입원 가료중입니다. 상기분야에 대한 선생님의 고진선처 부탁드립니다.

2017. 05. 23 이주홍 / 김민주 M.D.

Date Hour Signature of Attending Physician

Report of Consultation

C.C: soft tissue swelling (cystic nature)
on the suprapatella area (Rt. knee)

D: x 4 days

PHx: Trauma: 2015년 3월 8일 falling down
당시 abrasion on knee (ant. area) Rt. 있었다가 healing 되었다고 함

Aspiration: bloody cystic fluid (25cc) drained

Rec: 1. Compression elastic bandage apply
2. 1 wk 후 elastic bandage remove 해 주십시오

2017. 5. 23 여대세 M.D

등록번호	220 13 55	성별 M
성명	유 기 적	
주민등록	640205－1234567	

의사지시기록
Doctor's Orders

일 자	내 용	서 명
4.20	〈 Admission order 〉	
	1. NPO	
	2. Chest PA	
	skull series	
	C－spine AP & lat	
	3. CCS $\bar{c}$ diff $\bar{c}$ plt	
	4. S－electrolyte	
	FBS	
	5. U/A $\bar{c}$ micro	
	6. SMA (CK. LDH, TG, HDL－Chole)	
	7. RFT	
	8. PT/PTT	
	9. HBs Ag/Ab	
	10. EKG	
	11. ABGA	
	Preop order	
	12. NPO	
	13. Get op permission	
	14. Prep) P/C 2 pint after X－match	
	15. H/S 1L IV (OR용)	
	16. whole shaving	
	aseptic dressing on the scalp	
	17. foley catheter insertion	
	18. Send the patient to OR with chart & X－ray	
	Postop order	
	19. NPO	
	20. Postop) brain CT	
	21. Postop) chest PA	
	skull AP & lat	

의 사 지 시 기 록

일 자	내 용	서 명
	22. CBC ABGA 23. Check V/S $\bar{q}$ 15min x 2 $\bar{q}$ 30min x 2 if stable $\bar{q}$ 2 hrs 24. ABR $\bar{c}$ change position $\bar{q}$ 2 hrs 25. Routine TPR 26. O_2 3L/min inhalation 27. Head elevation 28. Apply both side frame 29. Phenytoin 500 mg $\bar{c}$ N/S 20cc #4 IV qid 30. Urantac 2Ⓐ #2 IV bid 31. Cefradin 4.0 #4 IV qid 32. Sagacin 2Ⓐ #2 IV bid 33. Acopex 8.0 #4 IV qid 34. Naloxane 4Ⓐ #4 IV qid 35. Botropane 6 mix to fluid IV qid 36. Dicknol 2Ⓐ #2 IV bid 37. 5% D/S 1L IV 38. 5% D/W 1L IV 39. N/S 1L IV	*Han*
4.21	40. Chest PA 41. CBC ASTRA ABGA qid 42. SMA 43. Thiopatol 125mg #1 IVx5(d) 44. Skull AP−lat x 2(d) 45. H/S 1L IV 46. 5% D/S 1L IV 47. post transfusion CBC 48. ABGA−post extubation	*Han*

의 사 지 시 기 록

일 자	내 용	서 명
4.23	49. N/S 1L IV 50. 3% Nacl 1L 51. sips of water → soft diet (oral feeding training) 52. D/C #29 32 53. phenytoin 250 mg $\bar{c}$ N/S 10ml #2 IV bid	*Han*
5.29	54. Discharge $\bar{c}$ disposition Depakin 1200 mg #2 PO bid 55. N/S OPD F/U (2주후)	*Han*

〈유 기 적〉

★ 유기적 차트를 읽고 맞는 것에 O표 하시오.

1 상기환자의 질병분류번호가 아닌 것은?

① S00.04, S09.7 ② S06.40, W13.6 ③ W13.6, S00.04
④ S06.80, W17.6 ⑤ S09.7, W13.6

2 의무기록 내용과 다른 것은?

① 오른쪽 경골(정강뼈) 뒷부분의 피부병변으로 피부과에 진료의뢰를 하였다.
② 약으로 급성 두드러기가 2일 동안 있었다.
③ 2015년에 추락으로 오른쪽 무릎에 타박상이 치유된 상태이다.
④ 오른쪽 무릎 위 연조직에 부종이 4일 동안 있었다.
⑤ 압박 탄력밴드 부착 1주일 후 제거하도록 권하였다.

3 환자의 GCS는 몇 점인가?

① 3점 ② 5점 ③ 6점
④ 11점 ⑤ 12점

4 수술분류가 맞게 짝지어진 것은?

① 01.59, 01.09 ② 01.24, 01.09 ③ 01.59, 41.31
④ 01.59, 02.07 ⑤ 01.24, 02.07

5 통계분석이다. 맞게 짝지어진 것은?

퇴원상태	㉮ 완쾌	㉯ 경쾌	㉰ 사망	
보험종류	㉮ 의료보험	㉯ 의료보호	㉰ 자동차보험	㉱ 산재보험
수술건수	㉮ 0	㉯ 1	㉰ 2	
마취	㉮ 전신, 전신	㉯ 전신, 척수	㉰ 전신, 국소	

① 나, 가, 나, 나 ② 나, 라, 다, 다 ③ 가, 나, 나, 가
④ 나, 가, 나, 가 ⑤ 나, 가, 가, 가

6 환자의 사고 당시 상황을 설명한 것으로 틀린 것은?

① 의식상실이 있었다. ② 오심, 구토가 있었다.
③ 코피를 흘렸다. ④ 귀에서 분비물이 흘렀다.
⑤ 목이 강직되었다.

7 입원당시 의사지시사항이 아닌 것은?

① 흉부, 머리 및 복부 x-ray를 촬영할 것 ② 교차시험 후에 농축혈액 2파인트를 준비할 것
③ 동맥혈가스분석 검사를 할 것 ④ 소변도뇨관을 삽입할 것
⑤ 심전도와 간염검사를 할 것

8 **수술 전후 의사지시 내용 중 맞지 않는 것은?**

① 수술동의서를 얻을 것
② 정맥주사용 하트만 1000cc를 수술실용으로 준비할 것
③ 침대에서 운동을 시키고 매 2시간 간격으로 체위변경해줄 것
④ 털을 깎고 무균 드레싱을 할 것
⑤ 2시간마다 안정하다면 15분마다 2회 활력징후 체크

9 **신체검진 중 신경학적 검사에 대한 내용으로 틀린 것은?**

① 발목의 간헐적 경련은 없음
② 양쪽 눈에 빛반사가 즉시 있음
③ 심부건반사는 정상 상태
④ 양쪽 눈의 동공의 크기가 같음
⑤ 운동신경은 정상이며 좋음 상태

10 **상기 의무기록의 약어이다. 원어가 옳지 않은 것은?**

① EVD: External ventricular drainage
② AJ: Ankle jerk
③ EOM: Extraocular membrane
④ ICH: Intracerebral hemorrhage
⑤ CBS: Clear breathing sound

07 척골동맥의 파열

Rupture of ulnar artery

표 1 • 동맥(artery)의 명칭

· carotid artery	경(목)동맥	· iliac artery	장골(엉덩)동맥
· brachiocephalic artery	상완두(팔머리)동맥	· axillary artery	액와(겨드랑)동맥
· hepatic artery	간동맥	· gastric artery	위동맥
· celiac artery	복강동맥	· renal artery	신(콩팥)동맥

1.1 결핵(Tuberculosis)

원 인: 결핵균, Mycobacterium tuberculosis에 의한 감염성 질환

증 상: 기침, 체중감소, night sweat(땀), hemophtysis(객혈), 가슴통증

진 단: X-ray 검사, PPD skin test

치 료: 항결핵 화학요법(Isoniazid, regampin)이 효과적

1.2 흉막(가슴막) 유출(Pleural effusion)

▸ 흉막강(가슴막강, pleural cavity)으로 액이 새어 나옴

2.1 처치 검사

▸ 심전도(Electrocardiogram): 심근의 흥분으로 인한 전류변화를 묘화(描畵)

▸ 심장의 자극 전도계(conduction system) 순서

동방결절(sinoatrial node; S-A node) → 방실결절(atrioventricular node; A-V node) → 방실속(A-V bundle)

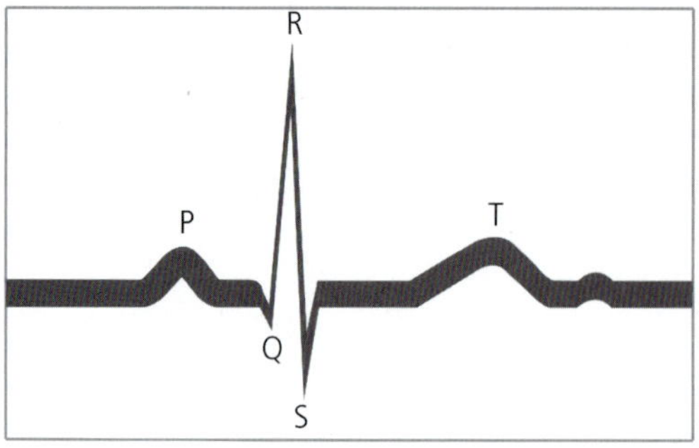

P wave: 흥분파가 심방으로 퍼져감(최초의 전기파)
QRS wave: 흥분파가 심실로 번져감
T wave: 전기적 회복과 심실이완

그림 1. 심전도(EKG)

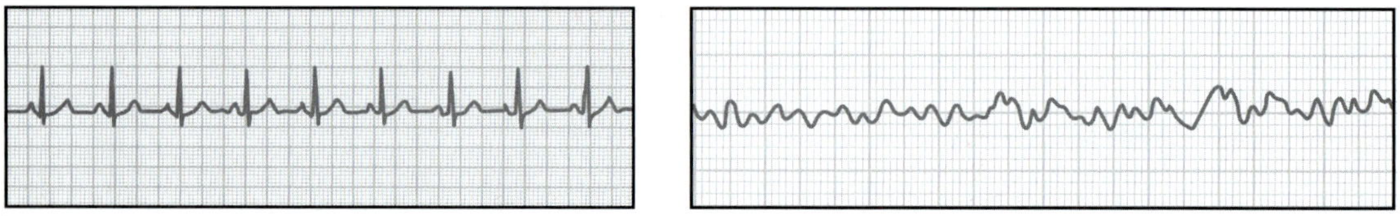

A. Normal sinus rhythm(NSR): 정상

B. 심실세동(ventricular fibrillation): 심장발작, 전기쇼크, 사망 시

그림 2. 정상과 비정상 심전도

폐기능 검사(Pulmonary function test; PFT)

- Spirometer(폐활량계)로 정상 상태에서 폐로 들어오고 나가는 공기의 양을 측정

결핵 검사(Tuberculin test)

- PPD와 같은 약물을 피부 표면에 여러 번 삽입 또는 진피내로 주사(Mantoux's test)
- 검사에 양성(positive)이면 결핵 감염중 또는 전 단계

동맥혈 가스분석(Arterial blood gas analysis; ABGA): 의사지시기록지

- 동맥혈의 산염기의 균형을 보는 검사
- 염기증, 알칼리증을 측정

표 2 • 손상 및 근골계 질환의 분류번호 비교

· S: 단일 신체부위와 관련된 여러 형태의 손상 분류	→ S00-S99	(최대 6자리)
· M: 근골격계 및 결합조직의 질환	→ M00-M99	
· T: 다발성 신체부위를 침범하는 손상	→ T00-T07	
체간, 사지 또는 신체부위의 상세불명 부분의 손상	T08-T14	
손상, 중독 및 외인의 기타 결과의 후유증	T90-T98	

예 1) Severe hemorrhage from ruptured pancreas, laceration of duodenum about 3㎜ with abdominal stabbed wound → S36.21, S36.440

복부자상, 췌장의 파열로 심한 출혈, 소장의 3㎜ 열상

파열(rupture) = 열상(laceration) = 외상성(traumatic) → 손상(injury)

예 2) Osteomyelitis of left distal femur → M86.95
대퇴골(넙다리뼈)의 골수염

예 3) Sequela of carbon monoxide intoxication → T97
일산화탄소 중독 후유증

S 코드

둘째자리(S.__) - **해부학적 부위별**
셋째자리(S__0.) - **손상의 유형**

- S__O. **표재성 손상**: 찰과상(abrasion), 수포(blister), 타박상 및 혈종 포함한 좌상(contusion), 개방성 상처없는 이물에 의한 손상
- S.__1. **개방성 손상**: 절단(cut), 열상(laceration), 천자상처(puncture wound), 이물질(foreign body)
- S.__2. **골절**:

표 3 • 폐쇄성 골절(closed fracture)		개방성 골절(open fracture)	
· simple fx	단순골절	· compound fx	복합골절
· comminuted fx	분쇄골절	· infected fx	감염성골절
· depressed fx	함몰골절	· missile fx	총탄성골절
· greenstick fx	약목골절	· foreign body fx	이물질골절
· impacted fx	매복골절	· puncture fx	천자골절

- S.__3. **탈구, 염좌, 긴장**: -열상, 염좌(sprain), 긴장(strain), 적출(avulsion)
  -외상성: 파열(rupture), 열상(tear), 아탈구(subluxation) 출혈성 관절증
- S__4. **신경의 손상**: -척수 및 신경 연속 병소
  -외상성(trauma): 신경의 분열, 척수내 출혈, 대마비, 사지마비
- S__5. **혈관의 손상**: 절단, 열상, 적출, 외상성 동맥류, 동맥성 혈종, 외상성 파열
- S.__6. **근육, 건의 손상**: 절단, 열상, 외상성 파열
- S.__7. **압궤 손상(crusing injury)**
- S.__8. **외상성 절단(traumatic amputation)**
- S.__9. **기타 손상**

2.2 진단 및 수술분류의 5자리

진단분류

▶ 근골격계 및 결합조직의 질환: **해부학적 부위**를 나타내 주는 분류

예) Thoracic spondylolysis M43.04
흉추(등뼈)의 척추분리증

▶ 개방성 또는 폐쇄성 골절 여부

예) Fracture of first cervical vertebra, open S12.01
제1경추골(목뼈)의 개방성 골절

▶ 두개강내, 흉곽내 및 복강내 **손상 시 개방창 동반여부**를 나타내 주는 분류

예) Subarachnoid hemorrhage by falling down injury from stairs at home S06.60, W10.0
외상성 지주막하(거미막하) 출혈, 집 계단에서 추락

▶ 질병이환 및 사망의 외인: **사건 발생 시** 수행된 **행위의 유형**을 나타내 주는 분류

예) Fracture of bimalleolar ankle, patient was a passenger and jumped from a moving train S82.820, V81.6
움직이는 기차에서 뛰어 내린 승객의 양측 복사 발목 골절

수술분류

▶ 38.8___

예) Ligation of ulnar artery 척골(자뼈)동맥의 결찰 38.83(해부학적 세부분류 추가)
↳ ulnar artery척골동맥의 결찰
[ulna(척골) = upper limb(상지)]

2.3 근골격계의 구성

▶ 뼈(bone) + 관절(joints) + 근육(muscles)

- 건/힘줄(tendon): 근육을 뼈에 부착시키는 결합조직 = 근육 + 뼈
- 인대(ligament): 뼈와 뼈를 묶은 결합조직 = 뼈 + 뼈
- 관절(articulation=joints): 뼈가 만나는 장소

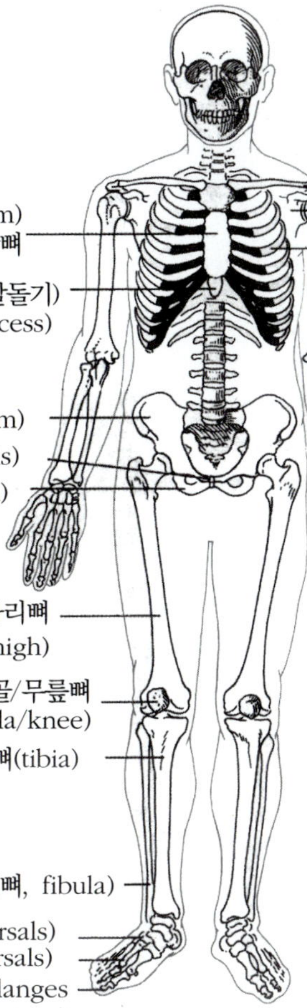

그림 3. 흉곽, 골반 및 사지의 뼈

표 4. 상지와 하지의 비교

상지/팔뼈(Upper limbs=extremities)	하지/다리뼈(Lower limbs=extremities)
▸ humerus(상완골/위팔뼈), ulna(척골/자뼈)	▸ femur(대퇴골/넙다리뼈), patella(슬개골/무릎뼈)
▸ radius(요골/노뼈), carpals(손목뼈)	▸ tibia(경골/정강뼈), fibula(비골/종아리뼈)
▸ metacarpals(손바닥뼈), phalanges(손가락뼈)	▸ tarsals(발목뼈), metatarsals(발바닥뼈)
	▸ phalanges of the toes(발가락뼈)

차트 용어

· Afebrile	무열성	· Finger	손가락	· Hyperesthesia	지각과민
· Irrigation	세척	· Laceration	열상	· Paresthesia	감각이상
· Pleural effusion	흉막삼출액	· Rubber drain	고무 배농관	· Rupture	파열
· Sedation	진정	· Volar = palm	손바닥	· Wrist	손목
		= dorsal			

약 어	원 어	
ABGA	Arterial blood gas analysis	동맥혈 가스분석(의사지시기록)
A-P	Anteroposterior	전후
AV, A-V	Atrioventricular	방실의
BT	Bleeding time	출혈시간
COPD	Chronic obstructive pulmonary disease	만성폐쇄성폐질환
CT	Coagulation time	응고시간
	Clotting time	응고시간
DIP	Distal interphalangeal(joint)	원위 지절간의(관절)
DOE	Dyspnea on exertion	노력성 호흡곤란
EKG, ECG	Electrocardiogram	심전도
FCU	Flexor carpi ulnaris	척측 수근 굴근
FDS	Flexor digitorum superficialis	천지굴근
LOM	Limitation of motion	운동 제한
PPD	Purified protein derivative	정제 단백질 유도체(결핵검사)
RBBB	Right bundle branch block(ECG)	우각 차단(심전도)
PID	Pelvic inflammatory disease	골반내 염증성 질환
MP	Metacarpal phalangeal(joint)	중수지절의(관절)
NBS	Normal breathing sound	정상 호흡음
NE	Neurological examination	신경계 검사
PT	Physical therapy	물리치료
RLL	Right lower lobe(lung)	우하엽(폐)
ROM	Range of motion	운동범위
RSR	Regular sinus rhythm(heart)	규칙적 동율동(심장)
RTC	Return to clinic	진료소 회송
SA, S-A	Sinoatrial	동방의
U/A	Urinalaysis	요분석, 소변검사
WNL	Within normal limit = G-F = intact = N-C	정상 범위내

등록번호	300 22 11	성별 M
성명	신 나 라	
주민등록	740203－1234567	

입 퇴 원 기 록
Admission and Discharge Record

주 소 : 대구시 남구 송현동 225				
출신지 :		직 업 :	전 화 :	
연고자성명 : 민순용		관 계 :	주 소 :	전 화 :
입원 : 2017 년 월 일 PS 과 병동 호	전과	20 년 월 일 과 병동 호		
퇴원 : 2017 년 월 일 과 병동 호		20 년 월 일 과 병동 호		
재원일수 :		20 년 월 일 과 병동 호		

최종진단명	분 류 번 호
주진단명 : Rupture of ulnar artery	
Laceration of Rt wrist & finger (2－5th)	
기타진단명 : tendon involvement	
Pulmonary tuberculosis $\bar{c}$ pleural effusion	
수술 및 처치명	
수술명 : Tenorrhaphy, myorrhaphy	
Ligation of ulnar artery	
기타수술 및 주요검사 : Debridement $\bar{c}$ long－arm splint	
Short arm splint	

치료결과 : 1. 완쾌 2. 경쾌 3. 호전안됨 4. 진단뿐 5. 가망없는 퇴원 6. 48시간내 사망 7. 48시간이후 사망	
퇴원형태 : 1. 퇴원지시후 2. 자의퇴원 3. 탈원 4. 전원	
병원감염 : 1. 수술후 2. 기타처치후 3. 비뇨기계 4. 호흡기계 5. 소화기계 6. 기타	
원사인 :	부검 : 예, 아니오
계속적 진료 계획	
없음있음 (약속일 20 년 월 일 시)	
담당 전공의 서명 : 민준화	담당 전문의 서명 : 성호양
의무기록 완성 : 20 년 월 일	의무기록사 서명 :

등록번호	300 22 11	성별	M
성명	신 나 라		
주민등록	740203-1234567		

퇴 원 요 약
Discharge Summary

1. Diagnosis : #1. Rupture of ulnar artery
#2. Laceration of FDS on Rt. 2-5th fingers and FCU with tendon involvement
#3. Pulmonary tuberculosis $\bar{c}$ pleural effusion

2. C.C : Pain on lacerated wound of volar aspect of Rt. wrist, in sutured state due to injury by drilling machine, yesterday.

3. P. E : Rt. wrist, sutured lacerated wound on the volar aspect (in 10cm length)
·LOM on flexion of Rt 2,3,4,5th fingers in M-P joint levels
·LOM on flexion of Rt wrist.
·Sensory defect: on ulnar aspect of Rt 4th finger and Rt 5th finger
·Pulsation on Rt ulnar artery (-)
but intact on Rt radial artery

4. X-Ray : RLL pulmonary tuberculosis, activity $\bar{c}$ pleural effusion
Lab : CBC U/A : WNL EKG : RBBB

5. Op. : (1) Teno-myorrhaphy & debridement in primary closure
(2) Ligation of ulnar artery
(3) Long-arm splint for 3wks, then short-arm splint

6. Discharge $\bar{c}$ medication
on POD#21 with short arm splint in situ $\bar{c}$ medication

7. Rec. : PT for finger exercise with current splint

Dr's sign Min

등록번호	300 22 11	성별	M
성명	신 나 라		
주민등록	740203－1234567		

병 력 기 록
History

키(Height):　체중(Weight):　체온(T):　맥박(P):　호흡(R):　혈압(B.P.):

C.C : deep laceration on volar aspect of Rt. wrist
(onset: 2017. 8. 5)

P.H. : 3 years ago (bleeding duodenal ulcer로 진단받음)

S.H. : Occupation : 기능공
alcohol, smoking : 약간

Past history : adulthood illness (−)
no op. or no drug abuse or drug allergy
DM (−)　asthma (−)　hypertension (−)　pul. Tb (+)

F.H.: his wife: PID로 치료중
his father : COPD
his mother : cataract, rheumatoid arthritis

P.I. : open wound of Rt. wrist and finger injury of ulnar artery

S/R : fever (−)
headache (−)
vomiting (−)
cough & dyspnea (+)
DOE (+)
sputum (+)
palpitation (−)

Kim

등록번호	300 22 11	성별 M
성명	신 나 라	
주민등록	740203－1234567	

신 체 검 진 기 록

Physical Examination

G/A : alert mental state, acute ill appearance

Head & neck : normocephaly

trachea, thyroid : WNL

shape : free

others : free

Eye : isocoria $\bar{c}$ Rt. light reflex no－icteric, not anemic

Ear & nose : free

Tooth & throat : grossly free

Hearts : RSR $\bar{s}$ ⓜ

Lung : NBS $\bar{s}$ ⓡ no deformity symmetrical exp.

Musculo－skeletal : Volar aspect of Rt. wrist, oblique laceration

Rt. 2－4 finger: M－P flexion ↓

DIP flexion : intact

Rt. wrist flexion : ↓

Ext. : WNL

N/E : DTR ++/++

Imp : deep laceration on Rt wrist

Plan : 1) Rt wrist A－P & lateral

2) CBC $\bar{c}$ hematocrit BT.CT

3) Op.: teno－arterio－neurorrhaphy

Kim

등록번호	300 22 11 성별 M
성명	신 나 라
주민등록	740203－1234567

경 과 기 록
Progress Notes

〈 Admission Note 〉

8.6 Admission via OPD

C/C : deep laceration on volar aspect of Rt. forearm.

·onset: 2017. 8. 5

·mode: drilling machine

Sutured in private clinic, transferred to our hosp.

P/E : Sutured wound on volar aspect, obliquely

·Rt. 2,3,4,5th fingers

M－P flexion : diminished

DIP flexion : intact

·Rt. wrist flexion : diminished

·hyperesthesia on innervated area of median and ulnar nerve

·Rt. hand circulation : intact

Imp : Deep laceration involved tendon, median nerve,
ulnar nerve and artery of Rt. wrist

Plan : Exploration Min

8.6 〈 Brief op. note 〉

1. Op. name : myorrhaphy & tenorrhaphy and ligation of ulnar artery
2. Operator : R_3 성호양
   R_1 민준화
3. Diagnosis & Op. findings
   1) deep laceration of volar aspect of Rt wrist
   2) severed structure injury
      ·flexor digitorum sublimis (2－5th finger)
      ·flexor carpi ulnaris
      ·ulnar artery
   3) intact : ulnar nerve and median nerve

경 과 기 록

일 자	내 용	서 명
	4. OP. procedures	
	1) under A/B & sedation	
	2) debridement & massive irrigation	
	3) ulnar artery ligated	
	4) ulnar nerve and median nerve intact	
	5) myorrhaphy by Daxon	
	tenorrhaphy by No. 5 silk	
	6) subcutaneous suture (No. 2 silk)	
	7) inserted rubber drain (×1)	
	8) skin suture (No. 3 silk)	
	9) applied long arm splint in wrist flexion	*Min*
8.7	POD #1	
	V/S : stable, afebrile	
	wound : slightly swelling	
	med. consultation : evaluation of pul. Tb	Min
8.10	POD #4	
	wound : slightly swelling and local heat	
	small discharge	
	removed rubber drain	*Min*
8.17	POD #11	
	wound : much subside of swelling & reddness	
	in good healing process	
	anti-Tb. medication continued	*Min*
8.25	POD #19	
	wound : complete cure	
	P/E : still persisted paresthesia on little and ring fingers, Rt. hand	
	Rec) : discharge and OPD care	*Min*
8.26	POD #20	
	change splint into short-arm neutrical splint	
	Rec) exercise in ROM, active	
	assisted on Rt. hand & fingers including wrist	*Min*
8.27	POD #21	
	discharge $\bar{c}$ medication	
	Rec) RTC on 8.29. 1998. for OPD care	
	PT for finger exercise $\bar{c}$ current splint	
	3 month later, med. OPD follow-up	*Min*

〈신 나 라〉

★ 신나라 차트를 보고 맞는 답에 O표 하시오.

1 환자는 기계에 의해 손상을 받아 오른쪽 척골동맥이 파열되어 수술을 받았다. 분류번호는?

① S65.7, 38.8 ② S65.06 38.83 ③ S55.06, 38.85
④ S65.02, 38.8 ⑤ S65.56, 38.83

2 오른쪽 손목과 손가락 열상에 대한 질병분류번호는?

① S06.91, S66.00 ② S61.0, S66.3 ③ S61.9, S66.8
④ S61.7, S66.10 ⑤ S69.7, S64.0

3 오른쪽 손가락건 열상에 대해 시행한 수술분류번호는?

① 83.64, 82.45 ② 83.64 ③ 81.96 ④ 82.45 ⑤ 86.59

4 환자가 받은 손상의 원인을 나타내 주는 분류번호는?

① W27 ② W20 ③ W23 ④ W28 ⑤ W31

5 가족력에 나타난 질환이 아닌 것은?

① J45.9 ② N73.9 ③ J44.9 ④ H26.99 ⑤ M06.99

6 심전도검사 결과 나타난 상태를 질병분류하면?

① I45.4 ② I45.1 ③ I45.9 ④ I44.3 ⑤ I44.6

7 내과에 협의진단 결과 확인된 진단명의 분류번호는?

① A16.0, J90 ② J90 ③ A15.1 ④ A15.6 ⑤ A16.5

8 수술 후 상태를 설명한 내용 중 맞는 것은?

① 수술 후 19일 되는 날 상처는 완전히 치유되었다.
② 수술 후 1일째 되는 날 미열이 있었다.
③ 배농관은 수술 후 11일째 되는 날 제거하였다.
④ 수술 후 19일째 되는 날까지도 여전히 오른손의 넷째, 새끼손가락에 점상출혈이 있었다.
⑤ 견인장치를 수술 후 20일째 되는 날 바꿔주었다.

9 퇴원요약지 내용과 다른 것은?

① 오른쪽 손목의 손바닥을 향한 쪽에 길이 약 10cm정도의 봉합한 열상이 있었다.
② 오른쪽 손목의 굴곡움직임에 제한이 있다.
③ 요골동맥도 파열되었다.
④ 부목을 댄 상태로 손가락 운동을 위한 물리치료를 받도록 권유하였다.
⑤ 수술 후 21일째 되는 날 부목을 댄 상태로 퇴원하였다.

10 과거력상 3년 전에 궤양 진단을 받았다. 그 상태의 분류번호는?

① K26.4 ② K26.3 ③ K28.3 ④ K26.9 ⑤ K28.4

01 척수병증 동반 추간판탈출증
Herniated intervertebral disk c̄ myelopathy

1.1 추간판탈출증(Herniated intervertebral disk; HID)

추간판탈출증의 정의: 디스크

- 추간원판탈출증은 소위 "디스크"로 알려짐
- 추간판이 돌출되어 요통 및 신경 증상을 유발하는 질환

수핵탈출증(Herniated nucleus pulposus; HNP) → 척추신경 압박: 질환 유발

- 어떤 원인에 의해 손상을 입으면서 추간판 내부의 젤리 같은 수핵이 탈출
- 주변을 지나는 척추신경을 압박함으로써 다양한 신경학적 이상증상을 유발하는 질환

추간원판탈출증 증상

- 다리가 저리고 허리 통증
- 추간원판의 수핵이 척추관으로 이탈되어(HNP) 척수신경근을 압박하여 통증
  - 좌골신경통(sciatica): 허리에서 다리아래 사이로 뻗치는 좌골신경의 통증
  - 요통(허리통증, Low back pain)
  - 목의 통증(Cervical pain)
- 심한 경우 신경에 손상
- 가장 빈번한 발생 부위는 L_4-L_5, L_5-S_1(HLD; herniated lumbar disc, 추간판 탈출) → M51.2

추간원판탈출증 수술

- **후궁절제술(Laminectomy)**
  - Lamina를 제거하여 협착된 신경을 넓혀 주는 방법
- **추간판절제술(Discectomy)**
  - 신경 또는 척수를 누르는 탈장된 디스크를 수술적으로 제거

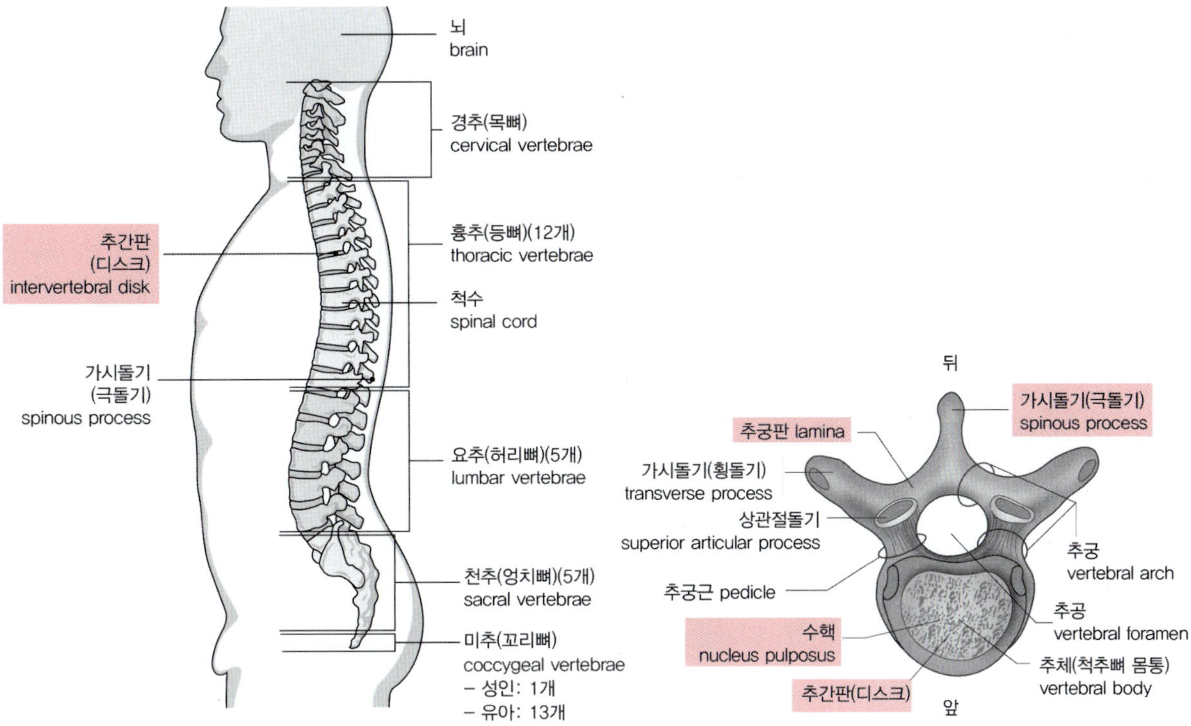

그림 1. 흉곽, 골반 및 사지의 뼈

2.1 폴리카테터(Foley catheter): 유치도뇨관 - 인공배뇨

폴리카테터의 의미

- 인공배뇨는 도뇨관을 요도(urethra)를 통해 방광(bladder)에 삽입
- 소변을 배출시키는 것: 인공배뇨

2.2 적혈구 침강 속도(Erythrocyte sedimentation rate, ESR)

- 적혈구 침강속도(ESR) 검사는 염증, 종양, 감염, 괴사 등을 알아내기 위한 검사
- ESR은 질병의 진행과정을 알려주는 신뢰감 있는 지표
- 정상치: 남성 10mm/hr 이하, 여성 20mm/hr 이하
  - ESR 상승: 임신중독증, 매독, 신장염, 폐렴, 류마티스성 관절염
  - ESR 저하: 울혈성 심부전, 저섬유소 혈증, 진성 적혈구 증가증

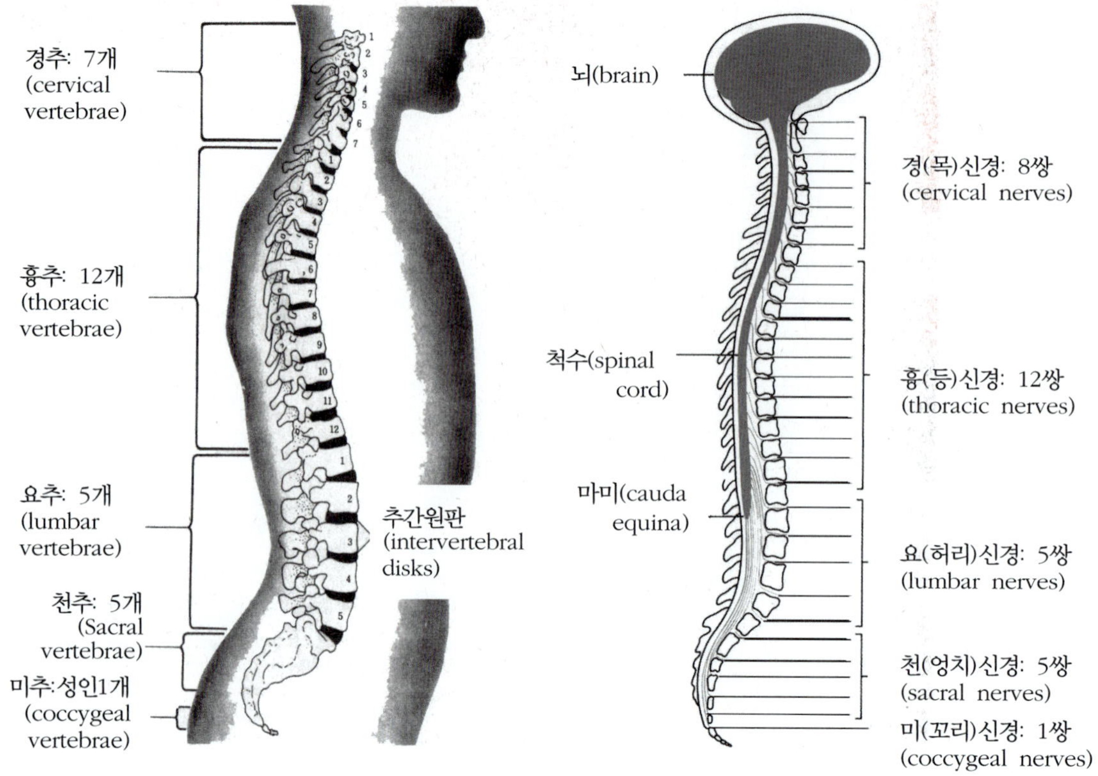

A. 척주(vertebral column)　　B. 척수신경(spinal nerve)

그림 2. 척주와 척수신경

표 1. 척주 및 척수신경의 비교

척주(Vertebral column): 근골격계			**척수신경(Spinal nerves): 신경계**	**31쌍**
• 경추/목뼈(Cevical vertebrae)	C1-C7	7개	• 경신/경/목신경(Cervical nerves)	8쌍
• 흉추/등뼈(Thoracic vertebrae)	T1-T12	12개	• 흉신경/등신경(Thoracic nerves)	12쌍
• 요추/허리뼈(Lumbar vertebrae)	L1-L5	5개	• 요신경/허리신경(Lumbar nerves)	5쌍
• 천추/엉치뼈(Sacral vertebrae)	S1-S5	5개	• 천신경/엉치경(Sacral nerves)	5쌍
• 미추/꼬리뼈(Coccygeal vertebrae)	평균 3~5개(성인 1개)		• 미신경/꼬리신경(Coccygeal nerves)	1쌍

중추신경계(Central nervous system; CNS)

↙ ↘

뇌(brain) + 척수(spinal cord) = 수막(뇌막, meninges)

말초신경계(Peripheral nervous system; PNS)

↙ ↓ ↘

Cranial nerves 뇌신경(12쌍)

1. 후각신경
2. 시각신경
3. 동안(눈돌림)신경: 눈운동
4. 활차(도르래)신경: 눈운동
5. 삼차신경(얼굴/혀/씹기)
6. 외전(가돌림)신경: 눈운동
7. 안면(얼굴)신경
8. 내이(속귀)신경
9. 설인(혀인두)신경
10. 미주신경: 목/내장
11. 부신경: 목/등운동
12. 설하(혀밑신경): 혀

Spinal nerves 척수신경(31쌍)

Autonomic nerves 자율신경

· 교감신경(Sympathetic nerves)
· 부교감신경(Parasympathetic nerves)

그림 3. 중추신경계와 말초신경계의 구분

3.1 철결핍성 빈혈(Iron deficiency anemia; IDA)

▸ 철(Fe)은 적혈구 내 있는 혈색소, 헤모글로빈(hemoglobin)의 가장 중요한 구성요소

▸ 철 부족 시 → 혈색소 생성 안됨 → 혈색소 없을 경우 → 적혈구 생성 안됨 → 빈혈 발생

3.2 무지외반증(Hallux valgus): 무지(Hallux, 엄지발가락)

▸ 무지외반증은 엄지발가락의 제1중족 발가락 관절을 기준

- 발가락쪽 뼈가 바깥쪽으로 치우치고 발뒤꿈치쪽 뼈는 안쪽으로 치우치는 변형

▸ 무지외반증은 선천적 또는 후천적으로 뼈가 변형되어 수술로 교정

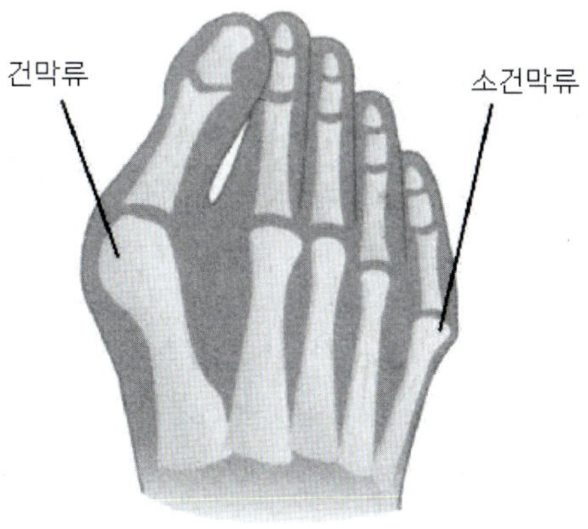

그림 4. 무지외반응(Hallux valgus)

차트 용어

· Acquired	후천적인	· Cough	기침	· Extension ↔ flexion	신전 굴곡	· Foley catheter	폴리카테터(소변배액) = 유치도뇨관
· Ambulation	보행/외래치료						
· Humidification	가습기	· Immobilization	고정	· Longitudinal ligament	종인대	· Medial border	내측 경계
· Motor	운동	· Myelopathy	척수병증	· Myopathy	근육병	· Neuropathy	신경병증
· Numbness	무감각	· Post neck	뒷목	· Posterior	뒤의	· Protrusion	돌출
· Radiculopathy	신경근병증	· Respiration	호흡	· Response	반응	· Retraction	견인
· Sensory	감각	· Severe pain	심한 통증	· Superior	상급의	· Teared	찢어진
· Thyroid artery	갑상선동맥	· Trachea	기관	· Tingling	저림 /얼얼	· Traction	견인
· Verbal	언어	· Ward	병동				

약 어	원 어	
ABR	Abolute bed rest	절대안정
AJ	Ankle jerk(=reflex)	발목반사
BJ	Biceps jerk(=reflex)	이두근반사
BR	Bed rest	안정
$\bar{c}$	With	동반
C4-5	Cervical vertebrae	경추/목뼈 4-5번
C5-6	Cervical vertebrae	경추/목뼈 5-6번
DTR	Deep tendon reflex	심부건반사(=깊은 힘줄 반사)
DW 5%	Dextrous Water 5%	5% 포도당 용액
EDBC	Encourage deep breathing and coughing	심호흡과 기침 격려
EMG	Electromyogram	근전도 검사
ESR	Erythrocyte sedimentation rate	적혈구 침강 속도
HIVD	Herniate intervertebral disc	추간판탈출증
HNP	Herniate nucleus pulposus	수핵탈출증
H/S	Hartman's solution	하트만 용액(1 L =1,000cc)
H/VAC	Hemovac	배액관
IDA	Iron deficiency anemia	철결핍성 빈혈
KJ	Knee jerk(=reflex)	무릎반사
LE	Lower extremities(=limb)	하지/다리
PRN	Whenever necessary	필요할 때마다
$\bar{q}$	Every	매
$\bar{s}$	Without	동반없이
SCM	Sternocleidomastoid	흉쇄유돌근
S-S	Saline solution	생리식염수
TJ	Triceps jerk(=reflex)	삼두근반사
U/E	Upper extremities(=limb)	상지/팔
VDRL	Venereal Disease Research Laboratory = VDRL: reactive(매독 있음) = VDRL: non-reactive(매독 없음)	매독검사

진 장 수 요약 차트

등록번호 : 35 42 86 이름 : 진장수

입원일 : 2017. 1. 10 퇴원일 : 2017. 1. 31 퇴원과 : NS

1/10 Diagnosi s: #1. C4-5-C5-6 HIVD $\bar{c}$ myelopathy
#2. Hallux valgus (acquired)
#3. lron deficiency anemia

C.C : Post neck pain
Lt. U/Ext tingling numbness remote O/S) 16-5
O/S) 내원 3주 전

P.I : 내원 한달 전 부터 post neck pain 있던 환자로 별다른 검사없이 지내오다 내원 3주 전부터 post neck pain & Lt. U/Ex. tingling numbness 증세가 악화되어 local Cx-CT & MRl check 결과 neck disc가 있어 OPD 통해 Adm.

N/E : Motor U/E : Hand graping power
Elbow flex / ext.
L/E : Knee flex / ext power (++/++)
Sensory : nearly intact
DTR BJ, TJ (++/++) KJ, AJ (++/++)

Cx-MRl
C4-5 C5-6 disc material protrusion, central to Lt.

Electrodiagnosis Report
Imp) No evidence of radiculopathy, neuropathy & myopathy *Kim*

〈Op. note〉

1/12 Preop Dx : C4-5 & C5-6 HNP, central to left rupture with cord compression
Postop Dx : Same as above
Name of operation : C4-5 & C5-6 discectomy with left anteromedial approach + interbody fusion with RABEA cages
(C4-5 : 6x12x14mm, C5-6 : 5x12x14mm)

진 장 수 요약 차트

등록번호 : 35 42 86 이름 : 진장수
입원일 : 2017. 1. 10 퇴원일 : 2017. 1. 31 퇴원과 : NS

Procedure & findings

Anesthesiologic method : G/A

Operative position supine position, shoulder roll bar 및 neck 밑에 roll bar를 받쳐 목을 약간 extension되게 함. Halter traction으로 7ℓb를 걸어 traction시킴

Skin incision : thyroid cartilage를 중심으로 SCM의 medial border를 따라 약 9cm의 linear incision을 가함

Main procedure: skin incision 후 Metzenbaum으로 platysma m.을 따라 박리 절개한 후 외측으로 SCM muscle과 carotid sheath를 내측으로 esophagus, trachea 및 strap muscle를 appe. retractor로 manual로 retraction함. 이 과정에서 sup. thyroid a.가 노출되어 이를 ligation 후 절개함. longus coli m.과 deep fascia를 확인 후 이를 blunt dissection으로 양측으로 벌리자 vertebral body와 disc space가 노출되어 disc space에 needle을 찔러 intraoperative C-arm으로 level을 확인함. 다음으로 C5-6 disc space에 No. 15 bladder로 incision을 가한 다음 disc forcep과 curret으로 disc를 cartilage and plate와 함께 대부분을 제거함. disc를 제거하자 좌측에서 teared posterior longitudinal ligament와 함께 탈출된 disc material이 있어 이를 blunt hook와 disc forcep을 이용하여 제거함. 다음으로 Kerrison punch로 remained PLL을 제거하여 decompression함. 이와 같은 방법으로 C4-5 disc material과 PLL을 제거하였는데 역시 PLL의 tearing이 있었고 이를 통해 탈출된 disc material이 C5-6보다 컸으며 보다 딱딱한 양상이었다. curret으로 나머지 disc를 제거하고 disc space에 sponge gelfoam를 packing함. 다음 intraoperative C-arm monitoring하에서 RABEA cages 삽입함. 수술시야에서 meticulous bleeding control 후 main procedure를 마침. *Park*

1/17 Ambulation start
현재 post neck pain & Lt. U/Ext
Tingling numbness
Sx improved state *Kim*

〈 Doctor's Orders 〉

1/10 〈 Adm Order 〉

1. Check V/S $\bar{q}$ 4hr
2. BR $\bar{c}$ philadelphia
3. GD
4. S-S enema, Proamine

진 장 수 요약 차트

등록번호 : 35 42 86 이름 : 진장수
입원일 : 2017. 1. 10 퇴원일 : 2017. 1. 31 퇴원과 : NS

5. C/O cir, motor, sensory
   F-NS20 1Ⓐ IV 1 gtt
   I-TPS 2Ⓐ
   I-PIRO 1Ⓐ IM q̄ 12hr

PRN) I-KTOR 1Ⓐ IM if severe pain
B-EPR 3T
B-SOMAL 3T] #3
Y-ALMA 3Ⓟ
CBC c̄ DC, ESR, CRP
24PF, U/A, EKG, chol P/A
Cx-series c̄ stress view
VDRL, viral marker 3종
HDL-Chol, ABO, Rh, x matching BT/CT *Yoon*

1/11 추) Cx MRI Ⓔ (by 김덕민 T/O)
1/12 추) EMG (PMR Consult)

〈 Preop order 〉

1/11 1. Get the op permission
2. NPO
3. Shaving the whole Cx area
4. NS10, SD10 IV
5. A-CEPA 4Ⓐ MIV
6. Prepare ABO, RH X-matching A-ISE 4Ⓐ
7. Send the pt to OR c̄ chart X-ray, MRI after foley Insertion when called
8. Halter traction 10ℓb philadelphia collar *Yoon*

〈 Postop order 〉

1/11 1. Check V/S q̄ 15min x 4
q̄ 30min x 2 & then stable q̄ 2 4hr

진 장 수 요약 차트

등록번호 : 35 42 86　　이름 : 진장수
입원일 : 2017. 1. 10　　퇴원일 : 2017. 1. 31　　퇴원과 : NS

2. ABR $\bar{c}$ Cx-immobilization
3. Check I/O
4. NPO
5. EDBC $\bar{c}$ humidification
6. O_2 2ℓ by NP
7. 5% DW 500cc IV
8. Remove foley catheter after fully awakening
9. Keep H/V, T/V function
10. Check out for motor, sensory, verbal response & respiration　　*Yoon*

〈 Nurse's order 〉

1/10 17:00　외래를 통해 걸어서 입원

1/10　S 목 아프고 팔 저려요
O No motor weakness
Lt) U/Ext tingling numbness (+)
grasping power 60%
ward, orientation given
20:00　philadelphia apply　　*Jung*

1/11 16:00　MRI check 하러 감　　*Jung*

1/12 17:30　OR에서 옴 A-VANCO 2Amp 보낸 것 사용하고 옴
O2 2ℓ/min inhalation 시킴
F/cath, H/VAC 걸치고 옴
ABR state $\bar{c}$ Humidifier apply, 심호흡 시킴.　　*Jung*

1/13 2:30　No fever & pain complain
6:30　Philadelphia collar keep, self voiding well　　*Jung*

〈진 장 수〉

★ 진장수 차트를 읽고 맞는 것에 O표 하시오.

1 **수술기록지 내용으로 옳은 것은?**

① 흉쇄유돌근을 외측연을 따라 9cm 정도 절개했다.
② 식도와 기관지 및 띠근육을 절개하였다.
③ 전종인대는 찢어져 있었다.
④ 상갑상선 동맥이 외부로 노출되었다.
⑤ 롤바를 받쳐 목을 약간 굴곡되게 하였다.

2 **환자의 상태에 대해 옳지 않은 것은?**

① 뒷목에 통증이 있었다.
② 신경근병증은 나타나지 않았다.
③ 왼쪽 경추장애 증상이 나타났다.
④ 타병원에서 목 디스크를 알고 내원했다.
⑤ 팔 다리의 굴곡과 신전에 이상이 있었다.

3 **의사지시사항으로 옳지 않은 것은?**

① 통증이 심하면 l-KTOR를 주도록 하였다.
② 수술 후 경추 고정과 절대안정을 취하도록 하였다.
③ 근전도는 시행하였고 성병검사는 실시하지 않았다.
④ 운동, 감각, 언어 반응 및 호흡을 확인하도록 하였다.
⑤ 가습기 사용과 깊은 호흡과 기침을 하도록 격려하였다.

4 **주진단분류로 옳은 것은?**

① M50.9
② M50.0+, G99.2*
③ 51.0+, G99.2*
④ M20.1
⑤ M51.8

5 **의사지시와 시행여부가 옳은 것은?**

① 환자는 의사의 지시대로 프로아민과 마니톨의 수액들이 투여되었다.
② 입원지시에 필라델피아를 하도록 했고 환자는 당일 저녁 7시에 시행했다.
③ MRI order는 11일에 있었고 시행은 13일 오후 4시에 실시하였다.
④ 11일에 근전도 검사의 협의진단을 의뢰하였고 당일 시행되었다.
⑤ 환자가 깨면 폴리도뇨관 제거를 지시했으나 병실에 폴리도뇨관 상태로 왔다.

6 **환자 상태의 의미로 옳지 않은 것은?**

① ESR 5mm는 감염증상이 있다.
② tingling은 저릿저릿한 감각이다.
③ 심부건반사가 ++인 것은 정상이다.
④ ambulation은 외래치료를 했다.
⑤ 상지의 신전능력이 ++은 정상이다.

03. 산부인과계

Obstetrics & Gynecology

I. 전체 차트 (Full Chart)

II. 요약 차트 (Summary Chart)

MEDICAL RECORD PRACTICE

01 아두골반 불균형
Cephalopelvic disproportion

1.1 골반협착

입구의 협착

▶ 정의

- 골반입구의 가장 짧은 전후경이 10.0cm 미만 또는 내골반횡경이 12.0cm 미만
- 대각결합형이 11.5cm 미만

▶ 태아에 미치는 영향

- 산류(caput succedaneum)
  - 골반협착으로 분만 중 가장 압박을 받았던 아두 부위에 산류 발생
  - 산류란 자궁경관입구에 바로 놓인 태아 두피 부분에 부종이 생겨 형성
  - 국소적인 종창
- 태아 두부의 주형(fetal head molding)
  - 강력한 자궁수축에 의해 태아의 두개골이 서로 겹치게 되는 현상
  - 대체로 태아에게 해롭지 않음
  - 정도가 심한 경우: 천막파열(tentorial tear), 혈관손상, 두강내 출혈 초래
- 제대탈출(prolapse nuchal cord)

출구의 협착

▶ 정의

- 보통 양측 좌골조면간경(interischial tuberous diameter)이 8cm 미만
- 골반출구의 협착 그 자체로 난산의 원인은 거의 없음(중간골반협착과 동반됨)
- 회음열상의 원인이 될 수 있음

▶ 중간골반의 협착

- 중간골반은 치골결합의 하부에서 좌골극(ischial spine)을 통과하는 제4~5천추골의 경계선
- 임상적으로 직접 중골반을 평가할 수 없음(영상적으로 가능)

- 골반의 형태 및 크기, 아두의 크기 및 중간골반 협착 정도에 따라 난산 가능성
- 골반입구의 협착보다 발생률이 높음
- 흔히 아두의 회정착(transverse arrest)의 원인
- 어려운 중간골반위 겸자분만이나 제왕절개술의 시행을 유발하는 요인

1.2 자궁벽(Uterine wall)

▶ 자궁(uterus)은 3층으로 구성
- 자궁내막(endometrium): 자궁(uterus)의 내측 점막(mucous membrane)
- 자궁근층(myometrium): 자궁(uterus)의 근육층(muscular layer)
- 자궁외막(perimetrium): 외부층, 막조직층(membranous tissue layer)

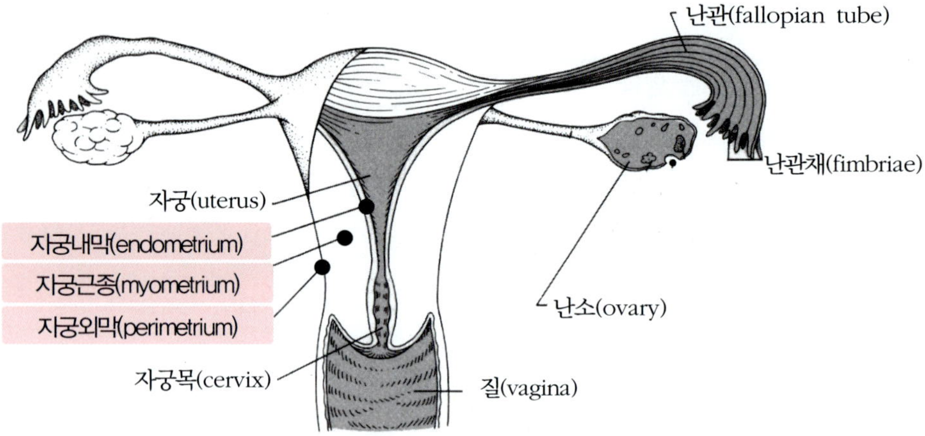

그림 1. 자궁벽(uterine wall)

2.1 제왕절개술(Cesarean section)

▶ 정상적인 질분만(vaginal delivery)이 어려운 경우, 복부절개를 통해 태아분만

시행

▶ 이상태위: 아두골반불균형, 얼굴태위(face presentation), 이마위(brow presentation) 등
▶ 태아 이상상태: 자간증, 전치태반, 태반조기박리 등

5大 제왕절개술(Cesarean section)의 적응증	
· cephalopelvic disproportion(CPD)	머리골반불균형
· abruptio placentae	태반조기박리
· fetal distress	태아곤란증
· very severe pre-eclampsia	매우 심한 자간전증
· Previous c/s status	이전 제왕절개

2.2 자궁무력증(Uterine inertia): IIOC(O34.3)

- 진통 시 자궁수축이 저하된 상태

3.1 전치태반(Placenta previa)

- 태반이 제 위치를 벗어나 자궁경 통로를 막음
- 자궁벽 아래쪽에 착상되어 분만 시 태아보다 태반이 먼저 나옴
- 산전모성 사망의 주된 원인

3.2 태반조기박리(Abruptio placentae)

- 태아가 만출되기 전에 태반이 박리되는 것

3.3 전자간증(Pre-eclampsia)

- 임신 20주 이상
- 임신의 고혈압성 질환
- 고혈압, 부종(edema), 단백뇨(proteinuria), 알부민뇨(albuminuria), 시력장애 발생
- 영양불량[특히 단백질(protein)]과 관련

태위의 종류

- **머리태위(cephalic presentation):** 분만 중 태아의 머리가 먼저 나오는 위치
  - 두정위(vertex presentation): 머리의 상부와 뒷부분
  - 안면위, 얼굴(face presentation)
  - 전액태위, 이마(brow presentation)
- **둔위/볼기·골반태위(Breech/pelvic presentation):** 분만 중 태아 엉덩이나 하지 일부가 먼저 나오는 위치
  - 엉덩이/볼기태위(complete breech presentation)
  - 족위, 발(footling presentation)
  - 슬위, 무릎(knee presentation)
- **횡위, 어깨(Transverse lie or shoulder presentation)**

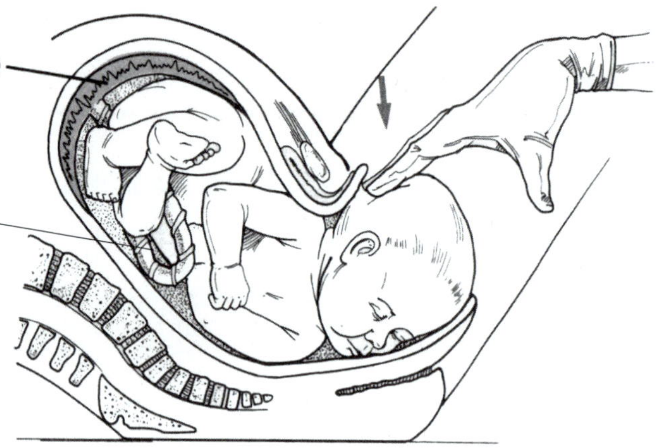

그림 2. 태아의 머리태위(cephalic presentation of the fetus): 정상분만

4.1 분만(Labor)

급산(Precipitate)

- 급속도로 진행되는 분만으로 보통 total stage 3시간 이내에 진행 분만

지연분만(Prolonged labor)

- 보통 18시간 경과해서 분만
- 초과시간: 초산부 24시간, 경산부 18시간

4.2 카테터삽입법, 도관법(Urinary catheterization)

- ▸ 유연한 관으로 된 기구를 요도를 통하여 방광으로 삽입
- ▸ 도관(catheter)의 사용
  - -소변 배액(drainage)
  - -방광으로 세척액(irrigation solution) 삽입
  - -방광 불릴 경우

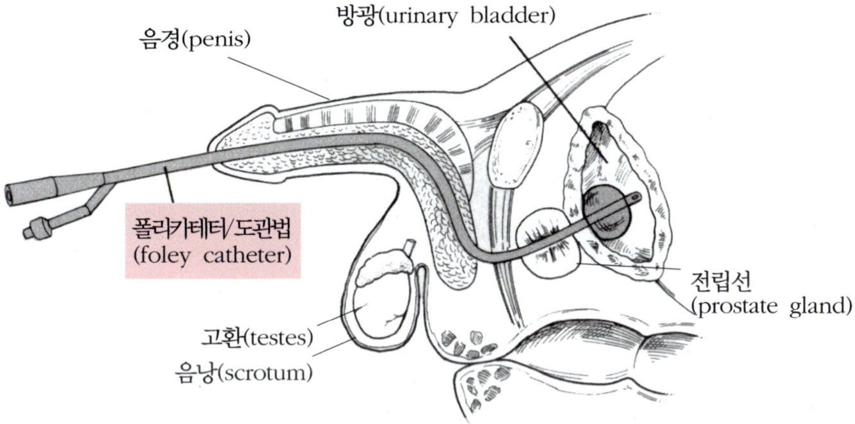

그림 3. 방광에 삽입된 폴리카테터(foley catheter)

출산력의 의미

G: Gravida(임신 횟수)　　P: Para(출산 횟수)

D: Dead(사망 수)　　A: Abortion(유산)　　L: Live(생존아 수)

- Parity 출산력 : ○ - ○ - ○ - ○
  - 만기분만 - 조산 - 유산 [자연 / 인공] - 생존아 [남 / 여]

예) ① G4 P2 L1 D1 A2

→ 임신 4회, 분만 2회, 생존아 1명, 사망 1명, 유산 2회

② Parity 출산력: 2 - 1 - 3 ┐ 1 - 1 ┐ 0
　　　　　　　　　　　　┘ 2　　　┘ 1

→ 분만 2회, 조산 1회, 유산 3회(자연유산 1회, 인공유산 2회), 생존아 1명(여자 1명)

⇨ 총 임신횟수: 5회(조산 1회 + 유산 3회 + 생존아 1명)

수술시 절개(Incision) 방법

- 정중절개법(midline incision): 신체의 정중선을 따라 긋는 절개선
- 측정중절개법(paramedian incision): 신체의 중심선에서 약간 우측 또는 좌측으로 평행 절개선
- 판넨스틸 절개법(Pfannenstiel's incision): 하부가 볼록하게 복부절개 → 여성생식기 수술
- 사근절개법(oblique inguinal incision): 샅부의 피부능을 따라 사선으로 긋는 절개법
- 맥버니 절개법(McBurney's incision): 장곡구에서 제대부를 향한 ⅓점에서 외사근과 평행 절개선 → 충수돌기 절제 시 사용
- 로키 또는 데이비스 절개법(Lockey or Davis incision): 맥버니 점 위에 수평 절개선 → 충수돌기 절제 시 사용

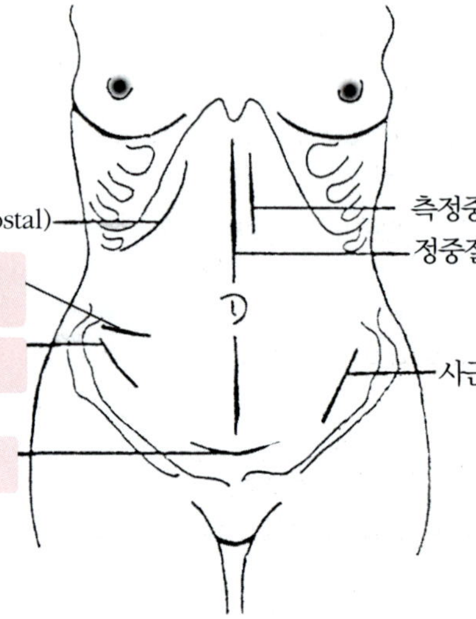

그림 4. 다양한 복부 절개법

중요 용어

· 오로(lochia) - 분만 후 1~2주 사이에 나타나는 질분비물	· 맥박수 정상: 1분에 60~80회 - 빈맥(tachy cardia): 1분에 맥박수 100 이상 - 서맥(brady cardia): 1분에 맥박수 60 미만

약 어	원 어	
BPM	Beats per minutes	분간박동
CPD	Cephalopelvic disproportion	머리골반불균형
EBL	Estimated blood loss	실추정량 ▸자연분만 과다출혈: 500ml 이상 ▸제왕절개 과다출혈: 1,000ml 이상
IIOC	Incomplete internal os of cervix	자궁경관 무력증
LOT	Left occiput transverse (position of fetus)	좌후두 횡위(태아위치)
38^{+3}wks	38weeks and 3days	38주 3일(임신)
PROM	Premature rupture of membranes	조기양막파열

등록번호	227 88 00	성별	F
성명	상 한 가		
주민등록	820703－1234567		

입 퇴 원 기 록
Admission and Discharge Record

<table>
<tr><td colspan="3">주 소 :</td></tr>
<tr><td colspan="3">출신지 : 직 업 : 전 화 :</td></tr>
<tr><td colspan="3">연고자성명 : 박연승 관 계 : 주 소 : 전 화 :</td></tr>
<tr><td>입원 : 2017년 11 월 9 일 과 병동 호</td><td rowspan="3">전과</td><td>20 년 월 일 과 병동 호</td></tr>
<tr><td>퇴원 : 2017년 11 월 18 일 과 병동 호</td><td>20 년 월 일 과 병동 호</td></tr>
<tr><td>재원일수 :</td><td>20 년 월 일 과 병동 호</td></tr>
</table>

최종진단명	분 류 번 호
주진단명 : CPD	
기타진단명 : Elderly primigravida	
Intrauterine pregnancy at 38^{+3}wks	
Leiomyoma with ischemic necrosis	
수술 및 처치명	
수술명 : Low flap transverse cesarean section	
myomectomy	
기타수술 및 주요검사 :	

<table>
<tr><td colspan="2">치료결과 : 1. 완쾌 2. 경쾌 3. 호전안됨 4. 진단뿐 5. 가망없는 퇴원 6. 48시간내 사망 7. 48시간이후 사망</td></tr>
<tr><td colspan="2">퇴원형태 : 1. 퇴원지시후 2. 자의퇴원 3. 탈원 4. 전원</td></tr>
<tr><td colspan="2">병원감염 : 1. 수술후 2. 기타처치후 3. 비뇨기계 4. 호흡기계 5. 소화기계 6. 기타</td></tr>
<tr><td colspan="2">원사인 : 부검 : 예, 아니오</td></tr>
<tr><td colspan="2">계속적 진료 계획</td></tr>
<tr><td colspan="2">없음·있음 (약속일 2017년 11월 22일 10시)</td></tr>
<tr><td>담당 전공의 서명 : 윤민국</td><td>담당 전문의 서명 : 한길영</td></tr>
<tr><td>의무기록 완성 : 2017년 11월 30일</td><td>의무기록사 서명 :</td></tr>
</table>

등록번호	227 88 00	성별	F
성명	상 한 가		
주민등록	820703－1234567		

산 과 기 록
Obstetric Record

Address : 서울시 송파구 잠실동 아시아선수촌 apt 1－601			Date of Birth 1982. 7. 3	Occupation(s) Premarital	present
Home phone 413－2233	Religion 기독교	Marital status Ⓜ W D	Date of Marriage 2015. 12. 4	회사원	회사원
Contact phone	Maternal Height (cm) 163	Education 21 yrs	Husband (or father of child) Date of Birth 1981. 2. 5	Height(cm) 180	Occu. 공무원

FH	MAT	PAT	Date Noted	Relative	Children or relatives /special schools
hypertension					
diabetes					
Twins					
Genetic disorder					
Other					

Medical / Surgical / Past history

Personal History	Yes	No	Personal History	Yes	No	Personal History	Yes	No
Op./Accidents		√	Rh fever/heart disease		√	Steroid therapy		√
Anes. difficulties		√	Chest conditions (Inc T.B.)		√	Other drugs		√
Blood transfusion		√	Anemia(<10g)		√	Smoking		√
Allergy(ds/drugs)	√		Rubella(cond./contact)		√	X－ray －pregnancy chest		√
Asymptomatic bacteriuria		√	Psychiatric disorders		√	－renal		√
						－ pelvimetry		√
UTI		√	Other serious illness		√	Anti D given		√
Kidney disease		√	Cone biopsy		√	Rubella vaccine given		√
Diabetes		√	Positive cervical smear		√	Infant(s) conges. abnorm		√
Endocrine disorders		√	D & C		√	LBW		√
G.T.T		√	Infertility investigations					

Comment

Obstetric History G_1 Po Lo Do A_2

Date	Place	Durn. (wks)	Norm ABN	Onset Norm Ind	Durn (Hrs)	Oxytoc drip	Delivery sp/inst/cs	3rd stage N/PPH/RP	Norm Abn	Bx Wt.(g)	LB SB PND
'17. 11.11	본원	38^{+3}	N		CPD		C/S			3150	CB

등록번호	227 88 00	성별	F
성명	상 한 가		
주민등록	820703－1234567		

산 전 기 록
Antenatal Clinic Data

Age	Height (cm)	Pre－preg Wt(kg)	Years Married	No. of Preg.	Live children	Abortions Spontaneous ab. Artificial ab.	No of Deaths: In uter	In 1Mo	From Mo To 1yr.	Consult
35	164	55	34	1	0	2				

LMP: 16. 2.16 EDC: 17. 11.24 PMP	Certain ☑ Uncertain ☐ Approx. ☐	pregnancy : planned ☑ unplanned ☐ Initially : pleased ☑ displeased ☐ ambivalent ☐ upset ☐ Now :	Pill	From	To
Usual cycle	Rhythm		Used ☐ Never used ☑		
Neg	Regular ☐ Irregular ☐		Other contraceptive measures IUD		

Bleeding since LMP	Significant medical history	Significant feature & recommend	
	Prenatal care: 본원 x 10회	abdominal pain (intermittent)	
		vaginal spotting	
		Cervical smear	Fetal movements
		Yes☐ No☐	Date of onset
		Result	Gestation of onset

General & pelvic exam at first visit

Normal	Yes	No	Normal	Yes	No	Normal	Yes	No		Yes	No	Investigations initiated: Specific	Other (X－ray, scan etc)
skin			Lungs			Abdomen			Vagina				
HEENT			Breasts			Extremities			Cervix				
Mouth			Nipples			Neurologic			Uterus				
Thyroid			Heart			Perineum			Adnexa				
Abdominal findings						Vulva			Rectal				
Uterine size/dates: ☐compatiable ☐smaller ☐larger													LBW
Pelvis ☐ Adequate ☐ borderline ☐ Inadeq ☐ clinical ☐ x－ray ☐													

Date 19	Urine ALB	SUG	KET	Wt (Kg)	B.P.	EDEMA	Gest Age	Fundal Ht.	Fetal pres－ent	F.H.	General health, drugs Investigations & results	R Weeks	Initial
3/26				58	100/35		5^{+3}				FHB⊖ G－sac⊖		
4/4				58	100/50		6^{+5}				FHB: 117bpm G－sac 1.66cm ≒ 6wks		
5/2				58	110/70		10^{+4}						

등록번호	227 88 00	성별	F
성명	상 한 가		
주민등록	820703－1234567		

분 만 요 약
Delivery Summary

Time : 17－11－9 4:00 PM Weeks Gest. 38^{+3} LNMP : 16－2－16
E.D.C : 17－11－24 Para. 0 (Living 0 Dead 0 Ab 2) Labor began : none Time & Date A.M. P.M Interval :
Fetus moving : ☑ Yes ☐ No. Show ☐ Yes, ☑ No
Bag of Water : ☑ Intact ☐ Ruptured Time & Date
A.M. P.M Blood: A+ Type: ☑ABO ☐AB, ☑Rh+ ☐Rh－, Serology☑－ Serology☐+   Chest X－Ray: ☑ Negative ☐ Positive: Date
Prenatal : Weight gain ☐No ☑Yes Hypertension ☑No ☐Yes Edema ☑No ☐Yes
Headache ☑No ☐Yes Bleeding ☑ No ☐ Yes
Other complications Elderly primigravidarum, myoma of uterus, CPD
PHx Type of Delivery Weight Gain Baby: Wt. Jaundice or Transfusion Complications
'17 current pregnancy ANC 본원 x 10회
BP 110/70 mmHg
PR 74 bpm
Hg/Hct 10.6/21.9
U/A (P/S) (－/－)
Med. Surg. Hist : '17. 6 Myoma of ut. Dx drug ANC at 본원
Family Hist. N－C
Physical Examination
General Condition : Not so ill looking app. M/D, M/N Body Wt. 55kg → 74Kg, Ht. : 163cm
Head : Not pale conj Not icteric sclera Far : N－C N & T : N－C
Thyroid : Not enlarged Teeth : N－C Denture : yes (no)
Lung : CBS $\bar{s}$ rales Heart : RHB $\bar{s}$ ⓜ
Abdomen : Ht. Fundus 33cm, Presentation : Vx Position:
Fetal Heart Sound : Location Rate : 142 bpm Character : Reg
Extremities : No pitting edema Varicosity : None
Pelvis : adequate
Remarks : EBW : 3200gm
Imp) Elderly primigravidarum
IUP at 38^{+3} wks $\bar{s}$ labor
Myoma of uterus
Signature *Han*

분 만 기 록
Delivery Record

By Dr. : G.Y. Han	Assistant : M. K. Yoon		
Date : 17－11－11 Time : 9 : 51 ☑ A.M. ☐ P.M.	Placenta Time 9: 53, AM	Length first stage hrs Labor end stage hrs	
Presentation : ☑ Scrubbed	☑ Draped	☑ Catheterized:	
Fetus Position : WT	Station: －3		
Anesthesia : ☐ Local ☐ Pudendal ☐ Caudal ☐ Spinal ☑ General	By G.Y.Hoon		
Type of Delivery LFT C/S ☑ Spontaneous ☐ Forceps: Low Mid Low－mid Type (Name)			
Other			
Placenta : ☑ Spontaneous	Crede: 800gm	Condition: grossly normal	
Blood loss : 600ml	Episiotomy : None	Midline LML	
Laceration : None			
Repair : Anatomically repaired c̄ CCGs, Vicryl, Silk, Nylon			
Medication (during delivery) : None			
Post－partum : Fundus	Blood pressure : 120/80mmg	Pulse : 78 bpm	
Infant : ☐boy ☑ girl	Wt. 3150gm	Length cm	Abnormalities ☑ No ☐ Yes
Positive Pressure : ☑ No ☐ Yes	Intubation : ☑ No ☐ Yes	Apgar Score : 7/1 min 9/5min	
Respiration : ☑ Spontaneous ☐ Assisted			
Immediate care : ☑ Cord	Eyes	☑ Gastric suction	☑ Brac & Prints
Remarks : BPD 10.5cm	C.L. = 60cm		

Discharge Examination

Date : 17－11－18	Puerperium : ☑ Normal ☐ Complications	
Breasts : Ample	Nipples : erect	Nursing : ☑ Yes ☐ No
Uterus : ☑ Normal involution ☐ Abnormal		
Lochia : ☑ Normal ☐ Abnormal		
Perineum : fair	Condition episiotomy or lac : clear	
Complications : None		
Remarks :		
Advise on family planning given : Yes		
		Signature : *Han*

진 통 기 록
Labor Record

2017	Time		Sign	Type R.V.	Presen–tation	Sta–tion	Dilata–tion	Effac–ement	Memb.	Contraction			Fetal heart		B.P	Pulse
M.D	A.M	P.M								Inteval	Dur.	Char–acter	rate	location		
11.9		6	*Yoon*	V	Vx		F.F	ST	I	−	none	−	142	+	110/70	74
11.10	10									−	none	−	144	+		
	6									−	none	−	142	+		
		12			Vx					−	none	−	146	+		
		6								−	none	−	144	+		
11.11	10									−	none	−	142	+		
	6			−	OR	−				−	none	−	140	+		
	9		*Yoon*	V	Vx	−3	FT	ST	I	−	none	−	142	+		

Explanations: Membrane status, medications, and other procedures − write in across labor record at time administered

At 4 : 00 PM on 17−11−9	Admitted to WARD
	Rec) H/D 1L IV
	Skin prep for C/S
	Yoon
At 9 : 00 AM on 17−11−11	A pt was sent to the OR $\overline{c}$ a chart & x−ray

등록번호	227 88 00	성별	F
성명	상 한 가		
주민등록	820703 − 1234567		

경 과 기 록
Progress Notes

〈 Admission Note 〉

11.9 본 35세된 G_1 Po Lo Do A_2 married 산모는 cephalopelvic disproportion Elderly primigravidarum, intrauterine pregnancy at 37^{+6} wks without labor, myoma of uterus imp하에 금일 dept of OB에 입원하였다. 산모는 평소 건강하였으며, IUP 37^{+6} wks로 EDC 17 − 11 − 24로 본원에서 ANC 받아 오던 중 Elderly primigravidarum 및 myoma 발견되어 LFT C/S 및 myomectomy 시행받고저 금일 dept of OB에 입원하였다.

PHx : G1 Po Lo Do A2
LNMP 16 − 2 − 16
EDC 17 − 11 − 24
GA 37^{+6}wks

No other M − S illness
FHx : N − C

Yoon

11.9 PHx : BP 110/70 mmHg PR 78 bpm
G/A : Not so ill looking app. M/N, M/D
alert M/S
Skin warm & dry
No abnormal skin rashes
Head & Neck supple
Not palpable LNs
HEENT Not pale conj.
Not icteric sclera
Heart & Chest: CBS $\bar{s}$ rales
RHB $\bar{s}$ ⓜ
ABD: Soft & distended
H.O.F 33cm
FHR ＋, 142 bpm, Reg
Ut. contraction: none

경 과 기 록

일 자	내 용	서 명
11.9	Pelvic exam : Pres : Vx Station : −3 Cx : F.T, soft memb : intact * myoma : Not palpable d/t pregnancy & it location of posterior portion Back x Ext. : No LOM No CVA tenderness No pitting edema Imp) Elderly primigravidarum, CPD IUP at 38^{+3} wks $\bar{s}$ labor Myoma of uterus	Yoon
	Plan) LFT C/S Possible myomectomy	
	Sono) 17−10−22 (IUP at 35^{+3}) : 3.67 x 3.85 cm sized myoma nodule on post wall of uterus 관찰	Yoon
	〈 OR Note 〉	
11.11	1. Name of operation Low flap transverse cesarean section myomectomy 2. Name of operator Operator: G.Y.Han M.D. 1st assistant: I.Q.Seo M.D. 2nd assistant: M.K.Yoon M.D. 3. Preoperation diagnosis : Cephalopelvic disproportion Elderly primigravidarum Myoma of uterus Intrauterine pregnancy at 38 wks without labor	Yoon

경 과 기 록

일 자	내 용	서 명
11.11	4. Postoperation diagnosis : Same as the above 5. Anesthesia : General anesthesia with endotracheal intubation 6. Operative findings and procedures 1) A low midline abdominal skin incision was made. 2) Entering the abdominal cavity, the uterus was enlarged to term size, both tubes and ovaries were grossly normal in size and shape. 3) Low flap transverse cesarean section was done. 4) A living female baby weighing 3,150gm with Apgar score of 1 ' −7 and 5 ' −9 (BPD 10.5cm) was delivered in LOT position at 9:15 AM on 17−11−11. Soon later, a placenta weighing 800gm was manually removed, of which finding was grossly normal. 5) A 3.0 x 2.0 x 2.0cm sized myoma was noted on posterior of uterus. 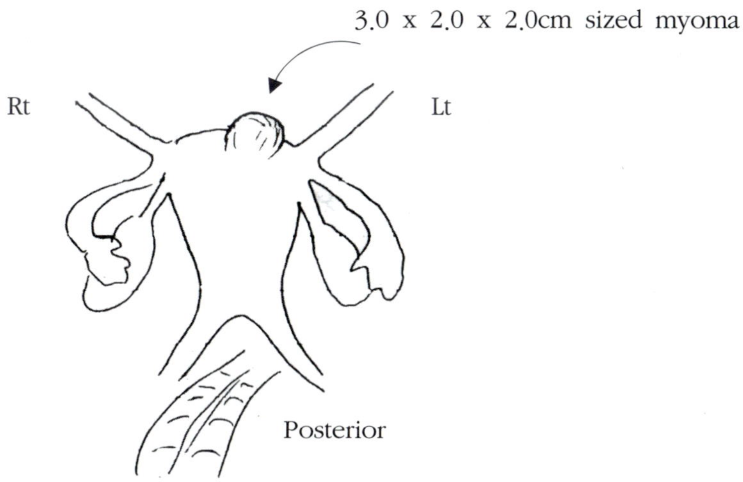 	Yoon

경 과 기 록

일 자	내 용	서 명
11.11	6) Myomectomy was done 7) On the manual exploration, the liver, stomach and intestines were grossly normal. 8) Anatomically repaired with CCGs, vicryl, silk and nylon. 9) EBL was about 600ml. 10) Neither gauze nor drain was inserted.	*Yoon*
11.11	〈 Immediate post op note 〉 Fully awakened from G.A Well functioning foley catheter Well running IV fluid. No active vaginal bleeding BP 120/80 mmHg PR 78bpm Not icteric sclera Not pale conjunctiva CBS $\bar{s}$ rales RHB $\bar{s}$ ⓜ	*Yoon*
	Imp) Immediate post op status Plan) Hydration & antibiotics Check I & O Check Hg/Hct on POD#1 Watch for vaginal bleeding	*Yoon*
11.12	S : Mild of site pain O : Wound infection (+) mild febrile status: 37˚C no active vaginal bleeding Hg/Hct : 10.2 / 30.0	

경 과 기 록

일 자	내 용	서 명
11.12	O : foley remove & good spont voiding CBS $\bar{s}$ ⓡ RHB $\bar{s}$ ⓜ A : POD #1 status P : Encourage cough & deep breathing Watch for vaginal bleeding Encourge early ambulation Op site dressing	*Yoon*
11.14	S : No specific complaints O : BT 36.8°C No active vaginal bleeding Hg/Hct : 10.1 / 30.1 Gas passed CBS $\bar{s}$ rales RHB $\bar{s}$ ⓜ A : POD #3 status P : Encourage more ambulation Watch for Vag. bleeding Op. wound care	*Yoon*

등록번호	227 88 00	성별	F
성명	상 한 가		
주민등록	820703 - 1234567		

병리조직보고서
Pathological Record*

접수일자: 17.11.11

조직명 및 검사부위

Uterus, myomectomy

Gross Description

The specimen consists of a 5x3.5cm sized relatively well-circumscribed and ovoid mass composed of grayish-while whorled with central reddish infarcted areas and myxoid change, clinically from the uterus.

황경수

Pathological Diagnosis :

Uterus, myometrium : Leiomyoma with ischemic necrosis

병리의사 : *Y. M. Kang*

〈상 한 가〉

★ 상한가 차트를 읽고 맞는 것에 O표 하시오.

1 최종진단명의 분류번호가 맞게 짝지어진 것은?

가. O33.9 나. O42.9 다. O34.1 라. O34.2 마. Z35.5 바. D07.3
사. D25.9 아. C54.2 자. R02 차. M8890/0 카. M8890/3

① 가, 나, 라, 마, 차 ② 나, 다, 바, 자, 차
③ 가, 다, 마, 아, 차 ④ 가, 다, 마, 차
⑤ 나, 다, 아, 자, 카

2 차트의 내용을 맞게 기재한 것은?

① 3,150gm의 정상체중으로 남아를 출산하였다.
② Apgar score는 1분에 9점과 5분에 7점으로 양호한 편이다.
③ 태반무게는 800gm이었으며 손으로 제거하였다.
④ 수술직후 플레 카테터의 기능이 제대로 되지 못했다.
⑤ 3.0×2.0×2.0cm 크기의 근종이 자궁 앞에서 보였다.

3 환자가 과거에 IIOC로 진단받아 Macdonald op.를 했다면 그 진단명과 수술명에 대한 분류번호는?

① O34.89, 67.69 ② O34.39, 67.5 ③ O34.40, 67.5
④ O34.30, 67.69 ⑤ O34.49, 67.69

4 ANC 중 환자에 대한 설명으로 틀린 것은?

① 피임방법은 배란주기법이었다. ② 간헐적으로 복통이 있었다.
③ 질출혈이 있었다 ④ 산전관리 횟수는 10회이다.
⑤ 분만예정일은 2017년 11월 24일이다.

5 수술 후 wound infection에 대한 분류번호가 맞는 것은?

① T81.4, Y62.0 ② O86.0, Y62.0 ③ T81.4
④ O86.0 ⑤ O86.0, Y60.0

6 Cesarean section을 시행하는 것과 관련이 없는 것은?

① PROM ② CPD ③ Previous cesarean section
④ Nuchal cord ⑤ Abruptio placenta

7 분만기록지에 대한 내용으로 틀리게 기재한 것은?

① 오로는 정상이다.
② 유두는 똑바로 세워져 있다.
③ 실추정량은 정상이며 맥박수는 빠른 빈맥이다.
④ 수술 시 사용된 봉합사는 CCG, silk, vicryl, nylon이다.
⑤ 회음은 양호하다.

8 **환자의 임신력이 맞게 기재된 것은?**

① 유산 1회, 사망 1명
② 임신 1회, 유산 2회
③ 분만 1회, 유산 2회
④ 사망 1명, 생존아 1명
⑤ 분만 1회, 생존아 2명

9 **환자의 혈액형으로 맞는 것은?**

① A, Rh+
② B, Rh−
③ AB, Rh+
④ O, Rh−
⑤ A, Rh−

10 **수술명에 대한 분류번호가 맞는 것은?**

① 74.1, 68.29
② 74.99, 68.29
③ 74.1, 68.9
④ 74.99, 68.9
⑤ 74.1, 68.6

02 쌍태아 36주 분만

Delivery at 36 wks c̄ twin

1.1 전치태반(Placenta previa)

- 태반이 제 위치를 벗어나 자궁경 통로를 막거나 자궁벽 아래쪽에 착상
- 분만시 태아보다 태반이 먼저 나옴
- 산전 모성사망의 원인
- 임신 8개월경 무통출혈이 가장 흔한 초기 증상
  - 완전(complete) 전치태반: 태반이 자궁구를 완전히 덮음
  - 변연성(marginal) 전치태반: 태반이 자궁구의 변연과 접해 있음
  - 부분(partial) 전치태반: 자궁구가 부분적으로 태반과 덮여 있음

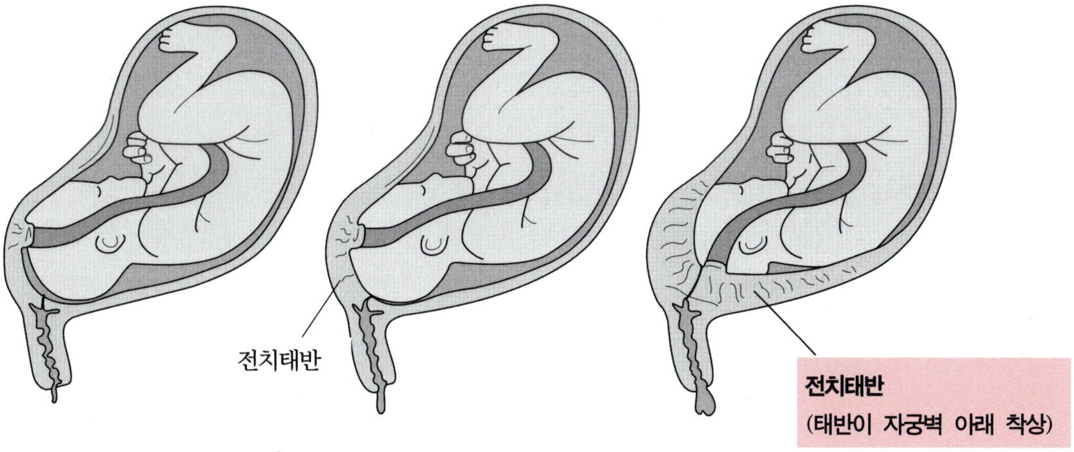

그림 1. 전치태반(Placenta previa) 발생과정

1.2 분만의 분류 및 방법

제왕절개술(Cesarean section): 복부를 통해 자궁을 절개하여 태아를 분만

표 1 • 제왕절개분만의 원인

모 체	태 아
•머리(아두)골반 불균형 •과거의 제왕절개 경험 •볼기태위(breech presentation) •내과적 합병증[예: PIH(임신성 고혈압)] •태반이상(예: 전치태반, 태반조기박리) •감염[예: herpes II virus(헤르페스 바이러스)]	•태아질식 •제대탈출 •태위이상(예: 볼기태위, 횡위) •태아기형(예: 뇌수종)

표 2 • 제왕절개의 유형

전통적 절개 (classic incision)	**하부절개**(lower segment incision)
•자궁을 수직으로 절개 •급작스런 분만, 횡위, 전치태반에 적용 •국소마취 시 적용 •임신 시 1~2%의 흉터파열과 소장의 유착이 발생되어 사용제한	•자궁하부절개는 수직절개 및 횡절개 가능 •횡절개 선호 - 혈액소실이 적음 - 다음 임신 시 자궁파열될 가능성 적음 - 절개 용이 - 절개부위로의 장관의 유착이 적음

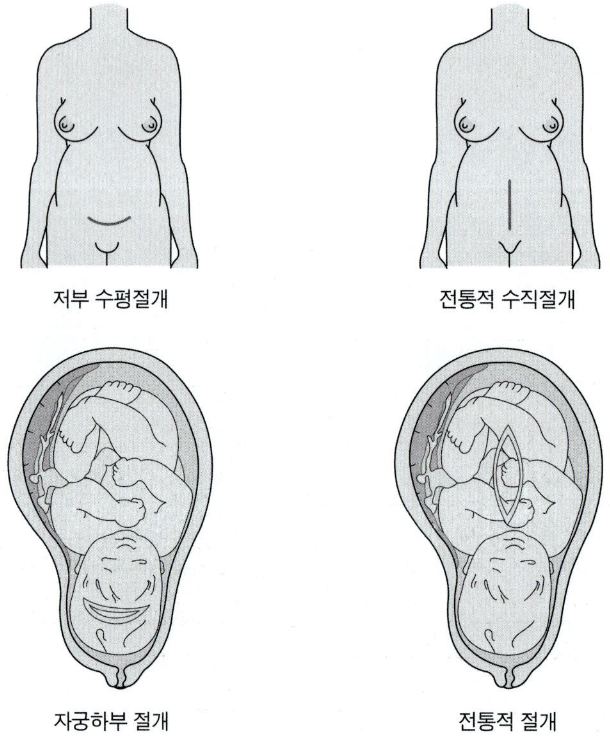

A. 자궁하부 절개　　B. 전통적 수직절개

그림 2. 자궁하부 및 전통적 수직절개

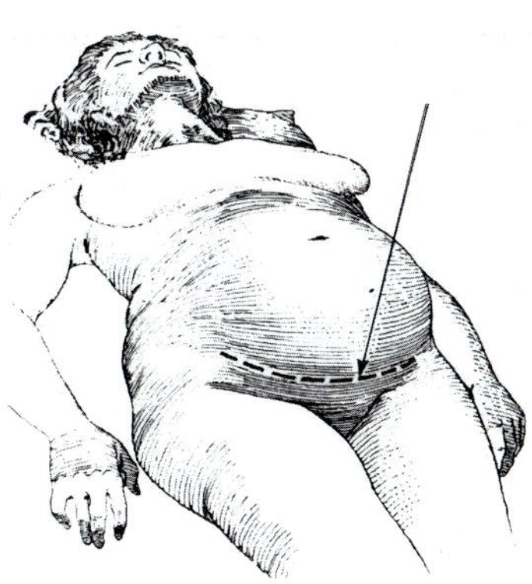

A. 복부 및 자궁하부

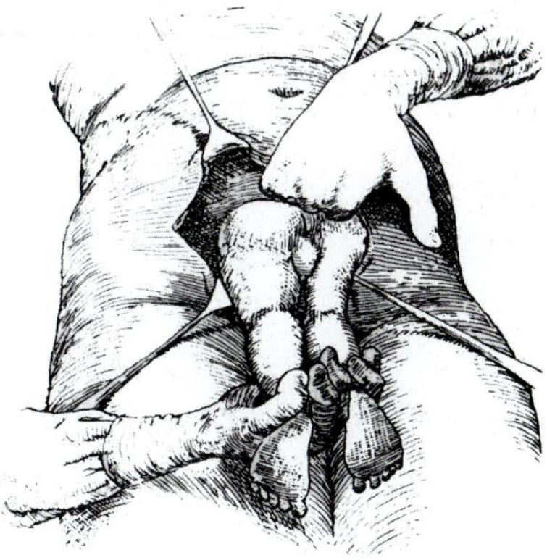

B. 태아만출

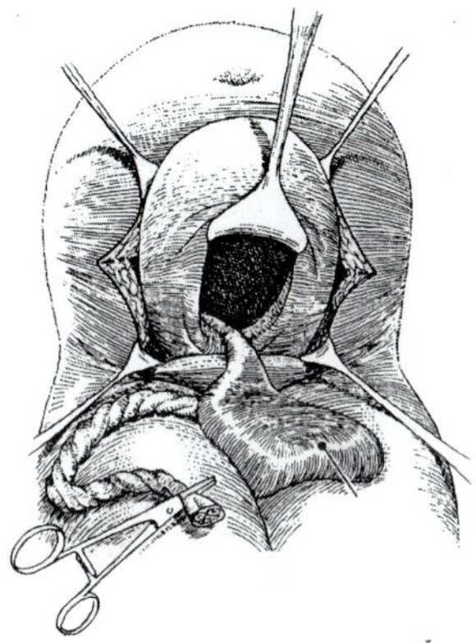

C. 태반만출

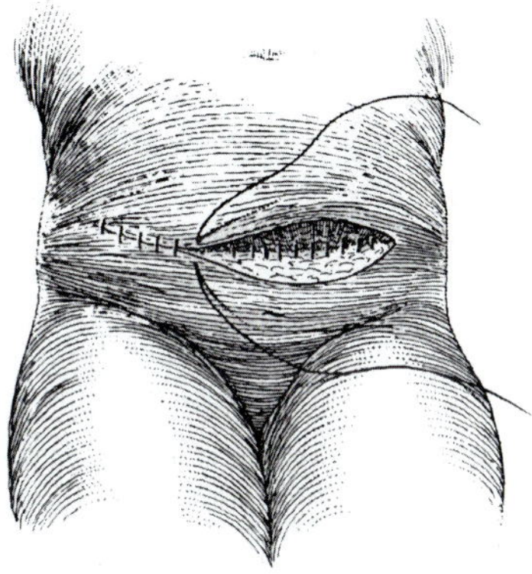

D. 복막봉합

그림 3. 자궁하부 제왕절개술(lower segment cesarean section)
(복부/자궁: 수평절개)

제왕절개술의 적응증

- 아두골반불균형(cephalopelvic disproportion; CPD)
- 자궁경관 무력증(incomplete internal os of cervix; IIOC)
- 태반조기박리(abruptio placenta)
- 태아 저산소증(fetal hypoxia)
- 횡위(transverse lie)
- 고령 초임부(elderly primigravida)
- 미성숙된 자궁목(unripened cervix)
- 완전전치태반(total placenta previa)
- 태아곤란증(fetal distress)
- 둔위(볼기태위, breech presentation)
- 자간전증(pre-eclampsia)
- 이전 제왕절개 상태(previous c/s status)

정상분만(Normal spontaneous vaginal delivery; NSVD)

- 질(vagina)을 통해 분만

분만의 4단계 분류

- 분만 1기(first stage of labor): 규칙적인 자궁수축의 시작~자궁경관이 완전 개대(열림)
- 분만 2기(second stage of labor): 자궁경관이 10cm 완전개대~태아만출, 태아만출 단계
- 분만 3기(third stage of labor): 태아의 만출 직후~태반(placenta)의 만출
- 분만 4기(fourth stage of labor): 분만후 1~2시간의 회복기

▶ 검사

- 자궁저 높이(Height of fundus; HOF)
  - 태아성장 및 임신기간 추정
  - 자궁저 높이 측정: 줄자를 이용, 치골결합 절흔~복부 중앙선~자궁저까지

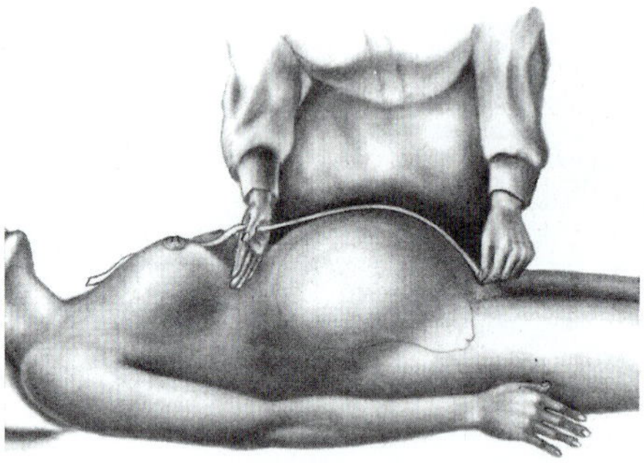

그림 4. 자궁 저부 높이 측정(HOF)

▶ 개대(Dilatation)

- 개대란 경관구 및 경관도관이 분만 1기 동안 증대 또는 확장되는 것
- 개대 확장: 1~10cm까지
- 염증 또는 수술로 인해 경관이 손상될 경우 경관확장이 지연됨

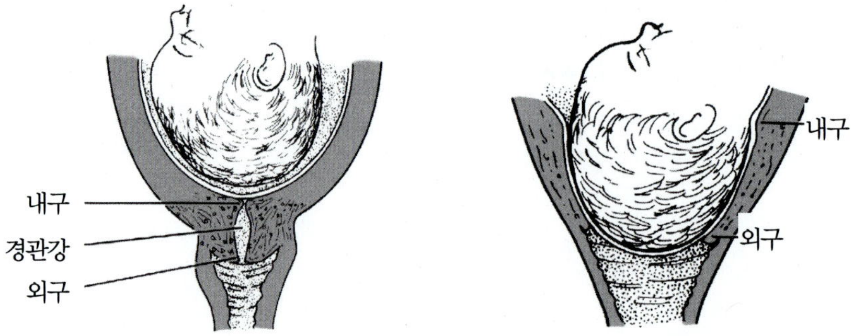

A. 분만 전 B. 분만 시: 완전 확장(10cm)

그림 5. 분만 전과 분만 시 개대확장 비교

▶ **부위마취**

- 음부신경 차단(pudendal block)
- 분만 2기 회음절개 시 사용
  - ▸ 자궁수축으로 인한 동통완화 효과 없음
  - ▸ 음핵, 대음순, 소음순 및 회음부위의 동통완화에 도움
- 회음부마취는 마취가 요구되는 10~20분 전에 주입
- 선진부가 경관 및 질 속 통과 시 음부가 확장됨
  - ▸ 이때 발생되는 질 및 회음부 동통 제거
- 음부신경은 S2~S4 신경을 통해 좌골극 끝 중간부위인 천좌골 신경 절흔까지 확대
  - ▸ 이 부분에 주사하여 음부신경 차단
- 음부신경 차단은 자연분만에는 효과있지만, 겸자분만에는 불충분

▶ **경부마취[Paracervical(uterosacral) block]**

- 희석된 국소마취제(1% procaine 5cc)로 경관 바로 외측에 있는 질 및 접하는 부분의 점막부위의 3시 및 9시 방향으로 주사
- 자궁수축으로 인한 동통 감소 효과
- 주사시기는 경관이 5cm 이상 개대된(열린) 후 실시
- 마취효과는 자궁하부 및 경관에서 질 상부 1/3까지 확장
- 경관개대 8cm까지 반복주사 가능

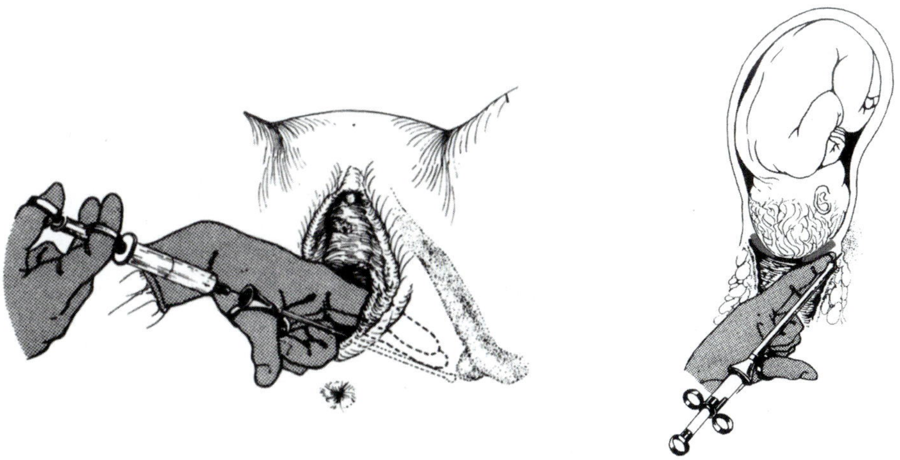

A. 음부신경마취(Pudendal block)
음부신경은 S2~S4 신경을 통해 좌골극 끝 중간부위인 천좌골 신경 절흔에 주사

B. 경부마취(Paracervical block)
경관 외측 질과 접하는 점막부위의 3시 및 9시 방향으로 주사

그림 6. 부위마취의 종류

▶ **회음절개술(Episiotomy)**

- 회음절개는 질 입구를 확장시키기 위한 절개
- 거대아, 급속한 아두의 만출, 선진부이상으로 회음열상 예방, 둔위 또는 겸자분만 시 시행

표 3 • 회음절개술의 형태

정중 회음절개술(median episiotomy)	중측방 회음절개술(medio-lateral episiotomy)
• 가장 많이 이용 • 쉽게 치유, 동통 적음 • 항문괄약근(3도 열상), 직장(4도 열상) 가능성	• 정중 회음절개술에 비해 출혈 많음 • 치유 어렵고, 동통 심함 • 3도 열상 가끔 발생(4도 열상 별로 없음)

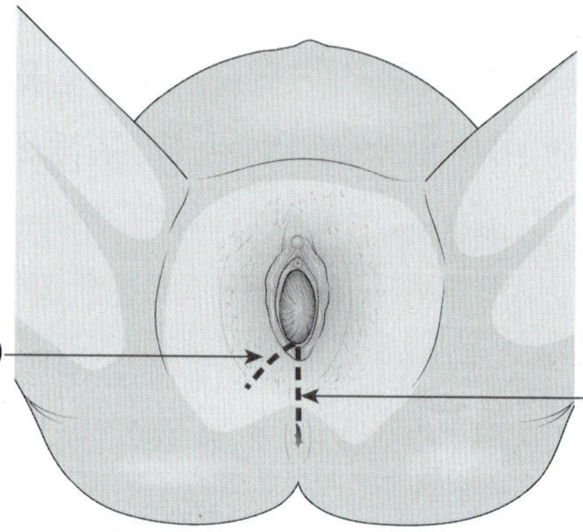

그림 7. 회음절개 위치 및 방향

▶ **열상(Laceration)**

- 태아 분만 시 회음, 질, 자궁 및 지지조직의 급성으로 손상
- 경관이 완전히 개대되기 전에 태아를 분만시킬 때 발생 가능성
- 봉합은 2도 열상 이상에서 실시
- 봉합 후 건열요법 및 더운물 좌욕 → 치유증진, 동통감소 및 감염예방

열상의 분류

• 제1도 열상: 질 점막 및 피부손상 국한 • 제2도 열상: 제1도 열상+회음체부의 손상	• 제3도 열상: 제2도 열상+항문괄약근 손상 • 제4도 열상: 제3도 열상+직장전벽의 손상

▶ **분만기전**

- **머리태위: 두정위(Vertex presentation)**
  - •자궁수축에 의해 선진부가 하강함에 따라 회음은 팽창됨
  - •수축 때마다 수의적으로 힘을 주어 아래로 밀어낼 때 아두가 질 입구로 나왔다가 수축이 사라지면 질 입구의 안쪽으로 들어가는 배림현상

☞ Ritgen's maneuver: 속도를 조절하기 위해 아두가 회음부를 밀어 질 개구부가 5cm 정도 열렸을 때 한 손에 소독수건 씌워 항문부위를 막으면서 미골의 회음부 통해 태아의 턱을 신전시킴

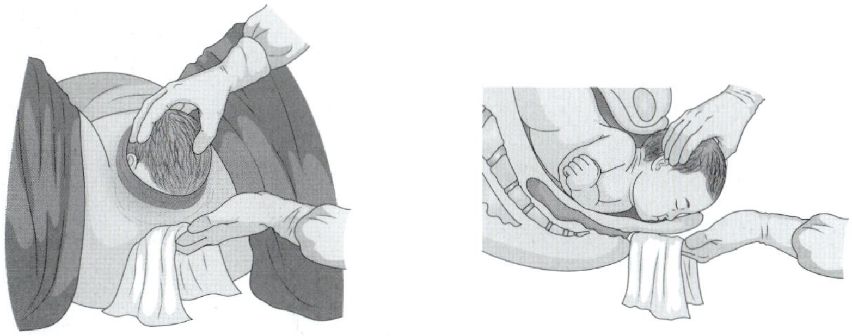

A. 아두 질(vagina) 입구에 보임 B. 아두 질 입구에서 나옴

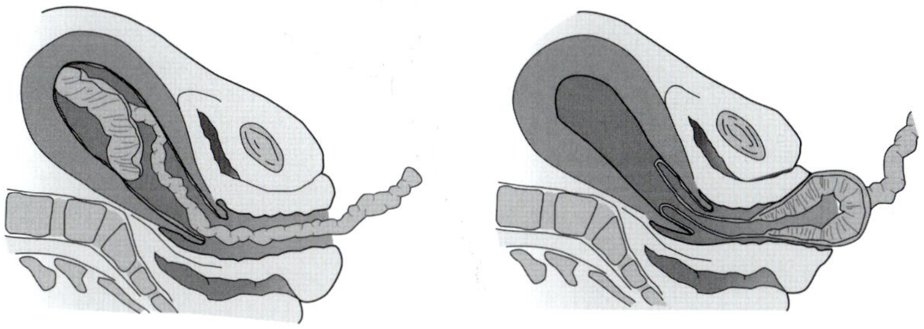

C. 태반박리 시작 D. 태반배출

그림 8. 정상분만: 두정위(Vertex presentation)

▶ 둔위분만(**볼기태위, Breech presentation)**

- 둔위(볼기태위)는 이상 선진부 중 가장 흔한 예
- 전분만의 3～4%, 조산의 25% 차지

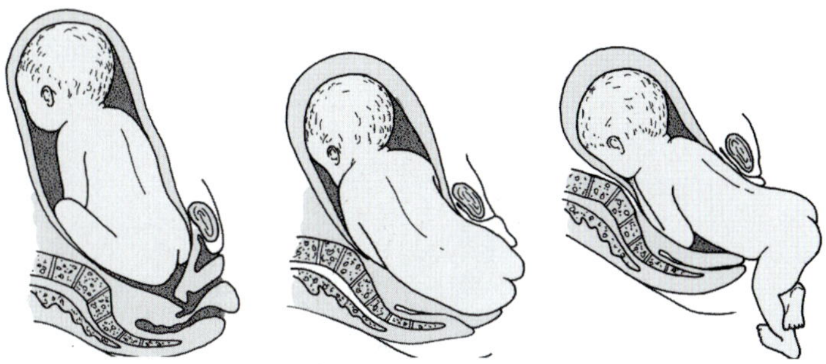

A. 분만진입 및 내회전 B. 측방굴곡 C. 외회전

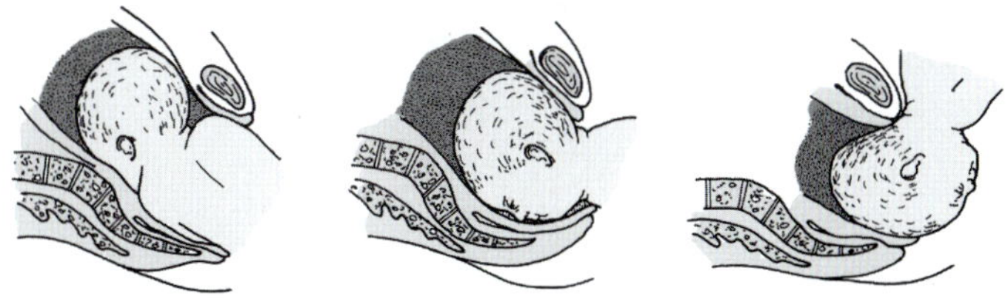

D. 어깨와 머리의 내회전 E. 안면회전 F. 아두만출

그림 9. 둔부태위(Breech presentation)

▶ **외측 머리회전(External cephalic version)**

- 외측두정회전은 외부조작으로 볼기태위에서 머리태위로 바꾸는 오래된 기술
- 제왕절개술을 하지 않기 위해 37주 이후와 진통 전에 실시
- 양극에 손을 얹어 부드럽게 둔부를 골반의 외측으로 회전
  - 아두는 반대방향으로 회전

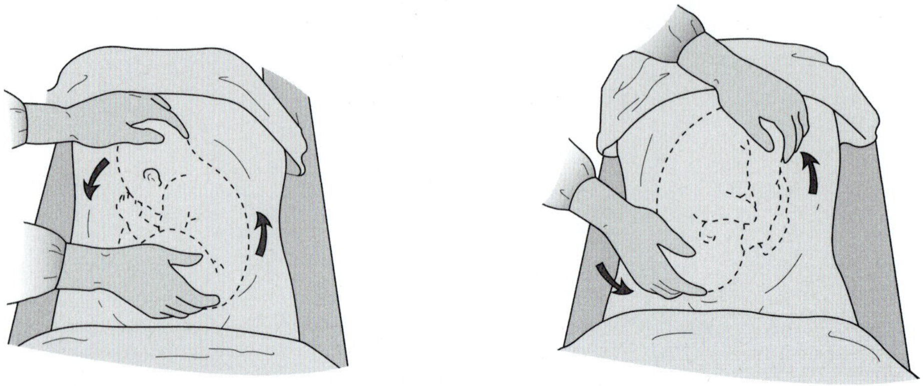

그림 10. 외측 두정회전술(External cephalic version)

겸자분만(Forceps-assisted birth)

- ▶ 산과적 겸자는 2개의 휘어진 스푼모양의 엽으로 되어 있음
- ▶ 가장 흔히 사용되는 겸자는 아두와 비슷하게 만곡된 모양
- ▶ 난산 시 분만 2기를 단축, 마취의 영향으로 산모의 만출노력이 약할 때 또는 산모가 위험 시 사용(예: 심장기능부전)
- ▶ 둔위(볼기태위) 또는 태아가 위험 시 사용(예: 태아질식, 선진부이상, 머리회전이상)

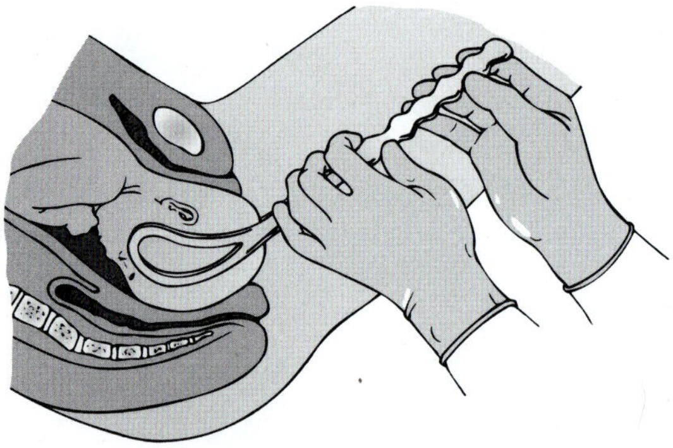

그림 11. 겸자분만(Forcep delivery)

흡인만출(Vaccum extraction)

- ▶ 컵모양의 흡인기를 이용하여 아두의 두피를 견인하여 태아를 분만

- 부작용 적어 많이 사용
- 흡인기는 불수의적인 자궁수축과 산모의 수의적인 노력에 견인을 가하므로 겸자분만보다 생리적인 방법
- 선진부가 두정위, 양막파열이 되어야 하며, 아두골반 불균형이 없어야 시행
- 산모는 쇄석위(lithotomy position) 상태에서 아두에 흡인 대고 아두의 하강 촉진
- 흡인기 적용이 30분 이상 지속 시 두피에 심한 손상 또는 두혈종 발생
- 필요하면 회음절개, 실패할 경우 겸자 또는 제왕절개분만
- 신생아 손상은 두혈종, 두피열상 등, 모체는 회음부, 질 및 경관열상 가능성

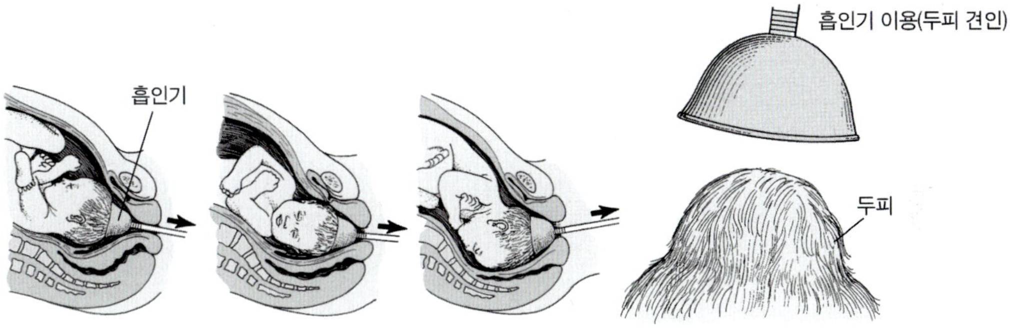

그림 12. 흡인만출(Vacuum extraction)

유도분만(Induction of labor)

- 유도분만은 인위적으로 자궁수축을 유도
- 모체 또는 태아상태에 따라 실시

  예) 임신중 고혈압(PIH), 당뇨병, 사산 및 지연된 임신 등

① 화학적 방법

- Prostaglandin(PGE_2)
  - PGE_2 gel은 경관내에 국소적으로 작용하여 경관을 부드럽게 하여 분만을 유도 시 사용
  - 경관이 부적당할 때 oxytocin보다 더 효과적
- Oxytocin
  - 불충분한 자궁수축으로 느리게 진행되는 분만과정을 유도 또는 촉진
  - 뇌하수체 후엽/내분비장기

② 물리적 방법

- Amniotomy(인공파막)
  - 경관의 상태가 적당한 조건하에서 자궁수축을 자극 시 사용
  - 분만은 양막파열 후 12시간 내 보통 시작
  - 인공파막은 oxytocin 유도와 함께 사용

2.1 다태임신(Multiple pregnancy)

표 4 • 일란성 및 이란성 쌍태

일란성 쌍태(identical pregnancy)	이란성 쌍태(dizygotic pregnancy)
• 하나의 난자로부터 발생된 쌍태 • 항상 동성(同性) • 신체적인 외모가 비슷 • 일란성 쌍태의 형성 – 착상부위(2개), 태반(2개): 난막 형성 – 내세포 분리 → 합쳐진 태반(1개), 양막 및 융모막(1개)	• 두 개의 난자로부터 발생된 쌍태 • 동성(同性) 또는 이성(異性) 가능 • 다른 형제나 자매보다 더 닮지 않음 • 수정란(2개), 착상부위(2개), 태반(2개) 양막(2개) 및 융모막(2개) 지님 – 단, 태반은 융합될 수도 있음

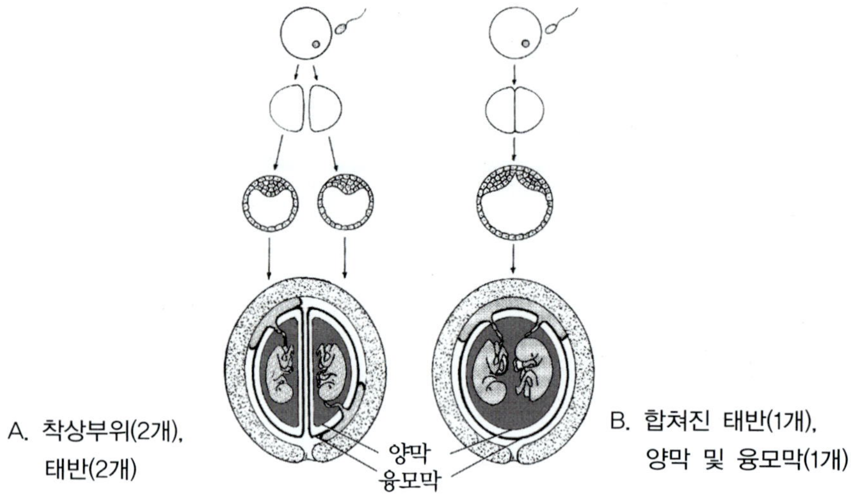

그림 13. 일란성 쌍태의 형성(A → B)

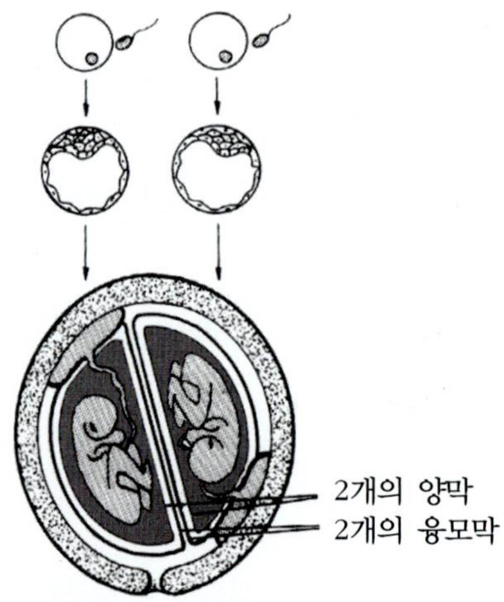

그림 14. 이란성 쌍태의 형성

수정란(2개), 착상부위(2개), 태반(2개), 양막(2개) 및 융모막(2개)

차트 용어

· Bulla	수포	· Cyanosis	청색증	· Demarcation	분획/경계구분	· Deep	깊은
· Engorgement	충혈	· Heel	발뒤꿈치	· Lochia	오로	· Omentum	대망
· Scanty	부족한	· Serosa	장막	· Surface	표면	· Woozing	삼출물

▸ lochia(오로): 분만 후 1주~2주 사이에 나타나는 분비물

▸ ♂: 남성, ♀: 여성

▸ Nitrazine test: · 검사지를 질내 분비물에 묻힘
· 색상을 표준색상도표와 비교
· pH가 6.5 이상 → 양막파열 의미

약 어	원 어	
AC	Abdominal circumference	복위
Am	Amenorrhea	무월경
A/S	Apgar score	아프가 점수법
	▸ **1분: 응급소생술, 5분: 태아의 사망률 및 이환율**	
EBL	Estimated blood loss	혈액손실 추정량
	▸ 과다출혈: 정상분만(500cc 이상), 제왕절개(1,000cc 이상)	
DF	Delivery floor	분만층 (ward/병동)
DOA	Date on admission	입원일
EDC	Estimated date of confinement	분만예정일
	▸ **최종월경일(LMP) – 3개월(또는 +9개월) +7일**	
FHR	Fetal heart rate	태아 심박수
FHT	Fetal heart tone	태아 심음
GA	Gross anomaly	육안이상
Hb	Hemoglobin	헤모글로빈/혈색소(빈혈검사)
HOF	Height of fundus	저부의 높이
I/O	Intake and output	섭취량 및 배설량
LMP	Last menstrual period	최종 월경일
L/P	Labor pain	분만진통
MS	Meconium stained	태변착색
NICU	Neonatal intensive care unit	신생아 중환자실
PIH	Pregnancy induced hypertension	임신성 고혈압
PP	Presenting part	분만방법(태위)
PROM	Premature rupture of membranes	양막 조기파열
RHB	Regular heart beat	규칙적인 심장음
ROM	Rupture of membranes(obstetrics)	양막파열
RR	Recovery room	회복실
S-S enema	Saline solution enema(procedure)	식염수 관장/처치
SSE	Soapsuds enema(procedure)	비눗물 관장/처치
V/S	Vital signs	활력징후

등록번호	200 66 33	성별	F
성명	빛 나 리		
주민등록	780507-1234567		

입 퇴 원 기 록
Admission and Discharge Record

주 소 : 서울시 관악구 신림 2동 101-7													
출신지 :		직 업 :			전 화 :								
연고자성명 : 조진민		관 계 :			주 소 :				전 화 :				
입원 : 2017년 4 월 23 일 OB 과 병동 호				전과	20	년	월	일	과	병동	호		
퇴원 : 2017년 5 월 22 일 과 병동 호					20	년	월	일	과	병동	호		
재원일수 :					20	년	월	일	과	병동	호		

최종진단명	분 류 번 호
주진단명 : Parity 36 wks $\bar{c}$ Twin	
기타진단명 : Lt. heel burn during Op.	
수술 및 처치명	
수술명 : Emergency C/S	
기타수술 및 주요검사 : Burn dressing	

치료결과 : 1. 완쾌 2. 경쾌 3. 호전안됨 4. 진단뿐 5. 가망없는 퇴원 6. 48시간내 사망 7. 48시간이후 사망	
퇴원형태 : 1. 퇴원지시후 2. 자의퇴원 3. 탈원 4. 전원	
병원감염 : 1. 수술후 2. 기타처치후 3. 비뇨기계 4. 호흡기계 5. 소화기계 6. 기타	
원사인 :	부검 : 예, 아니오
계속적 진료 계획	
없음·있음 (약속일 2017 년 6 월 1 일 시)	
담당 전공의 서명 : 남진호	담당 전문의 서명 : 박태영
의무기록 완성 : 2017 년 월 일	의무기록사 서명 :

등록번호	200 66 33	성별	F
성명	빛 나 리		
주민등록	780507-1234567		

퇴 원 요 약

Discharge Summary

Final Dx: PA 36 wks $\bar{c}$ L/P
$\bar{c}$ ROM
$\bar{c}$ Twin

Brief Hx.: Am. since 14/8.91
PN check at 본원 prof 박태영 → uneventful
2017/4/23 5:00(PM)부터 L/P있어 내원
2017/4/23 adm.
2017/4/23 Em C/S
Operator : 황달영
Anesthe : epidural
① ♂/ 1.65kg 8 : 34 (PM)
As (6 → 7 → 7) GA (−)
MS (−), O2 (+)
② ♀/ 2.19kg 8 : 35 (PM)
AS (7 → 8 → 8) GA (−)
MS (−), O2 (+)
P-op #2 Hb : 10.7 → 9.2
Lt. heel burn → burn dressing
2017/5/22 Discharge $\bar{c}$ uneventful
Rec) OPD F/U

Nam

등록번호	200 66 33	성별	F
성명	빛 나 리		
주민등록	780507-1234567		

병 력 기 록
History

Pt. 빛나리/39
P 1-O-
LMP : 2016/8/14
PMP : IR
30～45 d
EDC : 2017/6/21
DOA : 2017/4/23

C.C Am for 36 wks $\bar{c}$ L/P (6 PM 이후)
$\bar{c}$ ROM (2days ago)
$\bar{c}$ Twin (natural preg)

BHx 1. Am since 2017/8/14
2. PN check at local & our hospital (pf. 박태영)
: uneventful
3. USG at 2017/4/15(G-P 34^{+6} wk)
① head 1,649g ② head 2,072g
BPD 8.0 BPD 8.0
4. 2017/4/23 6 PM부터 시작된 L/P을 주소로 Adm. 함

PMHx : N-C

S/R : headache (−), diarrhea (−)
fever/chill (−/−), dyspnea /palpitation (−/−)
epigastric discomfort (−), blurred vision (−)
A/N/V/D/C (−/−/−/−/−)
oliguria (−), dysuria (−)

Choi

등록번호	200 66 33	성별	F
성명	빛 나 리		
주민등록	780507-1234567		

신체검진기록
Physical Examination

G.A	alert, intact
V/S	stable
HEENT	not anemic not icteric PTH (−/−), PI (−/−)
Neck	L/N (−), T/E (−)
Chest	CBS $\bar{s}$ ⓡ RHB $\bar{s}$ ⓜ
Abd	Soft protruted d/t preg. full term size
Back & Ext	CVAT (−/−) pitting (−)

Choi

등록번호	200 66 33	성별	F
성명	빛 나 리		
주민등록	780507-1234567		

경 과 기 록
Progress Notes

〈 Admission note 〉

4.23 8 PM (OB finding)

HOF 30cm

AC

FHT OK

PP breech

Cx alm

Os 4cm

ROM (+)

at 2017/4/21 저녁

Nitrazine test (+)

St −1~0

A : PA 36 wks $\bar{c}$ L/P

$\bar{c}$ ROM

$\bar{c}$ Twin

P : 1. Emergency lab

2. Toco cardiography

3. Emergency C/S *Nam*

9. PM

C/S was done

operator : R3 지순용/R4 홍도야

Assistant : R2 남진호/R1 박인서/In 강호인

Op name : C/S

(Low seg. trans. ut. incision)

4.23 baby : ① ♂/1.65kg

AS (6 → 7 → 7)

MS (−)

GA (−) : epigastric site retraction (+)

경 과 기 록

일 자	내 용	서 명
	② ♀/2.19kg AS (7 → 8 → 8) MS (−) GA (−) Immed post op : V/S 100/53−108 HOF umb. firm V/D rubra scanty	*Kim*
4.24	4 AM S : pain & tenderness on the Lt heel O : 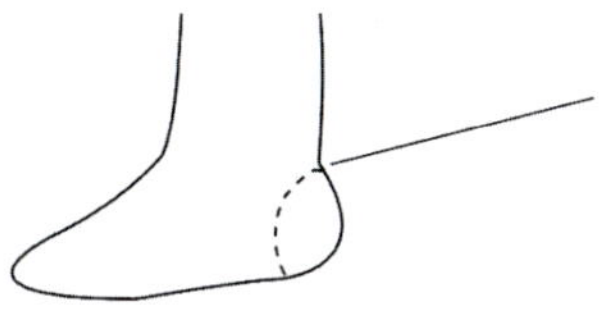 demarcation pain/tenderness (+/+) bulla (−) skin color: the same as others. A : Burn thermal (?) electrical (?)	
4.24	P : 1. wet dressing (x3) 2. 후시딘 ointment apply * For the operation bovie plate : 철판 (처음에 젖어 있어서 수술 시 작전 다시 갈아낌) 수술 후 환자가 다리가 저리다고 해서 양다리에 hot pack을 apply 해줬다고 함. 별로 뜨거운 온도는 아니었다고 함.	*Nam*
4.25	S : some improved pain on the heel O : black discoloration bulla (+) V/S : 130/90～140/90−118−38.8℃ HOF : umb. firm V/D : rubra scanty G/O : (+) Op. wd : clear CBC : 10.7−16600−286 K A : POD #2 $\bar{c}$ 2°burn $\bar{c}$ environmental factor에 의한 heat	

경 과 기 록

일 자	내 용	서 명
	P : 1. PS consult 2. Cooling by opening	*Nam*
4.25	− PS 회신 − electrical burn보다는 thermal burn 같습니다. pain sensation 있고 bulla 있어 2nd−degree burn 같습니다. hygiene으로 닦은 후 silvadene apply 하면 되겠습니다. (x2/Day) *Skin graft는 필요 없을 것 같습니다.	*Nam*
4.27	S : Breast engorgement (+) A : POD #4 $\bar{c}$ 2°burn P : 1. parlodel 1 Ⓣ po bid x 2 wbs 2. R − care	*Nam*
4.29	S : wd. site discomfort O : V/S − stable HOF : 1FB ↓ firm V/D : rubra scanty op wd : pus like material when squeezing 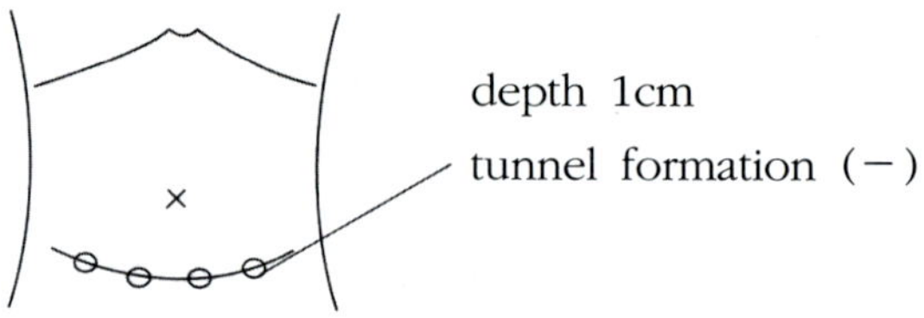 Breast engorgement (+) A : POD #6 $\bar{c}$ wd problem P : 1. wd. dressing (x3) 2. Anti start	
4.29	〈 Off duty Note 〉 Pt. 빛나리/39, F P : 1−0−0−2 [1 / 1] BHx : 1. 23/4 Admission 36wks $\bar{c}$ L/P $\bar{c}$ ROM (2days duration) $\bar{c}$ Twin (natural preg.)으로 와서 2. 23/4 Emergency C/S 시행하에 ① ♂/1.65kg AS (6 → 7 → 7) ② ♀/2.19kg AS (7 → 8 → 8)	

경 과 기 록

일 자	내 용	서 명

3. 29/4 POD #6 dressing 시 subcutaneous hematoma infection (?) 발견하고 dressing 함.

Problem : 1. wd. problem
2. Breast engorgement (+)
3. Lt. foot burn (2°)

4.29 Rec : 1. Dressing (x3/d)
2. Breast massage & parlodel medication encourage
3. Lt. foot burn dressing (x2/d)

4.29 〈 On duty Note 〉 *Nam*

Pt. 빛나리/39, F
P : 1－0－0－2 [1, 1]

S : 1. S/P Emergency C/S $\bar{c}$ Twin delivery
2. P－op wd problem
3. Lt. leg burn

O : 1. baby 4/23 ① ♂/1.65kg AS (6 → 7 → 7)
② ♀/2.19kg AS (7 → 8 → 8)
2. wd problem

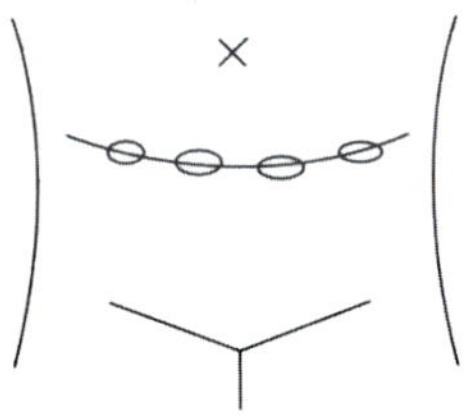

4곳 벌어짐 depth 1～2cm
discharge (±)
woozing (+)
pain (+)

3. Lt. leg burn
2001/4/25 PS consult : R/O thermal burn
pain sense (+)
2°degree *Nam*

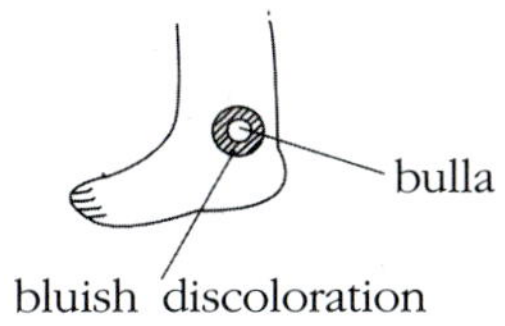

4.29 A : 1. Post C/S state (doing well except 2.3)
2. P－op wd prob.
3. Lt. leg 2°thermal burn

P : 1. P－op supportive Tx. NICU contact
2. wd daily dressing (x3/D)
by H_2O_2 & gauze drain

경 과 기 록

일 자	내 용	서 명
	3. ① burn dressing by hygiene & silvadine cr ② PS consult ③ antibiotic Tx cef − z 1.0g IM $\bar{q}$ 8hrs GM 80mg IM $\bar{q}$ 12hrs	*Nam*
5.3	S : op wd pain: tolerable burn wd pain: tolerable breast engorgement (+) O : op wd : discharge (−) woozing (−) gauze drain 중 improved state burn wd : stationary A : 1. Wd. problem 2. Breast engorgement 3. Lt. foot burn (2°) P : 1. daily dressing 지속 2. Breast massage 지속 3. PS reconsult	*Nam*
5.6	S : wd pain (+) syspepsia (+) O : 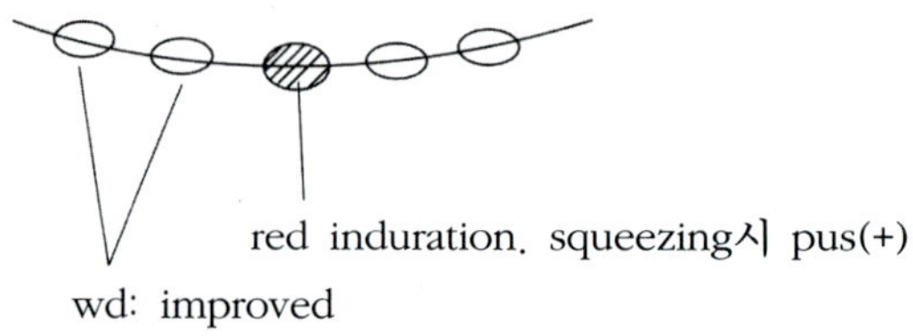 middle part of op wd에 pus collection (+) → stitch out ┐ was done wd reopening ┘ Burn wd : stationary A : P−op wd problem : pus collection으로 인해 wd 모두 벌려줌. P : 1. Dressing prn 2. resuture 3. 소화제 S : wd pain : improved dyspepsia : improved breast engorge : improved O : 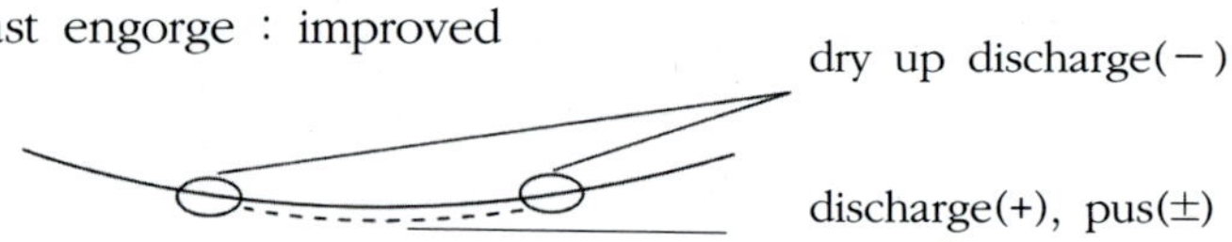	

경 과 기 록

일 자	내 용	서 명
	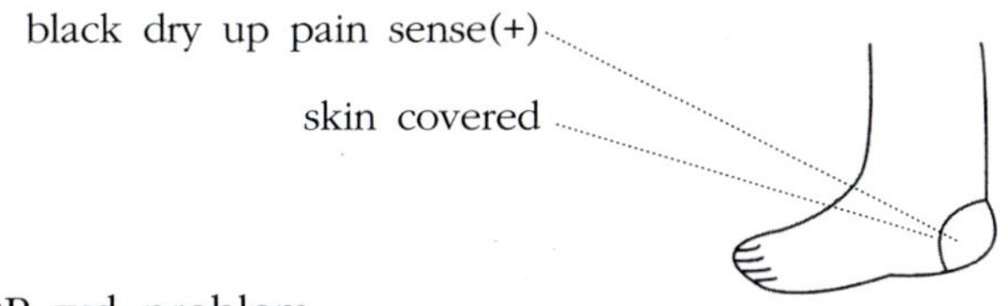	
	A : P−OP wd problem P : Dressing $\bar{c}$ H_2O_2 madecarsol powder	*Nam*
5.10	V/S stable HOF : 3 FB ↓ firm lochia : serosa scanty No oozing at OP wd & Burn site	*Nam*
5.17	S : wd pain (±) O : wd : clear, discharge (−) 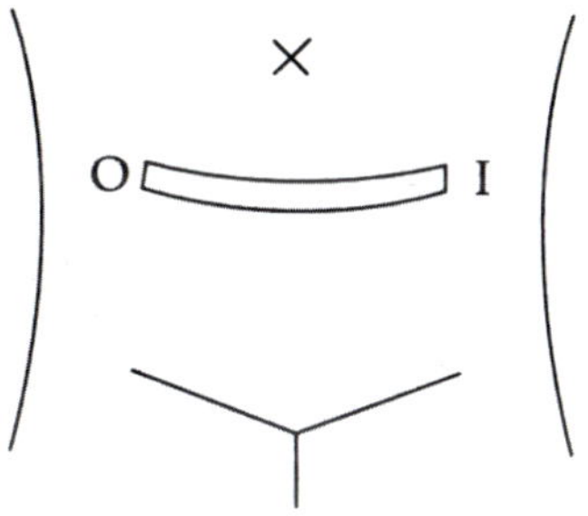 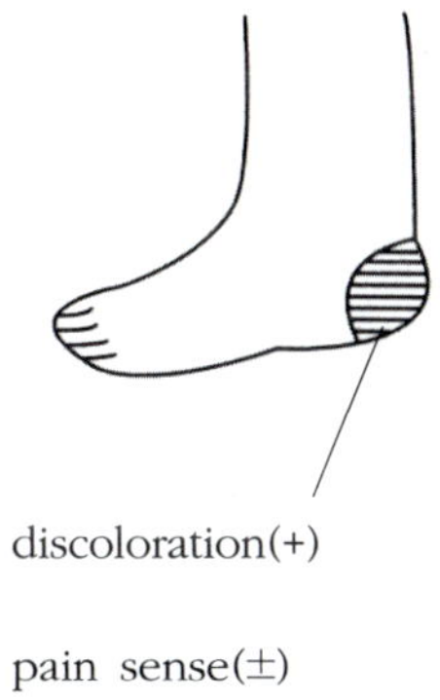 A : P−op wd problem: improved state P : continue daily dressing (x2)	*Nam*
5.20	S : wd pain (−) O : wd : discharge (−) much improved A : P. op wd : improved state P : continue daily dressing (x2)	*Nam*

등록 번호	200 66 33	성별	F
성명	빛 나 리		
주민 등록	780507-1234567		

수술 전 처치 및 간호상태 확인표

도착시간: __________ 수술예정 방번호: __________

확 인 내 용	간 호 단 위			수 술 부		
	예	아니오	해당무	예	아니오	해당무
환자확인				V		
수술서약서				V		
수술전 투약				none		
의치, 의안, 안경, 콘택트렌즈 제거				V		
장신구 제거(핀, 반지, 시계, 목걸이, 귀걸이)				V		
화장제거(입술, 볼연지, 매니큐어 등)				V		
환의만 입힌다(속옷 제거)				V		
혈액학적 검사				V		
뇨검사					V	
유치 카데타 삽입				V		
심전도				V		
금식				9시이후로 NPO		
수술부위 피부 준비				V		
위관 삽입						V
알러지(약물, 반창고 등)	유	무		유	무	
Embossing Card	유	무		유	무	
간호사 서명						

등록번호	200 66 33	성별	F
성명	빛 나 리		
주민등록	780507-1234567		

수 술 기 록
Operation Record

날짜 : 2017년 4월 23일 집도의 : T. Y. Pak M.D
제 1 보조의 : U. O. Lee M.D. 제 2 보조의 : J.H. Nam M.D.
참여간호사 : 순환간호사

Preoperative diagnosis	: PA 36 wks $\bar{c}$ twin $\bar{c}$ PROM $\bar{c}$ breech
Postoperative diagnosis	: Same as above
Name of operation	: Em. low transverse C/S

Findings & Procedures :

1. Ski n: pfannenstiel incision
2. Skin to peritoneum : free
3. Peritoneal cavity : bl (−), Ascites (−)
   Adh (+)
   1) Uterus: term sized
   2) Babies : ① ♂/1.65kg at 2: 30 (AM)
      AS (6 → 7) MS (−), GA (−), O_2 (+)
      ② ♀/2.19kg at 2: 31 (AM)
      AS (7 → 8) MS (−), GA (−), O_2 (+)
   3) Pl : "M" 930G/35cm, 40cm
4. EBL : Ca 700cc
5. Tf : Not done
6. Imm. postop status : stable
   ① L/N : retroperitoneal & inguinal: impalpable, enlargement (−)
   ② Omentum : free
   ③ Liver surface : free
   ④ Bladder & rectal mucosa : meta nodule impalpable

Biopsy Number : x 2 Surgical Bx.

수 술 기 록

OP. procedure

Under the epidural anesthesia, the patient was lain supine and the drapping was done as usual manner.

The pfannenstiel's skin incision was made and deeper into the peritoneum.

Entering the peritoneal cavity two pieces of abdominal tapes were inserted into each lateral gutters the low transverse uterine incision was made. The babies and placenta were delivered manually in succession. MTG 1Ⓐ was injected intramuscularly.

The uterine wall was closed layer by layer with interlocking suture continuous & gauze count. The abdominal wall was repaired in layers.

Date : 2017. 4. 23 Dictacted by J. H. Nam

등록번호	200 66 33	성별	F
성명	빛 나 리		
주민등록	780507-1234567		

의 사 지 시 기 록
Doctor's Orders

〈 Admission Note 〉

4.23

1. V/S $\bar{q}$ 1 hrs
2. BR
3. NPO
4. Check FHT & L/P $\bar{q}$ 30 min
5. Skin preparation
6. S－S enema
7. get op. permission
8. sent pt to DF
9. CBC(em), U/A(em) OP
   ABO, é BUN Cr, OT/PT
   EKG, Chest AP(p)

4.24

Postop. #1

1. V/S $\bar{q}$ 4 hrs
2. BR
3. NPO
4. I/O
5. Check HOF & V/S $\bar{q}$ 4 hrs
6. Remove foley at 9 : 00 (PM)
   → Check V/S 4 hrs later
   → IF (－) : cath
7. Abd binder

의 사 지 시 기 록

일 자	내 용	서 명
4.24	8. 5% DW 1L / V−P 1Ⓐ] miv (x1) 9. 5% DS 1L / V−P 1Ⓐ] miv (x1) 10. 5% DW 500cc IV 11. unasyn 1.5gm IV $\bar{q}$ 6 hrs(AST) 12. Tobramycin 60mg IM $\bar{q}$ 8 hrs 13. Reptilase 1Ⓐ IV $\bar{q}$ 12 hrs 14. methergin 1Ⓐ IM $\bar{q}$ 6 hrs 15. morphine 33mg via epidural cath. 16. 후시딘 연고 apply 17. wet dressing(x3/d) for 15min $\bar{c}$ saline 12: 34 (PM)	
5.15	Postop. #22 1. V/S $\bar{q}$ 8 hrs 2. BR 3. OBD 4. Check HOF & V/S $\bar{q}$ 8hrs 5. Abd binder 6. cefaclor 1Ⓣ / Bearse 1Ⓣ / FN 1Ⓣ / CPD 3.3mg] p.o tid self 7. feroba 1Ⓣ p.o bid 8. Burn dressing	
5.22	Postop. #22 1. V/S $\bar{q}$ 8 hrs 2. BR 3. OBD 4. Check HOF & V/S $\bar{q}$ 8hrs	

의 사 지 시 기 록

일 자	내 용	서 명
5.22	5. Abd binder ┐ 6. cefaclor 1Ⓣ │ Bearse 1Ⓣ │ p.o tid FN 1Ⓣ │ CPD 3.3mg ┘ self 7. feroba 1Ⓣ p.o bid 8. Burn dressing 9. Discharge	

등록번호	200 66 33	성별	F
성명	빛 나 리		
주민등록	780507-1234567		

분 만 간 호 기 록

분 만 전 기 록

날짜 시간	태아심음	진통간격	간호내용	배설	서명
4.23 8:00 (PM)	LLQ : 160xh U.U : 170xh	irre	transfer from 32 to 36 DF $\overline{c}$ chart on foot. Vg exam±4cm almost 진행되었음 monitor apply함. DF orientation함.		*Lee*
8:20 (PM)		20″$\overline{q}$ 1–0′	5% DW 1L IV start 함 hydrate 중임		*Lee*
8:30 (PM)	U.P : 166xh	20″$\overline{q}$ 1–2′	BT: 38℃, Dr. 박태영에게 Notify		*Lee*
8:50 (PM)	U.P : 150xh	25″$\overline{q}$ 2′ - 2′30″	FHR early decelerate 나타나고 있음. skin pre was done.		*Lee*
9:00 (AM) 9:05 (AM)	U.P : 155xh	25″$\overline{q}$ 2′ - 2′30″	Foley–cath insertion 함 carried C/S room by Dr. 박준		*Lee*

투약	날짜		시간 /서명	검사	날짜	종류	시간 및 서명
	4.23	5% DW 1L	8:20(P)인 8:55(P)인		4.23	Sono	8. 20(P)/인
	4.23	cefa–Z Crm ID HST	1mL			CBC, é, BUN/cr, OT/PT	8. 20(P)/인
		cefa–Z 1.0g $\overline{q}$ hrs IVS	9:00(P)/wh			Chest AP EKG	8. 20(P)/인

등록번호	200 66 33	성별	F
성명	빛 나 리		
주민등록	780507-1234567		

분 만 간 호 기 록

분 만 전 기 록							
회음절개	시 간		회음절개형			시행자	
분 만	시 간	2017. 4. 23 at 8:00	분만형	C/S		시행자	홍조
신생아간호	시행자	① 권인숙 ② 강성숙	성별	① ♂ ② ♀		체 중	① 1.63 ② 2.19
	1분내	① 6 ② 7	5분 후 아프가	① 6→7 ② 7→8		산소투여	①+ ②+
	첫소변	① - ② -	태 변	① not passed ② not passed			
	기형유무	① grossly free ② grossly free					
태반만출	소행술 실시 및 처치	epigastric site retraction No retraction L/S가 crack함 → NICU					
		심하게 있었으나 L/S는 clear함 → NICU					
	시 간	at 9:35 (PM)	태반만출형	M	소파여부		
	태반무게	930g	탯줄길이	35.40cm	시 행 자	황달구	
산모간호	Epidural Anesthesia was done.						
	Methergine 2Ⓐ IM injected at 9:35 (PM)						
	pad & Gauze count 맞음/RN 신주미						
검 사	종 류	시 간	서 명	종 류	시 간	서 명	

분 만 간 호 기 록

분 만 후 기 록							
날짜	시간	자궁저위측정	혈압	맥박	오로	간호내용	서명
4.23	11:00 (PM)	umb.firm	100/53	108	rubric scanty	C/S → R.R로 옴 H/S all infusion되어 H/S 1L connect 함. via F-bag yellow color 380cc op wd site에 sand bag apply & pain tolerable	
	11:15	35B↑: firm	110/75	108	rubric scanty		
	11:45	12B↑: firm	120/70	97	rubric scanty	chilling sense 호소함	
	12:15 (AM)	12B↑: firm	90/70	115	rubric scanty		
	12:40 (AM)					veno 1Ⓐ mixed 5% DW 1L Lt. heel: 계란크기의 skin lesion 있고 pain호소하며 Dr.황달수에게 Notify함.	
	4:30 (AM)					바셀린 dressing하고 관찰함. sand bag remove함. position change 안내하고 격려함. op wd site woozing 없음 BT: 38°C op wd pain: tolerable position change 잘함.	
	6:30 (AM)		130/90	108	rubric scanty	urination well F-catheter ≒ 1,400cc 5% DW $\bar{c}$ venol Ⓐ≒700 infusion	

등록번호	200 66 33	성별	F
성명	빛 나 리		
주민등록	780507-1234567		

간 호 기 록
Nurses Record

날 짜	시 간	내 용	서 명
4.24	6 : 30 (a)	11:00(P) ~6:00(a) I/O 1: Ⓟ 1300cc/Ⓤ 1400cc	
	7 : 40 (a)	HOF umb. form op. site pain mild하게 호소함.	
		5% DW $\bar{c}$ vero. Ⓡ inf. now	
	8 : 20 (a)	BT. 38.5˚C checked gas out 될 때까지 NPO 설명함	
	9 : 00 (a)	Lt. 발꿈치 알콜묻힌 소독 gauze 대어 줌. for cooling	
		BT 38.5˚C BT: 151/96mmHg, PR: 107회/min	
		vaginal discharge lochia rubric－scanty함.	
		Foley－cath patency 유지상태임.	
		Op wound pain mild하게 호소함.	
	11 : 00 (a)	op site pain 심하여 Notify to Dr. 구일동 &	
		Morphine 1Ⓣ + H/S mix하여 7cc 투여함.	
		though the epi－cath by Dr. 남진호	
	12 : 40 (a)	saline wet dressing applied on Lt. heel	
	12 : 58 (a)	wet dressing remove 후 인바도 크림 도포함.	
	2 PM	BP: 140/94mmHg. BT : 38˚4′ PR : 105회/min	
		lochia: rubric $\bar{c}$ scanty함. op wound pain: tolerable	
		6A~2P I/O Ⓟ 620cc/Ⓤ 1130cc(버림)	
		5% DW $\bar{c}$ veno 1Ⓣ: Ⓡ 80cc infusing now	
	2 : 40 (p)	5% DW 1L+ veno 1Ⓐ IV started 되어 inf 중임.	

등록번호	200 66 33	성별	F
성명	빛 나 리		
주민등록	780507-1234567		

신 생 아 검 진 기 록

Newborn Record

출생(0), 사산( ) 2017년 4월 23일 병록번호 24196－2
남, (여)
오전 (오후) 9:35 임신 36 주

Measurements at Birth

Weight 2190 gm OM ______ cm SOB ______ cm

Length ______ cm OF ______ cm SOB Circumference

CR ______ cm BP ______ cm ______ cm

Physical Exmination Birth

- Malformation Yes ( ), No (○) If yes, specify ______
- Skin appearance ______
- Abdomen ______
- Head neck ______
- Genital ______
- Eye & ENT ______
- Anus ______
- Lung ______
- Trunk & spine ______
- Heart ______
- Reflex ______

Care of Newborn

Interval between birth and initial respiratory movement : 2 min

Interval between birth and regular respiratory movement : 3 min

Apgar score 7 → 8 → 8

Cyanosis (+) Aspirated (−)

O2 administered (+) Duration (−)

Stimulants (−) Other drugs (−)

등록번호	200 66 33	성별	F
성명	빛 나 리		
주민등록	780507-1234567		

신 생 아 검 진 기 록

Newborn Record

출생(0), 사산( ) 2017년 4월 23일 병록번호 24196－1
남, (여)
오전 (오후:) 9:35 임신 36 주

Measurements at Birth

Weight 1650 gm　　OM_______cm　　SOB _______cm

Length _______cm　　OF _______cm　　SOB Circumference

CR _______ cm BP _______cm　　_______cm

Physical Exmination Birth

- Malformation Yes ( ), No (○)　　If yes, specify_______
- Skin appearance_______　　• Abdomen_______
- Head neck _______　　• Genital_______
- Eye & ENT _______　　• Anus_______
- Lung _______　　• Trunk & spine_______
- Heart _______　　• Reflex_______

Care of Newborn

Interval between birth and initial respiratory movement : 2 min

Interval between birth and regular respiratory movement : 3 min

Apgar score 6 → 7 → 7

Cyanosis	(－)	Aspirated	(－)
O2 administered	(+)	Duration	(－)
Stimulants	(+)	Other drugs	(－)

〈빛 나 리〉

★ 빛나리 차트를 읽고 맞는 것에 O표 하시오.

1 환자에 대한 설명으로 틀린 것은?

① 자궁저부 높이가 30cm였고, 4월 21일에 양막이 파열되었다.
② 여아의 체중은 2,190gm였고, Apgar score는 1분 내 7, 5분 후 8이었다.
③ 남아는 청색증이 있었으며, 첫 호흡개시가 2분이었다.
④ 왼쪽 다리의 화상으로 성형외과에 의뢰하였다.
⑤ 태아의 심장음은 정상이었고 가슴에 충혈이 있다가 호전되었다.

2 주진단 및 주수술에 대한 분류번호로 맞는 것은?

① O32.0, 74.1 ② O32.1, 74.1 ③ O32.2, 74,99
④ O32.3, 74.99 ⑤ O32.6, 74.1

3 경과기록지와 수술 전 처치 내용에 대해 맞게 기재한 것은?

① 입원 3일째 발뒤꿈치에 수포가 있었다.
② 입원 2일째 발뒤꿈치에 경계구분은 있었으나 압통은 없었다.
③ 5월 20일에 오로가 장막에 조금 분비되었다.
④ 수술 전 근전도 검사를 시행하였다.
⑤ 8시간마다 활력징후와 자궁저부 높이를 체크하였다.

4 수술 후 발생한 문제점에 대한 질병분류번호로 맞는 것은?

① T81.4, Y62.0 ② T81.4 ③ O86.0, Y62.0
④ O86.0 ⑤ O86.8, Y62.0

5 수술에 대한 설명으로 틀리게 기재한 것은?

① 방광과 직장 점막에 전이된 소결절이 촉진되었다.
② 피부는 판넨스티엘 절개를 하였으며, 추정치 실혈은 700cc였다.
③ 자궁벽은 interlocking 연속봉합을 하였다.
④ 복강은 출혈이 없었으며, 유착이 있었다.
⑤ 대망과 간표면은 정상이었다.

6 기타 진단명에 대한 질병분류 번호로 틀린 것은?

① O30.0 ② T25.2 ③ Y63.5
④ Y63.9 ⑤ O60.1

7 의사지시기록과 간호기록에 대한 설명으로 틀리게 기재한 것은?

① 수술 후 섭취량과 배설량은 1400/1300cc였다.
② 수술 상처부위에 모래 주머니를 대었다.
③ 수술청약서를 4월 23일에 받았다.
④ 식염수 관장을 했다.
⑤ 수술 상처부위에 삼출물은 없었다.

8 **Hb의 저하로 인한 질병분류번호로 맞는 것은?**

① D64.9 ② O99.0 ③ D70
④ D64.9, O99.0 ⑤ O99.1

9 **자궁하부 횡절개식 제왕절개를 할 때의 이점이 아닌 것은?**

① 출혈이 적다.
② 전치태반 시 사용하기 용이하다.
③ 다음 임신 시 자궁파열될 가능성이 적다.
④ 장 또는 장간막의 유착이 적다.
⑤ 절개가 용이하다.

10 **환자의 주소를 보고 최종진단명에 추가할 분류번호는 ?**

① Z37.2 ② Z37.3 ③ Z37.6
④ Z38.3 ⑤ Z38.4

03 자궁탈출
Prolapse uteri

1.1 탈출(Prolapse)

- 정상으로 있는 강(cavity)을 통해 장기(organ) 또는 장기의 근육성 막이 벌어져(bulging) 나오거나 탈출(prolapse)하는 것

1.2 자궁탈출(Uterine prolapse)

- 질구로 자궁(uterus)의 탈출

자궁질 탈출의 분류

- 불완전 자궁질 탈출(Incomplete uterovaginal prolapse): N81.2
  - 1도 자궁탈출(first degree uterine prolapse)
  - 2도 자궁탈출(second degree uterine prolapse)
- 완전 자궁질 탈출(Complete uterovaginal prolapse): N81.3
  - 3도 자궁탈출(third degree uterine prolapse)

치 료

- 질식전체자궁절제술(vaginal total hysterectomy; VTH)
- 질폐쇄술
- 맨체스터수술(Manchester operation)

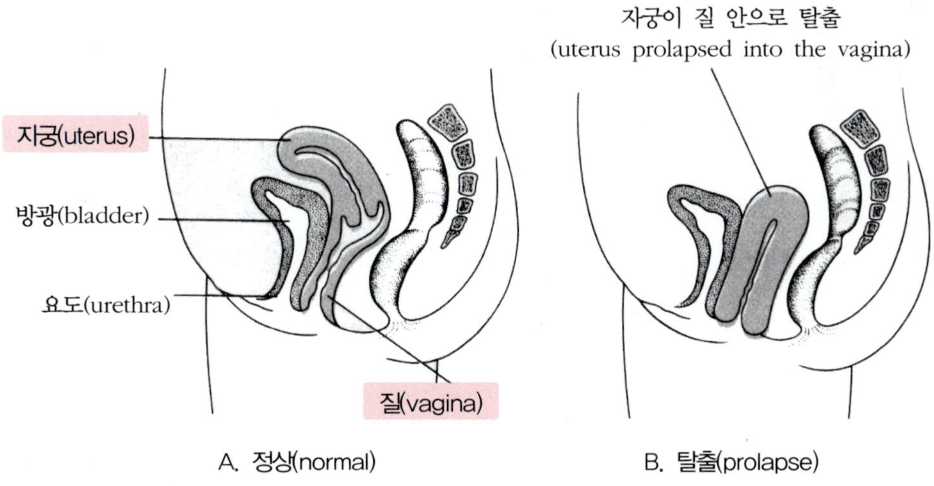

그림 1. 자궁탈출(prolapse uteri)

1.3 기타 탈출

- **직장류(rectocele):** 직장이 질쪽으로 돌출(protrusion)
- **방광류(cystocele):** 방광이 질(vagina)로 돌출
- **식도열공 헤르니아(hiatal hernia)**

  –가로막(diaphragm)의 식도 개구부를 통해 위가 종격동(mediastinum)으로 빠져 나옴
- **서혜(사타구니) 헤르니아(inguinal hernia)**

  –남성에서 장(intestine)의 일부가 서혜부위(groin region)의 아래 음낭(scrotal sac)으로 빠져 나옴

2.1 난소낭종(Ovarian cyst)

- 난소의 낭(sac, cyst) 내에 수분 축적

종양세포: 악·양성 구분 어려움 → 원발 장기: 난소(ovary)

- 낭선종(cystadenoma): D27, M8440/0

  –경계형 악성의 장액성 낭선종(serous cystadenoma, borderline malignancy)

  –D39.1, M8442/1
- 낭선종암종(cystadenocarcinoma): C56, M8440/3

유피낭종(dermoid cyst): 양성 낭성 기형종(benign cystic teratoma)

- 난소의 미성숙한 난자세포에서 발생
- 피부, 머리털, 치아, 연골 등 여러 종류의 세포로 구성

2.2 자궁내 피임장치(Intrauterine device; IUD)

- 수정란(fertilized egg)의 착상을 막음

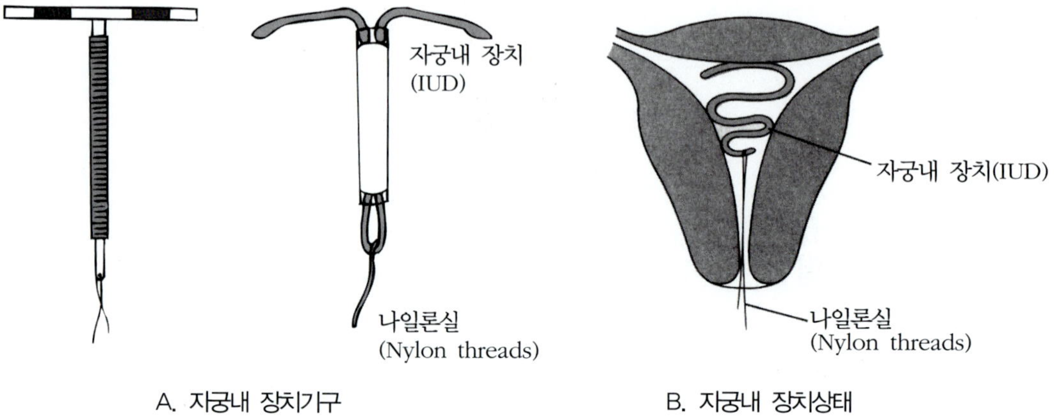

그림 2. 자궁내 장치(IUD)의 기구 및 상태

질병분류상 주의점

- 피임관리
  - 피임장치 삽입을 위해 내원 Z30.1
  - 피임장치의 기계적 합병증(전위, 돌출 등) T83.3
  - 피임장치 조사, 재삽입, 제거 Z30.5
  - 피임장치 존재 Z97.5
- 불임시술을 위한 입원 Z30.2

– Admitted for <u>displaced IUD</u>(IUD was removed) T83.3
전위된 자궁내 피임장치의 제거를 위한 입원(제거함)

– Admitted for <u>removal of IUD</u> in situ(IUD was removed) Z30.5
자궁내 피임장치의 제거

유사 용어

- 난소: ovary = oophoro
- 난관: uterine tube = fallopian tube = salpingo = tubal
- 자궁경부: cervico = trachelo
- 질: vagina = colpo
- 외음/회음: vulva = episio
- 자궁: hystero = uterus = metro

표 1 • 임상검사

구 분	검사항목	정상치	질 환
혈액검사 (hematology)	혈색소 (hemoglobin; Hb)	남: 13.0~17.0 g/dl 여: 12.0~16.0 g/dl	↑ 적혈구증다증 ↓ 빈혈
	적혈구 용적률 (hematocrit; Hct)	남: 36~54 g/dl 여: 36~47 g/dl	↑ 구토, 하리, 선천성심질환 ↓ 철결핍성 빈혈, 부종
	적혈구(RBC)	남: 20만~630만/mm^3 여: 400만~540만/mm^3	↑ 진성다혈증, 탈수, 쇼크 ↓ 각종빈혈, 수혈증
	백혈구(WBC)	4천~1만/mm^3	↑ 만성백혈병, 급성감염증 ↓ 재생불량성 빈혈, 과립수감소
일반생화학 검사 (biochemical)	AST(GOT, OT)	남: 37 U/L 이하 여: 31 U/L 이하	↑ 급성간염, 심근경색, 근질환, 악성종양, 폐쇄성 황달, 알코올성 간염 ↓ 간장괴사
	ALT(GPT, OT)	남: 40 U/L 이하 여: 31 U/L 이하	

차트 용어

· Atrophy	위축	· Displacement	전위	· Erode	부식
· Introitus	입구	· Metaplasia	화생/이형성	· 口; Os	구
· Parous	경산부의	· Protruding	탈출	· Staphylococcus	포도구균

약 어	원 어	
A-P repair	Anterior posterior repair	전후방 봉합
BS	Bowel sounds(abdomen)	장음(복부)
	Breath sounds(chest)	호흡음(흉부)
CBC	Complete blood count ‣ CBC 9.6/28.5/10.800 → 9.6(빈혈)	전혈구 조사(혈액검사)
CXR	Chest x ray	흉부 엑스레이
IUD, IUCD	Intrauterine contraceptive device	자궁내장치
LFT	Liver function test	간기능검사
M/D/N	Moderate, development, nutrition	발육 및 영양상태 적절
VTH	Vaginal total hysterectomy	질식전체자궁절제술

등록번호	233 55 66	성별 F
성명	이 태 양	
주민등록	660508－1234567	

입 퇴 원 기 록
Admission and Discharge Record

주 소 :					
출신지 :	직 업 :	전 화 :			
연고자성명 : 황인준	관 계 :	주 소 :	전 화 :		
입원 : 2017 년 8 월 30 일 Gyn 과 병동 호	전과	20 년 월 일 과 병동 호			
퇴원 : 2017 년 9 월 7 일 과 병동 호		20 년 월 일 과 병동 호			
재원일수 :		20 년 월 일 과 병동 호			

최종진단명	분 류 번 호
주진단명 : Prolapse uteri	
Cystocele	
기타진단명 : Lt. ovarian benign cystic teratoma	
수술 및 처치명	
수술명 : VTH	
Vaginal A－P repair	
Lt. oophorectomy	
기타수술 및 주요검사	

치료결과 : 1. 완쾌 2. 경쾌 3. 호전안됨 4. 진단뿐 5. 가망없는 퇴원 6. 48시간내 사망 7. 48시간이후 사망	
퇴원형태 : 1. 퇴원지시후 2. 자의퇴원 3. 탈원 4. 전원	
병원감염 : 1. 수술후 2. 기타처치후 3. 비뇨기계 4. 호흡기계 5. 소화기계 6. 기타	
원사인 :	부검 : □예 ☑아니오
계속적 진료 계획	
□없음 ☑있음 (약속일 2017 년 9 월 15 일 시)	
담당 전공의 서명 : 서무진	담당 전문의 서명 : 박동찬
의무기록 완성 : 2017 년 9 월 13 일	의무기록사 서명 : 유기인

등록번호	233 55 66	성별 F
성명	이 태 양	
주민등록	660508－1234567	

퇴 원 요 약
Discharge Summary

Final Dx. : Prolapse uteri, Cystocele, Rectocele
Lt. ovarian cystic teratoma

〈 Brief Op. Note 〉

Preop. Dx : Prolapse uteri, cystocele, rectocele, Ovarian cyst
Postop. Dx : Same as above
Op. name : VTH, A－P repair, Lt oophorectomy
Operator : L.U. Lee
Assist : M.J. Seo, Q.U. Kim, P.U. Yoo
Op. finding
Ut. : small, protruded
Vag. wall : relaxed, markedly
Rt. ovary : free
Lt. ovary : Cyst visible

Lab
Chest P－A : No active lesion in both lungs
Heart is not unusual
No pleural lesion is seen
EKG : W.N.L
CBC : 9.6－28.5－10.800
GPT/GOT/r－GPT 35/30/57
Culture : Staphylococcus
Complication
Wound infection

Park

등록번호	233 55 66	성별 F
성명	이 태 양	
주민등록	660508 - 1234567	

병력 및 신체기록

History & Physical Examination

일 자	내 용	서 명
	Adm. Date: 2017. 8. 30 C.C. : Protruding mass through vagina (Du: 10년) P.I. : 10년 전부터 above C.C. 있어 proper Tx. 위해 입원 PHx : OB/Gy G_5 P_1 L_1 Do A_4 Menopause 48 yr. old 5년 전 길을 건너다 택시에 부딪혀 Depressed skull Fx. of parietal 있어 cranioplasty $\bar{c}$ graft 받음 FHx : N - C S/R : No specific problem P/Ex G/A Acute ill, alert M/D/N H/N Normocephaly except post op. scar Isocoric (+/+) Not anemic, not icteric No thyroid enlargement Chest Sym. expansion CBS $\bar{s}$ ⓡ RHB $\bar{s}$ ⓜ Abd Soft & flat Normal B.S No organomegaly No tender point Pelvic 2°degree uterine prolapse Imp) Prolapsed uteri (2°degree)	*Yoo*

등록번호	233 55 66	성별 F
성명	이 태 양	
주민등록	660508－1234567	

경 과 기 록
Progress Notes

일 자	내 용	서 명
8.30	〈 Resident Admission Note 〉 C.C　Protruding mass through the introitus 　　Frequency (Du : 25yrs) P.I　10년 전부터 상기 C/C로 내원 　　G5 P1 L1 D0 A4 at home delivery 　　Menopause : 48yr old 　　No DM,　No HT,　No pul. tbc 　　평소 anxiety & palpitation 있다고 함 　　No chest pain history P.E　V/S　stable 　　G/A　not so ill 　　　alert 　　　M/D/N 　　H/N　isocoria $\bar{c}$ L/R (+/+) 　　　not anemic 　　　not icteric 　　　supple neck 　　Chest　CBS $\bar{s}$ ⓡ 　　　RHB $\bar{s}$ ⓜ 　　Abdomen　soft 　　　not tender 　　　not distended 　　　audible B.S 　　　no palpable mass 　　Extr.　free 　　N/Ex　free 　　Pelvic exam. 　　　vag. outlet: markedly relaxed 　　　Ut. : small, displacement of ICUD 　　　Cx : atrophic 　　　Protruding to introitus 　　　　Imp) Prolapsed uteri 　　　　　Cystocele	R_1 *Seo*

경 과 기 록

일 자	내 용	서 명
8.30	〈 Chief pelvic exam. note 〉	
	Ut. : Subnormal sized, movable	
	Cx : Sl. eroded on both lip	
	Parous Os.	
	Imp) 1. Prolapsed uteri 2°	
	2. Cystocele	
	〈 Brief Op. Note 〉	
8.31	Op. time : 8.31 9 : 53 − 11 : 00	
	Pre−op Dx : Prolapsed uteri, cystocele & rectocele	
	Lt. ovarian cyst	
	Displacement of IUD	
	Post op. Dx : SAA	
	Op. name : VTH, A−P repair	
	Lt. oophorectomy	
	Removal of IUD	
	Operator : L.U. Lee	
	Assist : M.J. Seo, Q.U. Kim, P.U. Yoo	
	G/A, EBL, U/O – not check	
	Op. finding	
	Ut : small, protruded through introitus	
	Vaginal wall : relaxed, markedly	
	Rt. ovary : free	
	Lt. ovary : cyst visible	R_1 *Seo*
9.1	POD #1	
	V/S stable	
	Clear breathing sound	
	Pain Op. site	*Seo*

경 과 기 록

일 자	내 용	서 명
9.2	POD #2 Improve pain V/S stable Keep F－cath	*Yeo*
9.3	POD #3 B/T 37.6℃ Improve pain Diet change	*Yeo*
9.4	POD #4 Op wound infection : culture (+) Voiding sense (－)	*Yeo*
9.6	POD #6 Removal F－cath Wound dressing	*Yeo*
9.7	POD #7 Wound clear Self voiding (+)	*Yeo*

등록번호	233 55 66	성별	F
성명	이 태 양		
주민등록	660508－1234567		

수 술 기 록
Operation Record

Date: 2017년 8 월 31 일　　Surgeon: L.U.Lee
1st. Ass't: M.J. Seo　　2nd. Ass't.: Q.U.Kim
Scrud nurse:　　Circ nurse:

Preoperative diagnosis : Prolapse uteri, rectocele, cystocele
Lt. ovarian cyst

Postoperative diagnosis : S/A

Name of operation : VTH, vaginal A－P repair, Lt. oophorectomy

Findings

Uterus: small, protruded through the introitus.
Vaginal wall: moderately relaxed.
Lt. ovary: small cyst visible
Rt. ovary and both tubes: intact

Procedures

With the patient in the lithotomy position, under the general anesthesia the perineum was surgically prepared. And then Foley catheter was insertion.

A circular incision was made around the portion about 2cm from the external os and the vaginal wall elevated and dissected and the bladder was advanced.

And then the anterior peritoneal reflexation was entered and silk suture was placed on the anterior peritoneum for identification. And then the posterior peritoneal sac was opened between the uterosacral ligaments and sutured to the posterior vaginal wall with #1－0 CCG.

The uterosacral ligaments and cardial ligaments were clamped, cut, sutured and ligated with #1－0 CCG. The uterine vessels on either side were clamped divided, sutured and ligated with #1－0 CCG. And the uterine fundus was grasped with tenaculum and brought anteriorly and then the round ligaments were clamp, cut, sutured and ligated with #1－0 CCG. The right tube and ovarian ligament was clamped, cut, sutured and ligated with #1－0 CCG. The left infundivulopelvic ligament was clamped, cut, sutured and ligated with #1－0 CCG. And the relaxed anterior vaginal wall was dissected and vaginal mucosa was approximated with interrupted sutures of #2－0 CCG. Posterior repair was done as same method. The superficial perineal skin was repaired with #3－0 CCG.

Tissue of path : ☑ Yes ☐ No　　Drains
Dictated/Written by L.U.Lee　　Surgeon's signature *Seo*

등록번호	233 55 66	성별 F
성명	이 태 양	
주민등록	660508－1234567	

병리조직검사보고
Pathological Record

Postoperative diagnosis: Prolapse uteri
Name of operation: VTH, Lt. oophorectomy

Reports :

The specimen consists of an entire uterus, left cystic ovary, and several pieces of vaginal wall.
The uterus measures 6.5 x 3.0 x 2.0cm in size and 20g in weight.
The external os shows whitish and fine nodular appearance.
The endometrial cavity and endocervical canal measure 3.0cm and 2.0cm respectively.
The thickness of endometrium and myometrium measure 0.3cm and 0.8cm respectively.
Two sections from cervix, and two sections from endometrium and myometrium are embedded. Blocked in A & B.
The left ovary measures 5.0 x 4.0 x 1.5cm in size and 10gm in weight.
Yellowish Rochitansky tubercle shows multiple calcification.
Representative sections are embedded. Blocked in C & D.
The vaginal wall measure 5.0 x 1.0 x 0.3cm in the largest one.
Representative sections are embedded. Blocked in E.

Dx : Myometrium, no pathologic diagnosis, hysterectomy of endometrium, proliferative phase, hysterectomy of cervix, uterine, cervicitis, chronic with squamous metaplasia, hysterectomy of ovary, left, benign cystic teratoma, oophorectomy of vaginal wall, hyperkeratosis

Han

〈이 태 양〉

★ 이태양 차트를 읽고 맞는 것에 O표 하시오.

1 최종진단명이 Prolapse와 관련된 분류번호는?

① N81.2 ② N81.1 ③ N81.3
④ N81.4 ⑤ N81.9

2 환자의 내용과 옳지 않은 것은?

① 자궁의 무게는 20g이었다. ② 폐경시기는 48세이다.
③ 환자는 다뇨, 빈뇨의 증상이 있다. ④ 골반 신체조사 시 자궁경은 위축되고 부식되었다.
⑤ 발육과 영양상태는 적절하였다.

3 Cystocele, Rectocele에 대한 분류번호는?

① N81.1 ② 70.8 ③ 70.50 ④ 70.79 ⑤ 70.52

4 상기 환자의 임상검사와 방사선 검사에서 정상이 아닌 것은?

① LFT ② CBC ③ EKG
④ CXR ⑤ OT/PT

5 최종진단명에 추가될 수 있는 진단명의 분류번호가 맞게 조립된 것은?

가. B15.9 나. N87.9 다. N85.8 라. N72
마. F45.3 바. N94.8 사. F48.9

① 가, 사 ② 다, 라 ③ 마, 바
④ 나, 라 ⑤ 바, 사

6 자궁탈출에 대한 적절한 치료방법으로 옳은 것은?

① Manchester op. ② TAH. ③ Oophorostomy
④ Tubal ligation ⑤ Oophoropexy

7 과거병력에 대한 분류번호로 옳은 것은?

① 02.07 ② V03.1 ③ S02.0
④ V01.0 ⑤ V09.2

8 상기 환자의 ICUD에 대한 분류번호로 맞는 것은?

① Z30.1 ② Z30.5 ③ Z97.5
④ T83.3 ⑤ T83.6

9 환자의 난소의 상태를 잘 나타내는 분류번호는?

① C56.1 ② D07.3 ③ D27.1
④ D39.19 ⑤ C79.61

10 수술 후 합병증이 발생하였다. 이에 대해 맞게 짝지어진 것은?

① T81.4, Y60.0, B95.8 ② T85.8, Y65.2
③ T83.6, Y61.0, A49.0 ④ T81.4, Y62.0, B95.8
⑤ T81.4, Y62.0, A49.0

04 태아곤란증 동반 임신 43주

IUP at 43^{+4} wks c̄ fetal distress

1.1 전자간증(Pre-eclampsia)

▸ 임신 20주 이후에 발생되는 단백뇨, 부종을 동반한 고혈압, 시력장애

자간전증의 분류

▸ **경도 전자간증(mild pre-eclampsia):** O14.0
- 혈압상승(140/90 mmHg 이상)
- 체중증가(0.9kg 이상/week)
- 손과 안면 부종
- 무균배뇨검사결과 단백뇨(trace 또는 +)

▸ **중등도 전자간증(moderate pre-eclampsia):** O14.0

▸ **중증 전자간증(severe pre-eclampsia):** O14.1
- 혈압(160/110 mmHg 이상)
- 심한 단백뇨(3+ 또는 4+)
- 뇨량의 감소, 부종, 시력장애 초래

처 치

▸ 안정요법, 식이요법

▸ 체중측정, 뇨검사, 혈액검사, 수분섭취량 및 배설량 측정

▸ 진정제, 이뇨제, 혈압하강제 등의 약물요법과 수액요법

▸ 중증 자간전증은 진정제 사용

1.2 자간증(Eclampsia)

▸ 임신에 의해 발생

▸ 악화된 고혈압의 간헐적이고 강직성 경련인 급성질환

2.1 임신성 고혈압(Pregnancy induced hypertension; PIH)

- 단백뇨 혹은 부종이 없는 경우
- 단백뇨 혹은 부종이 있는 경우: 경도 자간전증, 중증 전자간증

2.2 Leopold's Maneuver

- 산모의 복부촉진으로 산전진찰 때마다 반복
- 제1수기~제4수기
- 태위, 태세, 태향, 골반진입, 여부하강정도여부 및 다태아 등 진단

2.3 Nitrazine test

- 양수인지의 여부를 가리는 리트머스 용지와 같은 산부인과에서 사용하는 검사지

표 1 • 임신기간 및 출생 시 체중

임신기간		출생 시 체중	
•37주 미만	조기(Pre-term)	•1,000g ~ 2,500g 미만	저체중 출산아(low birth weight)
•37주 이상 ~ 42주 미만	**정상(Term)**	**•2,500g ~ 4,500g 미만**	**정상아(mature infant)**
•42주 이상	주기 후(Post-term)	•4,500g 이상	예외적으로 큰 아기 (exceptionally Large baby)

표 2 • 산과 및 신생아의 비교

분 류	산 과	신생아*
•구분 용어 •질병분류번호 •필수분류번호	•분만(delivery) • 【 O 】 •분만결과: Z37.___(출생아/사산아) → 주의) IUP at 33weeks 임신 33주 (미분만 시 번호부여 안함)	•출생(born, birth) • 【 P 】 •출생: Z38.___ (병원내/병원외)
•37주 미만 •42주 이상 •2,500g 미만 •4,500g 이상	•조기분만(pre-term) : O60 •주기 후 (post-term) : O48 •체중미달(light-for-dates) : O36.5 •체중과다(large-for-dates) : O36.6	•조산아(pre-term) : P07.3** •만기 후(post-term) : P08.2 •체중미달(light-for-dates) : P05.1 •체중과다(large-for-dates) : P08.0

*신생아: 출생 ~ 4주(28일)이내
- 신생아 사망: 출생~28일(4주)이내 사망

**조산아(P07.3): 28주 ~ 37주 이하
- 주산기 사망: 임신 20주 이상+신생아 28일(4주 이내) → 사망

3.1 임신과 관련된 용어 비교

- 자궁내 임신(정상 임신부위): intrauterine pregnancy(IUP)
- 자궁내 기구, 피임기구: intrauterine device(IUD)

- 난관(자궁관) 임신(tubal pregnancy): 자궁외 임신(ectopic pregnancy) = 유산
- 난관(자궁관)결찰술(tubal ligation): 여성 불임술 ↔ 정관절제술(vasectomy): 남성 불임술

- 산욕기(puerperium): 분만 직후~6주 이내
- 산욕열(puerperal fever): 분만 24시간 후~10일 이내, 체온이 38℃ 이상 2번 올라감

3.2 산과 계산방법

- **분만예정일(Estimated date of confinement; EDC)**
  - 월(月): 최종월경일의 월수 + 9 또는 월수 − 3
  - 일(日): 최종월경일의 제1일 + 7

  예) 분만예정일의 계산

  최종월경일: 2017년 6월 24일 − 26일(계산 시 첫날 기준)

  → 6−3=3월 또는 6+9=15=3월(15월=12월/1년+3월)

  24+7=31일 [답: 분만예정일 2018년 3월 31일]

- **자궁저부 높이(Height of fundus; HOF)**
  - 자궁저부 높이(cm) × 2/7 = 임신월수
  - 자궁저부 높이(cm) × 8/7 = 임신주수

4.1 호흡곤란증후군(Respiratory distress syndrome; RDS)

- 일명 유리질막병(초자막 질환, hyaline membrane disease; HMD)
- 미숙아(premature)의 호흡기 문제
- 폐조직 내면의 단백질 결핍은 폐허탈(collaps of lung)의 원인

4.2 아프가 채점법(Apgar score; A/S): 총 10점

- 영아의 신체상태를 측정하는 점수제도
- 출산후 1분 후 또는 5분 후에 측정
  - 1분: 응급소생술, 5분: 태아의 사망률과 이환율
- 5개 항목
  - 심박동률(heart rate), 호흡(respiration), 색깔(color), 근육강도(muscle tone), 자극에 대한 반응(response to stimuli)
- 0~10점 부여
  - Apgar 점수가 낮은 신생아 진료 요구

4.3 태아감시(Fetal monitoring)

- 진통 중에 태아의 심박동률을 기록하는 전기기구를 이용

혼란 용어 비교

- elderly(초로의, 고령) - early(조; 早)
- nevus(모반; 피부/양성종양) - nervus(신경)
- cheilo(입술) - celio(복부=laparo) - chiro(손)
- hepatoma(간암) - hematoma(혈종)
- melanoma(흑색종; 피부/악성종양) - melena(혈변)
- hystero(자궁=uterus=metro) - history(병력)
- oozing(삼출/분비) - squeezing(짜내는)

4.4 질병분류상 주의점

제왕절개술(Cesarean section)

① **제왕절개분만의 종류**

- 선택적 제왕절개 분만(elective C/S): O82.0
  - 입원 전후에 미리 제왕절개분만이 예정
- 응급 제왕절개 분만(emergency C/S): O82.1
  - 제왕절개 분만이 예정되어 있지 않았음
  - 산모의 상태에 의해 제왕절개 분만
- 제왕자궁적출술(cesarean hysterectomy): O82.2
  - 자궁적출술과 제왕절개 분만이 동반

② **제왕절개술 진단 및 수술분류**

－수술명: Lower segment transverse C/S (자궁하부 제왕절개) 74.1(첫번째 제왕절개 분만)

－진단명: Previous C/S(이전 제왕절개술) O34.22
수술명: Repeated C/S(반복 제왕절개술) 74.1

▸ 산과: 분만, 미분만, 유산, 산욕기 → [O] 번호부여

예) 수술 후 열상 T81.2 Y60.0

제왕절개 중 방광 열상(bladder laceration) O71.5 Y60.0

차트 용어

· Dehiscence	터짐	· Elderly primipara	고령 초산부	· Nulliparous	미경산	· Oozing	삼출
· Presenting part	선진부	· Serous	장액의	· Squeeze	짜내다	· Uterine involution	자궁수복/회복

약 어	원 어	
AC	Abdominal circumference	복위
AFV	Amniotic fluid volume	양수량
A/S	Apgar score	아프가 채점법
BOW	Bag of water	양수낭
BST	Bedside testing	침상검사
EBL	Estimated blood loss	출혈손실 추정량
EDC	Estimated date of confinement	분만예정일
EFW	Estimated fetal weight	추정 태아체중
FBS	Fasting blood sugar	공복 시 혈당
FHT	Fetal heart tone	태아 심음
HOF	Height of fundus	(자궁)저부 높이
IUD	Intrauterine device: contraceptive	자궁내 기구: 피임기구
IUP	Intrauterine pregnancy	자궁내 임신(정상 임신부위)
LML	Left mediolateral(episiotomy)	좌측 중외측(회음절개술)
LMP	Last menstrual period	최종 월경일
N & A	Normal and active	정상활동
PIH	Pregnancy induced hypertension	임신성 고혈압
PMP	Previous menstrual period 예) LMP 마지막 생리일 3월 20일 PMP 직전 생리일 2월 20일	직전 월경일
PP	Presenting part	태위
RHB	Regular heart beat	정상 심박동
RML	Right mediolateral(episiotomy)	우측 중외측(회음절개술)
RUQ	Right upper quadrant	우상 1/4분획
WA	Ward ambulation	병동보행

등록번호	120 33 00	성별 F
성명	전 완 승	
주민등록	861126－1234567	

입 퇴 원 기 록
Admission and Discharge Record

주 소 : 전북 이리시

출신지 : **직 업** : **전 화** :

연고자성명 : 양수주 **관 계** : 주 소 : 전 화 :

입원 : 2017 년 12 월 3 일 과 병동 호	전과	20 년 월 일 과 병동 호
퇴원 : 2017 년 월 일 과 병동 호		20 년 월 일 과 병동 호
재원일수 :		20 년 월 일 과 병동 호

최종진단명	분 류 번 호
주진단명 : IUP at 43^{+4} weeks $\bar{c}$ fetal distress	
$\bar{c}$ severe pre－eclampsia	
기타진단명 : $\bar{c}$ elderly primipara	
$\bar{c}$ DM	
Wound dehiscence	
수술 및 처치명	
수술명 : Lower segment transverse c/section	
기타수술 및 주요검사	

치료결과 : 1. 완쾌 2. 경쾌 3. 호전안됨 4. 진단뿐 5. 가망없는 퇴원 6. 48시간내 사망 7. 48시간이후 사망

퇴원형태 : 1. 퇴원지시후 2. 자의퇴원 3. 탈원 4. 전원

병원감염 : 1. 수술후 2. 기타처치후 3. 비뇨기계 4. 호흡기계 5. 소화기계 6. 기타

원사인 : 부검 : 예, 아니오

계속적 진료 계획

없음·있음 (약속일 2017 년 12 월 17 일 시)

담당 전공의 서명 : 지승자	담당 전문의 서명 : 정동춘
의무기록 완성 : 2018 년 1 월 19 일	의무기록사 서명 : *Park*

임산부 입원기록

Admission Note of Obstetrics Patient

Unit No. ____________

Name 전 완 승 Age 31 Para 0−0−0−0 Registered, not Registered
Time of admission at 1: 50 am **pm** 12. 3 2017 Private Doctor ______________
Time of examination at 1: 50 am **pm** 12. 3 2017
LMP 2017. 2. 20 PMP ____________ EDC ____________ Duration of preg. ____________ Wks

Last Delivery Baby's size
Type Baby's condition Any abnormality
Position Baby's weight
Duration

Antepartum Course
Antepartum Care: **recieved**, not recieved uneventful or eventful
If eventful, describe in detail
Others

Labor symptoms prior to admission
Pain started at 5 am **pm** 12.2
Show at ________ am pm ________
Membrane ruptured spontaneously at ________ am pm ____________
Bleeding

Examination prior to admission by outside doctors (Yes, **No**)
When
Where
Diagnosis
Treatments (in detail)

Condition on admission
General condition B.P. 200/120 Pulse 98 / min Body weight 92 kg
Heart *NL* Lungs *NL* Height 160 cm
Pain character Urine alb. ______
Abdominal findings
H.O.F ________ cm A.C. ________ cm Pelvic Mensurations
F.H.T 140/min Fetal position : Cephalic •External pelvis
Internal examination Interspines Intercrests Intertrochanters
Cx: effacement PE B.D.
dilatation 1FB R. ob. _____ L. ob. _____
rigid or soft •Internal Pelvis
P.P. Vx C.D. __ Biischial __ Sacrum __
B.O.W. Coccyx ___ Ischial spines ___
Station −3 Pubic arch : Side walls :
Soft parts wide converg.
Other findings narrow parallel
ave diverg.
•Evaluation of pelvis

Impression
1. IUP at 43^{+4} wks
2. $\bar{c}$ pre. eclampsia
3. DM

Dispositions
1.
2.
3.

Doctor's sign 박숙우

퇴 원 요 약
Discharge Summary

Name : 전완승 Age : 31 Para : 0-0-0-0
Date of admission : 12.3 Date of discharge : 12.12
Date of delivery : 12.5 Duration of hospitalization
Discharge diagnosis : IUP at 43^{+4} wks $\bar{c}$ pre-eclampsia, DM
Presentation & Position : Cephalic (0) Breech ( ) Transverse ( )

Type of delivery :
1. Spontaneous
2. Forceps (Outlet, Low, Mid, High)
3. Vacuum extraction when the os dilated in cm. succeeded or failed.
4. Version & extraction
5. Breech extraction (Partial, Total)
6. Cesarean section (Classical, Extraperitoneal, Low cervical transverse or longitudinal)
7. Cesarean section plus hysterectomy (Total, subtotal)
8. Destructive procedure
9. Others

Episiotomy : ☐Yes ☑No Median ( ) R.M.L ( ) L.M.L.( ) Suture
Mode of placental delivery : Spontaneous ☐(Schultze, Duncan) Manual ☑
Laceration : Cervix, Vagina, Perineum (1st, 2nd, 3rd), sutured with silk or catgut
Stimulation ☐ Induction ☐
Analgesia & anesthesia : ☑Yes ☐No Type : General Drug :
Baby : 1. (single), twin, others 2. Sex : female 3. Wt. : 4.8
4. term, overterm, premature, immature 5. alive, dead(when why)
Placenta : Wt. 750 Size : normal, abnormal
Cord : (Normal) Abnormal Length : 47 cm
Complications : Mother ( ) Baby ( )
Total duration of labor : (3) hrs.
Estimated blood loss : 700 cc

Mother's condition	on admission	on discharge	
blood pressure	200/130	150/100	
edema	+	+	
visual disturbance	−	−	
eye ground	−	−	
urine protein		−	−
weight	−	−	
hemoglobin	12.4	11.3	

Present baby's condition : 1. discharge with mother ( ) remains in nursery ( )
2. Poor, fair, (good) Wt. 4.8 Length: 46.2

Recommendation :

등록번호	120 33 00	성별 F
성명	전 완 승	
주민등록	861126 − 1234567	

병 력 기 록
History

키(Height) : 체중(Weight) : 체온(T) : 맥박(P) : 호흡(R) : 혈압(B.P.) :

C/C : Amenorrhea for 43^{+4} wks
evaluation for PIH & DM

P/I : 상기 31세 nulliparous pt는 상기 c/c으로 delivery 위해 본원 admission

P/H : '15년 1월초 김내과에서 DM 진단받음

ROS : N − S

P/Ex : G/A well being
HEENT not anemic
not icteric
Chest CBS $\bar{s}$ ⓡ
RHB $\bar{s}$ ⓜ
Abd normoactive B.S
no tender point
B/Ext CVAT (−/−)
pitting edema (+/+)

Imp) IUP at 43^{+4} wks
$\bar{c}$ pre − eclampsia & DM

Int. 박 국 수

등록번호	120 33 00	성별 F
성명	전 완 승	
주민등록	861126 - 1234567	

경 과 기 록
Progress Notes

일 자	내 용	서 명
	〈 Admission Note 〉	
'17.12.3	C/C Amenorrhea for 43^{+4} wks Evaluation for PIH & DM	
	P/I 상기 31세 nulliparous woman은 early preg.부터 G.A 35wks까지 김철 OBGyn에서 antenatal care받았는데 elderly primigravida DM있어 큰 병원 recommend 받고 G.A 35wks에 본원 OBGyn OPD visit, 내원일('17.12.3)(GA 43^{+4} weeks) check한 BP. 150/90으로 높아 PIH & DM evaluation 위해 금일 OPD 거쳐 admission('17.11.9 내과에서 DM control 위해 admission recommend했으나 환자 개인사정으로 refuse) P/Hx '15.1월 external genitalia에 itching sensation있어 김철 OBGyn visit: DM evaluation recommend 받고 김내과 visit. DM 진단받고 weight & diet control 권유받음	
	OB (Mense Hx) Para: 0 - 0 - 0 - 0	
12.3	LMP : '17. 2. 20 PMP : '17 1월 Mense : R / 30d / 6 - 7d / profuse Dysmenorrhea : (-) Leukorrhea : scanty foul oder(±) Menarche : 18yr Marriage : '11 ROM (+) at '17/12/1 오후 Nitrazine test (+) Contraception : none PAP smear : '15 negative 김철 OBGyn. ROS : lower abd. pain (-) uterine contraction (-) dizziness (-) headache (-) RUQ or epigastric pain (- / -) dyspnea (-) blurred vision (+)	

경 과 기 록

일 자	내 용	서 명
12.3	P/Hx GA obesity (slightly): BW: 92kg V/S 200/130 − 90/min − 37℃ HEENT Normocephaly not anemic anicteric Chest: symm CBS $\bar{s}$ Ⓡ RHB $\bar{s}$ ⓜ Abd: HOF: 37cm AC: 110cm FHT: 150/min 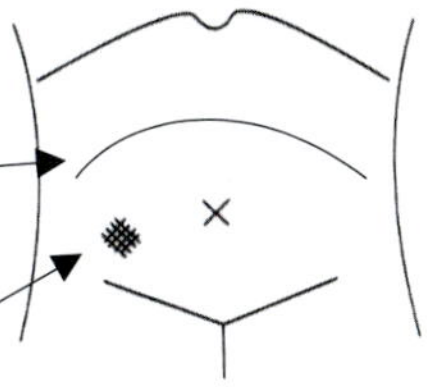 Back/Ext: CVA tenderness (−/−) Severe pre−tibial pitting edema (+/+) (Leopold's Maneuver) 1st: fundus에서 large. nodule body 촉진됨 2nd: Lt. site: Hard, resistant structure is felt (back) Rt. site: numerous nodulation were felt. 3rd: body was not movable → engaged 4th: Lt hand is arrested sooner than the other by a rounded body Rt. hand descends more deeply into the pelvis Imp) IUP at 43^{+4} wks $\bar{c}$ PIH $\bar{c}$ DM Plan) 1. ABR 2. BP control 3. BST monitoring 4. Fetal monitoring 5. Induction of labor Initial labs) Chest PA: no active lung lesion EKG: WNL CBC :13.2/39.1 − 9460 PLT: 252 x 10^3 UA: protein: trace BUN/Cr: SGOT / SGPT: 12/0.7 21/19 Pelvic sono) '17. 12. 3 P.P: Cephalic Pl: Lt. lat wall AFV: ample EFW: 2.832 kg	지승자

경 과 기 록

일 자	내 용	서 명
'17.12.5	〈 Brief op. note 〉 1. Op. name: Lower segment transverse c/section 2. Operator: Prof. 홍준구, 양호주, 이동수, 지승자 3. General epidural anesthesia 4. Pre. op. Dx.: IUP at 43^{+4} wks c̄ fetal distress c̄ severe pre－eclampsia c̄ elderly primipara c̄ DM 5. Post op. Dx: Same as above 6. Op. findings 1) Pfannenstiel skin incision 2) Uterus : Normal full term sized & grossly free 3) Lower segment transverse uterine incision 4) Amniotic fluid, thick meconium stained 5) Female 4.8kg 46.2cm fetus was delivered c̄ cephalic presentation at 8 : 06 AM (AS 5 → 8) 6) Placenta : "M" removal defect 7) Immediate postpartum uterine contraction : good 8) Both adnexa & other pelvic organs : grossly free 9) EBL : 1000 cc 10) Cx : none	지승자
12.7	〈 POD #2 〉 S : gas out (+) self voiding (－) breast pain (+) headache (－) blurred vision (－) O : V/S : 140/90 － 88/min － 37.8℃ Breast : tenderness (+) enlargement (+) Abd. : Op. wound: clear CBC : 11.6/34.6 － 16990 c̄ PLT : 195 x 10^3 UA, protein trace glucose (－)	지승자

경 과 기 록

일 자	내 용	서 명
12.7	P : 1. Breast massage & expression of milk → Bromocriptine medication 2. Keep foley cath. 3. Hydration 4. Apply ice pack 5. BP control 6. General measures 7. FBS & PP 2hrs check 8. DM diet 1600 cal #4	지승자
12.9	〈 POD #4 〉 S : headache (−) blurred vision (−) O : V/S: 140/90 − 86/min − 36.6℃ Breast: enlargement (−) abd.: op. wound serous oozing overlaping suture site 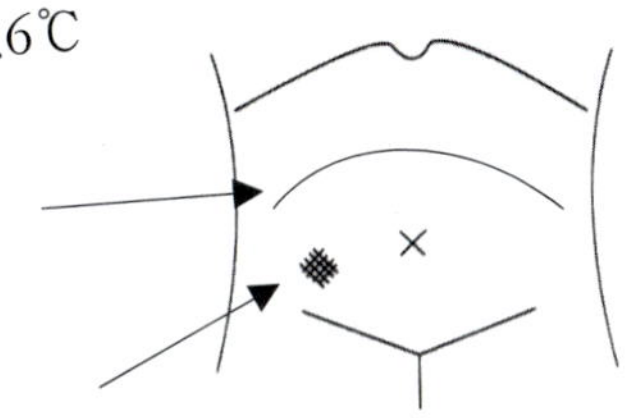 P : 1. wound dressing 2. B.P. control 3. W.A	지승자
12.10	〈 POD #5 〉 S : Op. wound pain (+) O : V/S 150/90 − 88/min − 36.6℃ Abd. op wound : serous discharge (+) → squeezing & dressing CBC : 11.3/34.6− 10950 UA : protein trace 10−29 WBC / HPF P : 1. Apply hot pack on lower abdomen 2. Wound dressing 3. General measures 4. BST monitoring	지승자

경 과 기 록

일 자	내 용	서 명
12.12	〈 Discharge note 〉 1. Post op. course : uneventful 2. Uterine involution : good 3. Op. wound: wound dehiscence 4. Labs CBC : 11.3/34.6 − 10950 UA : protein trace VDRL : N−R HBsAg/Ab : −/+ Bun/cr SGOT/SGPT : 12/0.7 21/19 FBS PP 2hrs 5. Cx. wound dehiscence 6. NA 2weeks later 7. recommend : General measures	지승자

등록번호	120 33 00	성별 F
성명	전 완 승	
주민등록	861126-1234567	

협의진료기록
Consultation Record

Request For Consultation To Dr. 내과 맹준무 선생님께

Summary of Present Findings

상기 산모는 IUP at 43^{+4}weeks $\bar{c}$ PIH, DM으로 Induction of labor 중입니다 '17. 11. 9, '17. 11. 14 선생님께서 OPD에서 consult 보셨던 산모로 DM control 에 대해 consult드리오니 고진선처 바랍니다. 감사합니다.

2017. 12. 4 a.m.
Date Hour p.m.

Prof. 유도민/지승자 M.D.
Signature of Attending Physician

Report of Consultation

Opinion and Recommendation

〈 Dept of IM 〉

현재 혈당은 C/S에 문제 없습니다.
현재대로 manage하시고 수술 시에는 BST monitoring하여 주십시오.
delivery 후 다시 F/U시켜 주십시오.

2017. 12. 4
Date Hour

맹준무 M.D.
Signature of Attending Physician

등록번호	120 33 00	성별 F
성명	전 완 승	
주민등록	861126-1234567	

협의진료기록
Consultation Record

〈 내과 맹준무 선생님께 〉

선생님께서 보셨던 산모입니다.
금일 fetal distress있어 emergency c/section 했습니다.
follow up consult 드리오니 고진선처 바랍니다.
감사합니다.
* 현재 severe pre-eclampsia로 $MgSO_4$ mixed fluid (25gtt/min) infusion 중입니다.

2017. 12. 5 Prof. 유도민/지승자

〈 Dept of IM 〉

현재 혈당은 문제 없으며 non-DM 환자에 준해서 manage하십시오.
($\bar{c}$ BST × 4/day)
환자 oral intake 시작되고 stable해지면 FBS/min F/U시켜 주십시오.
감사합니다.

2017. 12. 5 맹준무 M.D.

Date Hour Signature of Attending Physician

등록번호	120 33 00	성별 F
성명	전 완 승	
주민등록	861126－1234567	

협의진료기록
Consultation Record

Request For Consultation To   Dr. 내과 맹준무 선생님께

Summary of Present Findings

for follow up
선생님께서 보셨던 산모입니다.
현재 DM diet 1600 cal #4 1day 중입니다.
FBS : 136 ┐
PP 2hrs : 268 ┘ 입니다.
follow up consult 부탁드리오니 고진선처 바랍니다.

2017. 12. 9   a.m.
Date   Hour p.m.

Prof. 유도민/지승자 M.D.
Signature of Attending Physician

Report of Consultation

Opinion and Recommendation

〈 Dept of IM 〉

Daonil $\frac{1}{2}$ⓣ #1 po ac 30' (at morning)으로 주시고 3일 후 FBS/PPh
F/U하여 주십시오.
감사합니다.

2017. 12. 9
Date   Hour

맹준무 M.D.
Signature of Attending Physician

등록번호	120 33 00	성별 F
성명	전 완 승	
주민등록	861126－1234567	

응급검사
Emergency Laboratory

검 체: Serum

발행일시: 171021 보고자: 성동유 보고일시: 171021 1521

검 사	결 과	정상 범위	단 위
Glucose	170	70 － 110	
BUN	9	7 － 25	
Creatinine	0.8	0.7 － 1.7	
Na	134.4	135 － 145	
K	3.8	3.5 － 5.5	
CI	104.5	98 － 110	
Color	yellow	0 － 0	
Sg	1.020	1.003 － 1.03	
PH(UA)	5.0	5 － 8	
Protein(UA)	3 positive	0 － 0	
Glucose(UA)	negative	negative	
Ketone(UA)	1 positive	negative	
Urobilinogen	10X	0 － 0	
Bile	negative	negative	
Blood	3 positive	negative	
Nitrite	negative	negative	
Micro scopy			
Micro1	many RBC	0 － 0 /HPF	
Micro2	1－4 WBC	0 － 0 /HPF	

검 체: Serum

발행일시 : 171021 보고자 : 성동유 보고일시 : 171021 1631

검 사	결 과	정상 범위	단 위
Na	140.6	135 － 145	
K	4.5	3.5 － 5.5	
CI	106.1	98 － 110	

등록번호	120 33 00	성별 F
성명	전 완 승	
주민등록	861126－1234567	

수 술 기 록
Operation Record

Date: 2017년 12월 5일 Surgeon: 홍준구
1st Ass't: 양호주 2nd. Ass't.: 이동수
Scrud nurse: Circ nurse:

Preoperative diagnosis : IUP at 43^{+4} wks with fetal distress
severe pre－eclampsia
elderly primipara
DM

Postoperative diagnosis: S/A

Name of operation : Lower segment transverse C－section

Findings and Procedures

1. Pfannenstiel skin incision & scar revision.
2. Uterus: Normal full term sized and grossly free.
3. Lower segment transverse uterine incision
4. Amnionic fluid: clear
5. Female 4.8kg, 46.2cm fetus was delivered with cephalic presentation at 8:06 am A/S 5 at 1 minute and 8 at 5 minute.
6. Placenta: Manual removal without defect
7. Immediate postpartum uterine contraction: Good
8. Repair of the uterus :
   1) Inner layer: Running suture with 1－0 CCG.
   2) Outer layer: Running suture with 2－0 CCG.
   3) Pelvic peritoneum: Running suture with 1－0 CCG.
9. Both adnexae and other pelvic organs: Grossly free.
10. Repair of the abdominal wall :
    1) Peritoneum: Running suture with 1－0 CCG.
    2) Rectus muscle: Running suture with 1－0 CCG.
    3) Rectus fascia: Running suture with 1－0 Vicryl.
    4) Subcutaneous tissue: Interrupted suture with No.3 silk.
    5) Skin: Subcuticular suture with 3－0 Prolene.
11. E.B.L.: About 800cc
12. Complication: Absent

Tissue of path.: Yes ☐ No ☑ Drains Yes ☐, No ☑
Dictated/Written by 지승자 Surgeon's signature 홍준구

〈전 완 승〉

★ 전완승 차트를 보고 맞는 답에 O표 하시오.

1 **환자의 입원시 상태와 관계가 없는 것은?**

① 시력장애를 호소하였다. ② 하지에 심한 부종이 있었다.
③ pap smear 검사시 단백질이 발견되었다. ④ 혈압이 200/130으로 높았다.
⑤ 복부둘레는 110cm였다.

2 **상기 환자는 Emergency c/section 하였다. 그 이유는?**

① 중증의 전자간증 ② fetal distress ③ DM
④ early primigravida ⑤ PIH

3 **내과에 협의한 결과 얻어지는 진단명을 옳게 분류한 것은?**

① O24.9 ② O24.3 ③ O24.4
④ E14.79 ⑤ E11.9

4 **환자가 C-section하던 중 bladder laceration이 되었다면 이에 맞는 분류번호는?**

① O71.5, Y60.0 ② T81.2, Y60.0 ③ S37.21, Y60.9
④ O71.5, Y65.2 ⑤ O71.5, Y62.0

5 **Leopold's Maneuver란 무엇인가?**

① 양수강내에 조영 물질을 주입하여 태아의 상태와 태반의 위치를 확인한다.
② 분만과정으로 제1기에서 제3기로 분류한다.
③ 태아와 태반의 병적 상태를 직접 관찰하고 생검과 태아의 적혈구를 채취하여 진단한다.
④ 산모의 복부촉진으로 태위, 태세 및 골반진입 등 산전진찰 때마다 반복한다.
⑤ 영아의 신체상태를 측정하는 점수제도이다.

6 **경과기록 내용과 관계가 없는 것은?**

① '15년 1월 local 산부인과에서 DM 진단받고 체중과 운동을 권유받았다.
② Pelvic sono한 결과 presenting part가 두위였다.
③ 수술 후 4일째 수술부위에 장액이 분비되어 다음날 squeezing하였다.
④ 자궁의 위치가 제자리로 복고되고 있다.
⑤ 12월 1일 오후에 Nitrazine test를 하였다.

7 **수술건수와 재원일수가 맞게 짝지어진 것은?**

① 1건, 9일 ② 2건, 9일 ③ 1건, 11일
④ 2건, 11일 ⑤ 1건, 10일

8 주진단명과 기타 진단명들을 옳게 분류한 것은?

a. O36.6	b. O14.1	c. Z35.5	d. O68.1	e. O33.5
f. O48	g. P20.9	h. O11	i. O75.0	j. P08.0

① a, b, c, d, e ② a, b, c, f ③ c, d, g, h, i
④ a, c, e, g, i ⑤ c, e, g, j

9 환자의 수술한 부위가 dehiscence되었다. 옳게 분류한 것은?

① T81.3, Y65.2 ② T81.0, Y60.0 ③ O90.0, Y65.2
④ O90.1, Y65.2 ⑤ O90.0, Y60.0

10 주수술명을 옳게 분류한 것은?

① 74.99 ② 74.1, 86.59 ③ 74.99, 86.59
④ 74.1 ⑤ 74.91

05 난소암 Ovarian cancer

1.1 난소암(Ovarian cancer)

- 난소의 악성종양: C56
- 높은 치사율
- 복부 덩어리(mass)로 진전된 단계에서 발견 - 초기 무증상
- 진단 시 골반을 지나 전이
- 전이성 암: Krukenberg's tumor → M8490/6, C79.69(난소의 속발성)
- 치료: 난소 및 난관(자궁관)절제술, 화학요법, 방사선요법

표 1 • 난소종양(Ovarian tumor)*의 분류

낭포성 종양(Cystic ovarian tumor)	충실성 종양(Solid ovarian tumor)
• 대부분 양성: 6배 많음 • 낭선종 – 장액성 낭선종(serous cystadenoma) – 점액성 낭선종(mucinous cystadenoma)	• 양성(20%): 섬유종(fibroma), 협막세포종 • 악·양성중간(20%) – 과립협막세포종 – 미분화세포종(dysgerminoma) • 악성(60%) – 낭선종 암종 ‣ 장액성 낭포선암종(serous cystadenocarcinoma) ‣ 점액성 낭포선암종(mucinous cystadenocarcinoma) – 악성기형종(malignant teratoma) – 태아성암(embryonal carcinoma) – 융모막암종(choriocarcinoma): 장기(placenta, 태반) – 전이성 암

*난소종양(ovarian tumor)=브레너 종양(Brenner tumor)

난소암의 병기분류

- **Stage I: 난소에 국한된 종양**

  – Ia: **한쪽** 난소에 국한(무복수, 난소평면에 종양이 없음, 피막 깨끗)

  – Ib: **양쪽** 난소에 국한(무복수, 난소평면에 종양이 없음, 피막 깨끗) - Ia 동일

  – Ic: Ia기나 Ib기(난소 표면에 종양, 피막 파열, 복수, 복강내 세척으로 악성세포)

▶ **Stage II: 골반내 전이, 한측 또는 양측 난소에 국한된 종양**

- IIa: 자궁 혹은 난관으로 전이
- IIb: 다른 골반조직으로 전이
- IIc: IIa 또는 IIb(난소표면에 종양, 피막 파열, 복수, 복강내 세척으로 악성세포) - Ic 동일

▶ **Stage III: 한쪽 또는 양쪽 난소의 종양이 골반을 넘어 복강내로 전이, 후복막 또는 서혜부 임파절에 양성**

▶ **Stage IV: 원격전이, 한쪽 또는 양측 난소 종양**

표 2 • 종양표지자(Tumor Marker)

검사항목	정상치	질 환
CA-125	35U/ml 이하	• 난소암, 자궁경부암, 자궁내막염
CA19-9	37U/ml 이하	• 소화기암: 위암, 직장암, 췌장암, 담도암

1.2 화학요법(Chemotherapy) 분류번호

▶ 세포독성 약물치료(cytotoxic drug therapy) 99.25

어휘

복막(Peritoneum)

- 벽측복막과 장측복막으로 구분(이 사이의 공간이 복막강)
- 복막의 변형
  - 장간막(mesentery), 결장간막(mesocolon), 대망(greater omentum)

소망(Lesser omentum)

- 위와 십이지장의 두장막층이 합쳐진 것
- 간으로부터 십이지장을 분리

대망(Greater omentum)

- 위의 장막층이 형성하는 주름
- 소장(작은창자)와 횡행(가로)결장의 전면을 덮음
- 후복벽의 벽측복막에 부착

2.1 자궁근종(Myoma of uterus): 유섬유종(Fibroids)

▶ 정의: 자궁내의 양성종양

▶ 발생부위: 장막하조직(subserosal), 벽내의(intramural), 점막하조직(submucosal)

▶ 치료: 근종절제술(myomectomy), 자궁적출술(hysterectomy)

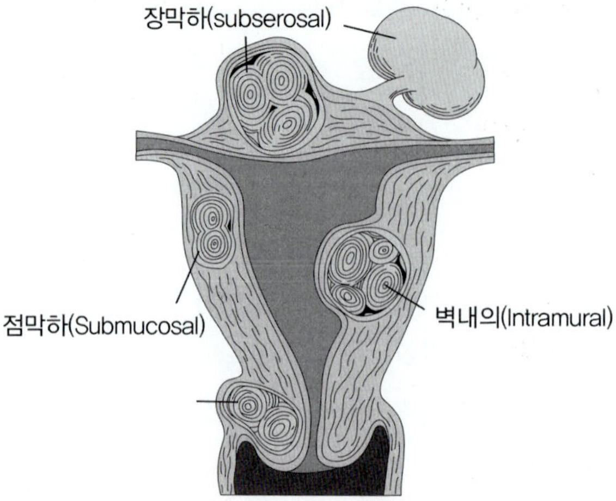

그림 1. 유섬유종(fibroids)

2.2 자궁내막증식증(Endometriosis)

- **정의:** 자궁내막조직이 비정상적인 부위에서 발견
  - 비정상적 부위: 난소, 맹낭(막힌주머니, cul-de-sac), 골반 복막, 소장
- **증상:** 월경통, 골반통, 불임증, 이상 성감증(dyspareunia)
- **원인:** 자궁내막 조각이 자궁관의 입구(lumen)를 통하여 복강내로 역류되어 들어감
- **치료:** 통증완화 및 월경주기 조절약제, 자궁내막 조직의 외과적 절제

3.1 유방암(Breast cancer)

- **정의:** 유선(milk glands)과 유관(milk ducts)에서 발생하는 악성종양
- **전이순서:** 인접한 겨드랑이(axilla)의 임파절 → 피부 → 흉벽(가슴벽, chest wall)
- **림프절 전이 시:** 뼈, 간, 폐 및 뇌 등의 장기로 전이 용이

유방암의 진단

- **방사선 및 초음파 검사**
  - 무증상 및 병변이 미세한 초기
  - 유방촬영술(mammography), 초음파검사, 진찰소견
  - 90% 진단 가능
- **미세침을 이용한 세포암 검사(fine needle aspiration cytology)**
  - 병변이 의심되는 부위에 주사침을 찔러 넣어 세포를 흡입하여 검사

▶ **조직생검(biopsy)**

- 의심되는 부위의 종괴나 조직을 국소 또는 전신마취하에 제거
- 동결조직검사를 통해 확진

수술방법

▶ **덩어리 절제술(lumpectomy)**

- 종양이 작은 경우
- 덩어리(lump)를 제거하고 유방은 남겨두는 수술
- 방사선요법 병행: 수술 후 잔여 종양세포 소멸

▶ **단순 또는 유방전절제술(simple or total mastectomy)**

- 유방전체를 제거하는 수술
- 겨드랑이 림프절 절제: 유방의 전이여부 파악

▶ **변형조치유방절제술(modified radical mastectomy)**

- 유방, 임파절 및 인접한 흉벽의 근육(pectorals)을 절제하는 수술
- 겨드랑이 림프절의 종양 발견 시: 약물치료 병행(재발방지)

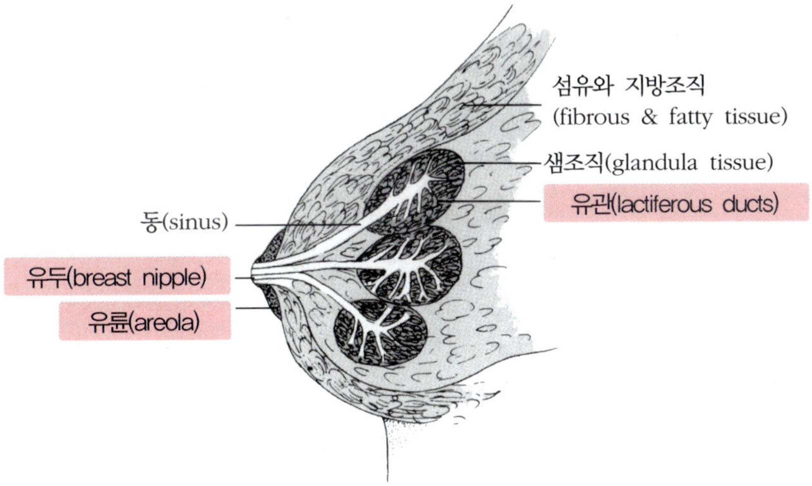

그림 2. 유방의 구조

출산력(Parity)

$$2 - 0 - 1\left[\begin{smallmatrix}0\\1\end{smallmatrix}\right. - 2\left[\begin{smallmatrix}1\\1\end{smallmatrix}\right.$$

분만력 조산 유산 생존아

- 임신력: 유산(1) + 생존아(2) = 3번

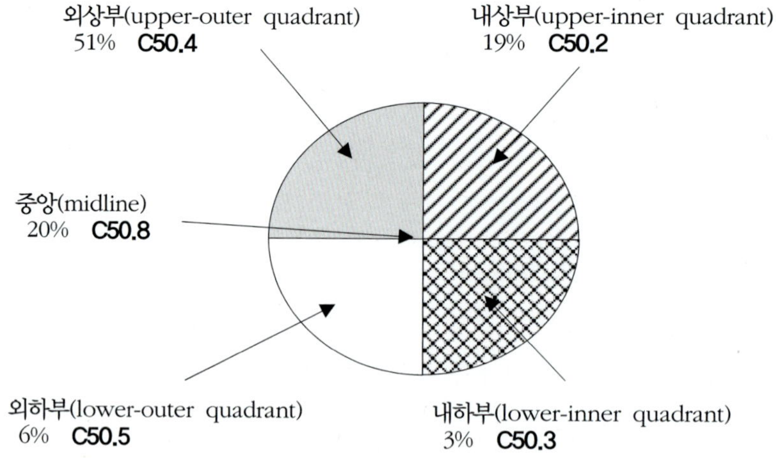

그림 3. 유방암 발생부위 (C50.__)

차트 용어									
·Abscess	농양	· Adhesion	유착	· Antibiotic	항생제	· Ascites	복수	· Bladder	방광
·Disinfection	소독	· Exercise	운동	· Infection	감염	· Inguinal	서혜부의	· Injury	손상
·Mammography	유방 촬영술	· Obstruction	폐색	· Peritonitis	복막염	· Retro-peritoneal	후복막의	· Transfusion	수혈
·Tubal	난관/자궁관 = salpingo = fallopian tube = uterine tube							· Ureter	요관

약 어	원 어	
BSO	Bilateral salpingo-oophorectomy	양측 난관(자궁관)-난소절제술
CA-125	Tumor marker	종양표지자: 암 진단사용
	‣ 상피성 난소암에서 증가하는 항원(정상치: 2~48U/ml)	
CEP	Cyclolphosphamide, epirubicin, cisplatin	복합 항암화학요법
DAMA	Discharge against medical advice	자의퇴원
GY	Gynecology	부인과
LOS	Length of stay	재원일수/단입법
	‣ 퇴원일–입원일	
NFSD	Normal forcep spontaneous delivery	정상 겸자분만
PCDS	Para cul-de-sac(space)	맹낭(막힌주머니) 주위(공간)
TAH	Total abdominal hysterectomy	전체복부 자궁절제술
T/L	Tubal ligation	난관(자궁관) 결찰
WNL	Within normal limits	정상범위내의

등록번호	130 22 66	성별 F
성명	한 승 리	
주민등록	710103－1234567	

입 퇴 원 기 록
Admission and Discharge Record

주 소 : 서울시 강남구 대치동 12－1				
출신지 :	**직 업** :	**전 화** :		
연고자성명 : 주기진	**관 계** :	주 소 :	전 화 :	
입원 : 2017 년 11월 14 일 OB/GY 과 3 병동 2 호	전과	20 년 월 일 과 병동 호		
퇴원 : 2017 년 11월 24 일 OB/GY 과 3 병동 2 호		20 년 월 일 과 병동 호		
재원일수:		20 년 월 일 과 병동 호		

최종진단명	**분 류 번 호**
주진단명 : Ovarian Cancer Ic	
기타진단명	
수술 및 처치명	
수술명 : TAH $\bar{c}$ BSO	
기타수술 및 주요검사 :	

치료결과 : 1. 완쾌 2. 경쾌 3. 호전안됨 4. 진단뿐 5. 가망없는 퇴원 6. 48시간내 사망 7. 48시간이후 사망	
퇴원형태 : 1. 퇴원지시후 2. 자의퇴원 3. 탈원 4. 전원	
병원감염 : 1. 수술후 2. 기타처치후 3. 비뇨기계 4. 호흡기계 5. 소화기계 6. 기타	
원사인 :	부검 : 예, 아니오
계속적 진료 계획	
없음있음 (약속일 년 월 일 시)	
담당 전공의 서명 : 이장승	담당 전문의 서명 : 윤축복
의무기록 완성 : 2017 년 11 월 26 일	의무기록사 서명 :

등록번호	130 22 66	성별 F
성명	한 승 리	
주민등록	710103－1234567	

퇴 원 요 약
Discharge Summary

Final dx : Rt. abd. tumor

C.C : Rt. abd. tumor

Brief Hx :

1. 2017. 11. lower abd, discomfort & fullness (+)
   → Local OB & Gyn. visit
   USG : pelvic mass R/O ovary, malignancy
   ∅ 10.4 x 8 x 6.8
2. 2017. 11. 7 our hospital pf 윤축복 OPD visit
   CA － 125 〉 439
3. Explo － lapa 위해 adm.

Hospital course :

1. 2017. 11. 15 Op.
   Operator : Pf 윤축복
   Op name : TAH $\bar{c}$ BSO
   Anesthesia : General
   Op findings : skin : low middline incision
   peritoneal cavity : adh (+), ascites ≒ 300cc (bloody)
   ut : AVF. sl enlarged : movable
   adhesion to Rt. ov. mass
   Adn : Rt. ovary : over goose egg sized
   solid & cystic cancerous mass
   ruptured
   Lt. ovary : hen's egg sized, irregular
   margin mass
   L/N : impalpable
   omentum, liver surface bladder: free
   Appe : free (Not done)

Dr.'s Signature *Lee*

퇴 원 요 약

일 자	내 용	서 명
	Patho : papillary serous cystadeno Ca. Bilat. ovary Grade II/III $\bar{c}$ extracapsular extension Ut. : chronic cervicitis peritoneal cytology : papillary adeno ca. metastatic 2. 2017. 11. 17 : CBC : 16600－12.0－280 K 3. 2017. 11. 21 : CBC : 8400－12.0－333 K Mammo 〉 WNL 4. 2017. 11. 23 : CEP #1 BSA : 1.67m^3 cyclophosphamide : 1000mg Epirubicin : 100mg cisplatin : 83.5mg 5. 2017. 11. 24 : postchemo lab CBC : 8600(87.9%)－11.5－351 K OT/PT : 22/25 BUN/Cr : 8/0.7 6. 2017. 11. 24 : Discharge $\bar{c}$ Uneventful Rec) OPD f/u Prechemo. lab	*Lee*

등록번호	130 22 66	성별 F
성명	한 승 리	
주민등록	710103－1234567	

경 과 기 록
Progress Notes

11.14 〈 Admisson note 〉

A : 46

P : 2－0－ 1 ┐ 0 － 2 ┐ 1
　　　　　　┘ 1　　　┘ 1

LMP : 2016, 11. 7

PMP : Ⓡ

LD : ‘03 NFSD

T/L : 12 years ago

C.C Rt. abd. tumor

PHx 1. Prev. healthy

2. 2 M ago lower abd. discomfort & fullness (+)

→ local visit (송기영 OB & Gyn)

USG : Pelvic mass ovary tumor

R/O malignancy (¢ 10.4 x 8 x 6.8cm)

3. 11. 7 our hospital pf. 윤축복 OPD visit

CA－125 〉 439

4. Explo－lapa. 위해 adm.

PMHx DM (－), Tbc (－), HT (－)

OP Hx (－)

FHx

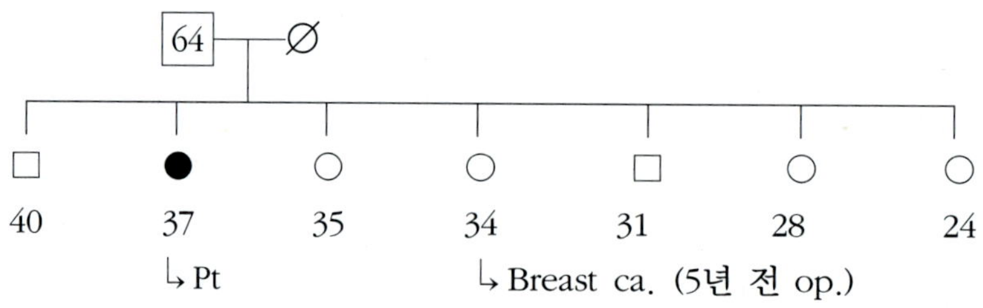

경 과 기 록

일 자	내 용	서 명
S.R	headache (−), dizziness (−), fever (−), chill (−) dyspnea (−), palpitation (−), cough (−), sputum (−) epigastric pain (−) A/N/V/D/C/M (−/−/−/−/−/−) oliguria (−) freg (−) reddish urine (−)	
P.E	G/A : alert intact V/S : 130/90−80−36.4℃ HEENT : Normo ceph. $\bar{s}$ scar L/R (++/++) isocoric prompt. not anemic, anicteric Chest : symm. exp. $\bar{s}$ retraction RHB $\bar{s}$ ⓜ CBC $\bar{s}$ ⓡ Abd. : soft. flat T/RT (−/−) B.S : OK Back & Extr. : CVAT (−/−) P/C/C (−/−/−) Gyn. exam : Ut. : AVF n.s movable, nontender Adn : Rt − large first sized cystic mass sl. tender. not movable Lt − neg. Cx : NS, NE Ass : Rt abd. tumor R/O malignancy Plan : explo−lapa.	*Lee*

경 과 기 록

일 자	내 용	서 명
11.15	〈 Op note 〉	
	Operator : Pf 윤춘복	
	Op name : TAH $\bar{c}$ BSO	
	$\bar{c}$ omental Bx.	
	Pop. Dx : Ovarian Ca. Ic	*Lee*
11.17	POD #2	
	S : G/O (+)	
	self voiding : well	
	O : V/S – stable	
	Wound : clear, well adapted	
	CBC : 16600 – 12.0 – 280 K	
	V/D : (–)	
	A : POD #2 doing well	
	P : R – care	
	chemo Tx.	R1 *Lee*
11.19	POD #4	
	S : No specific complaints	
	O : V/S : stable	
	Wound : Clear, well adapted	
	Patho : papillary serous cystadeno ca.	
	bilat. ovary, grade II/III	
	$\bar{c}$ extracapsular extension	
	V/D : (–)	
	Breast exam : No mass palpable	
	A : POD #4 doing well	
	P : 1. Wound dressing	
	2. Chemo Tx	
	Washing cytology 〉 metastatic adeno ca.	*Lee*

경 과 기 록

일자	내용	서명
11.21	POD # 6 S : No specific complaints O : V/S : stable Wound : clear well adapted CBC : 8400 − 12.0 − 333 K V/D : (−) Breast exam : No palpable mass A : POD #6 doing well P : S/O tomorrow	*Lee*
11.22	POD #7 S : No specific complaints O : V/S : stable S/O : was done Wound : well adapted Mammo 〉 WNL A : POD #7 doing well P : CEP #1 tomorrow	*Lee*
11.23	POD #8 (CEP #1〈 D1〉) S : No specific complaints nausea : (−), vomiting : (−) O : V/S : stable A : POD #8 CEP #1 〈 D1 〉 P : Post chemo. lab. tomorrow & discharge	*Lee*
11.24	〈 D2 〉 S : Nausea (−), Vomiting (−) O : V/S : stable RHB $\bar{s}$ ⓜ CBC $\bar{s}$ ⓡ A : POD #9 CEP #1 〈D2〉 P : discharge $\bar{c}$ prechemo lab OPD F/U R1 *Lee*	

등록번호	130 22 66	성별 F
성명	한 승 리	
주민등록	710103－1234567	

Chemotherapy Flow Sheet for Gyn. Malig. & TRO

Dx. (stage): Ovary ca. Ic Ht. 164cm

Wt. 68kg B.S: 1.67m³

Date/Mo/Yr	11. 23								
Regimen(#/cycle)									
CEP									
cyclphospamide									
epirubicin									
cisplatin									
Transfusion									
Antibiotics									
Analgesics									
Pain									
Bleeding									
Infection									
N/V									
Mouth									
G.I.									
Skin/Hair									
Eye/Ear									
Pulmonary									
Urinary									
Hb/Hct									
WBC									
Platelet									
BUN/Cr									
SGOT/SGPT									
β－HCG									
Chest X－ray									
Radiation									
Surgery									

등록번호	130 22 66	성별 F
성명	한 승 리	
주민등록	710103 - 1234567	

방사선 검사 보고서
X - Ray Report

11. 21 Mammography

No focal masses or clustered microcalcifications
are visible

결 론 : There is no specific mammographic evidence of malignancy

판독의사 : 현명인

등록번호	130 22 66	성별 F
성명	한 승 리	
주민등록	710103 – 1234567	

수 술 요 청 서

환자성명: 이승진

수술 또는 검사: explolaparotomy

본인은 본인(또는 상기환자)에게 행하여질 수술, 검사 및 이에 수반되는 바의 필요성과 그 내용, 의학상 일반적으로 예상되는 합병증과 후유증에 대하여 금일 (윤축복) 의사로부터 자세한 설명을 들었으며, 본 수술, 검사로써 불가항력적이거나 일반적으로 야기될 수도 합병증 또는 후유증, 환자의 특이체질로 인한 우발 사고가 있다는 것을 충분히 이해하면서 귀병원에 상기 수술 또는 검사를 실시하여 줄 것을 본 서면으로 요청하며 이에 따른 일반적인 후유증이나 합병증에 대하여 민 · 형사상의 제소 또는 이의를 제기하지 않을 것을 자필서명, 날인으로 서약합니다.

2017. 11. 14

* 환자, 친권자 또는 보호자 *

과 명 : 산부인과

주 소 : 서울시 송파구 잠실동

의사명 : 윤축복

성 명 : 서남우

* 입 회 자 *

주 소 : 서울시 송파구 잠실동

성 명 : 서남우

* 미성년자이거나 환자가 심신의 장애로 본인 서명이 불가능할 때에는 친권자나 보호자가 서명한다.

병 원 장 귀하

수술기록요청서

내 용
6시간 ↓ 2시간 30분~3시간 ↓ 2시간 ↓ 병실 마취 전신마취 ↳ 약 부작용 : 쇼크, 두드러기 기도 손상 > 이빨 마취지속 1. Blood → transfusion 2. Infection → peritonitis, abscess antibiotic disinfection 3. Adhesion → exercise 4. Bladder, ureter injury 5. Intestinal adhesion, intestinal obstruction 수술시도 끝 조직검사 양성 ⇒ 조직 악성

등록번호	130 22 66	성별	F
성명	한 승 리		
주민등록	710103-1234567		

수술전 처치 및 간호상태 확인표

2017년 11월 15일

도착시간 ______ 수술예정 방번호 18

확 인 내 용	간 호 단 위			수 술 부		
	예	아니오	해당무	예	아니오	해당무
환자확인	+			∨		
수술서약서	+			∨		
수술전 투약	+			none		
의치, 의안, 안경, 콘택트렌즈 제거	+			∨		
장신구 제거(핀, 반지, 시계, 목걸이, 귀걸이)	+			∨		
화장제거(입술, 볼연지, 매니큐어 등)	+			∨		
환의만 입힌다(속옷 제거)	+			∨		
혈액학적 검사	+			∨		
뇨검사	+			∨		
유치카데터 삽입		+			∨	
심전도	+			∨		
금식	+			∨		
수술부위 피부 준비	+			∨		
위관 삽입		+	−		∨	
알러지(약물, 반창고 등)	유	무		유	무	
Embossing Card	유	무		유	무	
간호사 서명						

등록번호	130 22 66	성별 F
성명	한 승 리	
주민등록	710103－1234567	

수 술 기 록
Operation Record

Date: 2017. 11. 15　　Surgeon: C. B.Yoon

1st Ass't: I.H.Park　　2nd Ass't: J.S.Lee

Scrub nurse: 주민음　　Circ. nurse: 도민진

Operative Diagnosis : Ovary Ca. Ic

Anesthesia : GEA

Name of operation : TAH + BSO

Operative findings & Procedure :

1. Skin : low midline incision
2. Skin to peritoneum : free
3. Peritoneal cavity : adh (+), bl (+)
   asc (+) ≒ 300cc
   ① Uterus : AVF. sl. enlarged, movable, adhesion to Rt ovary mass
   ② Adnexa : Rt. ovary : over goose egg sized
   solid and cystic cancerous mass
   － ruptured
   Lt. ovary : hen's egg sized. irregular margin mass
   Tube: free
   ③ PCDS : bloody ascites (≒ 300cc) with partial obstruction
   Appe : Normal (Not done)
   ④ L/N : retroperitoneal & inguinal: impalpable, enlargement (－)
   ⑤ Omentum : free
   ⑥ Liver surface : free
   ⑦ Bladder & rectal mucosa : meta nodule impalpable
4. EBL : ca. 200cc
5. Tf : not done
6. Immediate : postop. state: stable

Biopsy Number
Requested examination] 2 Surgical Bx.

Date 2017년 11월 15일　　Described by : *Lee*

등록번호	130 22 66	성별 F
성명	한 승 리	
주민등록	710103－1234567	

병리학적 보고서

Pathological Report

Accession N.: s 2017－1283

Specimen received: 2017. 11. 15

Gross : Examined (JHO)

Clinical impression : Right adnexa mass

Specimen received fresh is an entire uterus with both adnexa in continuity.

The uterus weight 125gm and measures 8.5x4.5x3cm. The outer surface of the uterus is smooth and glistening. On section along the uterus. the uterine cavity measures 4x2cm and endocervical canal measures 3cm in length. On serial section there is not intramural mass.

The right ovary is previously ruptured mass, measuring 11x5.5x3.5cm and weighing, 149gm.

The protruding mass material is pinkish gray, granular, and solid. The remaining right ovarian tissue change into cyst. On serial section, the mass is friable and central whitish yellow area is noted. The mass is attached to ovary, dark greenish fluid is expelled. The inner surface of the ovary is granular and multiple nodule is noted.

The left ovary measures 4x2x1.5cm. There is a large mass at the surface of the ovary. The mass is 4x3x2.5cm. The outer surface of the mass is pinkish yellow and focal hemorrhagic. On serial section, the mass surface is variegated showing yellowish whited, solid and marginal necrosis.

The omentum, peritoneum and mesentery are not submitted, Representative sections are embedded. 〈Slide Key: A－D: Right ovary, E, F: LO(1), G. H: LO(2)〉 Micro(8HE)

Diagnosis :

Ovary and salpinx, bilateral adnexectomy :

Papillary serous cystadenocarcinoma, ovary, grade II/III,
with extracapsular extension

Uterus, total hysterectomy :

1. Chronic cervicitis
2. Proliferative endometrium

2017. Mo. 11. D. 18　　　Signature of Pathologist : 박찬호 M.D.

등록번호	130 22 66	성별 F
성명	한 승 리	
주민등록	710103－1234567	

세포학적 보고서
Cytology Report

Accession N.: s 2017－1288

Specimen received: 2017. 11. 16

Diagnosis : Peritoneal washing, cytology and cell block :
Papillary adenocarcinoma, metastatic

2017. Mo. 11. D. 19

Signature of Pathologist : 박찬호 M.D.

〈한 승 리〉

★ 한승리 차트를 읽고 맞는 것에 O표 하시오.

1 주진단명 및 주수술명에 대한 분류번호로 옳은 것은?
① C56,0, M8460/3, 68.4, 65.61
② C56,0, M8460/3, 68.6, 65.51
③ C57.8, M8140/6, 68.4, 65.61
④ C57.8, M8260/2, 68.4, 65.4
⑤ C56,9, M8460/6, 68.6, 65.61

2 가족력에 대한 설명으로 옳은 것은?
① 특별한 기재사항이 없다.
② 환자의 언니가 유방암 수술을 5년 전에 받았다.
③ 부여할 질병분류번호는 Z80.3이다.
④ 환자는 5녀 2남 중 막내딸이다.
⑤ 어머니는 64세이다.

3 환자의 통계분석에 대한 설명으로 옳은 것은?
① LOS는 11일이다.
② biopsy는 2번이다.
③ 암환자이며, 수술은 2번이다.
④ DAMA했다.
⑤ 재원일수는 12일이다.

4 환자의 입퇴원기록상에 첨가할 수 있는 질병분류 번호로 연결된 것은?
① N72, N85.8, C78.5
② N72, C78.6, 99.25
③ N73.0, C78.5, 99.25
④ N73.0, C78.6, 99.28
⑤ N85.8, N73.0, 99.28

5 환자의 출산력에 대한 설명으로 옳은 것은?
① 사산 1명, 조산 1명의 기왕력이 있다.
② 아들, 딸이 각각 1명이며, 총 임신 수는 3번이다.
③ 유산을 2번, 총 임신 수는 4번이다.
④ 유산 2번, 사산 1명에 살아있는 아이는 2명이다.
⑤ 조산은 1명, 유산 2번이다.

6 12년 전에 시행한 T/L에 대한 분류번호로 옳은 것은?
① 66.39
② 47.19
③ 85.41
④ 85.44
⑤ 66.51

7 환자에 대한 설명으로 옳게 기재된 것은?
① 유방촬영술결과 악성 증거가 없다.
② 복강내 유착 및 300cc 가량의 복수가 있으며, 혈액은 섞여 있지 않다.
③ 수술 중 총실혈량은 약 300cc였다.
④ 수술 중 후복막 및 서혜부(사타구니) 림프절이 촉진되었다.
⑤ 왼쪽 난관(자궁관)에 달걀 크기의 불규칙한 덩어리가 있었다.

8 수술 전 처치로 환자에게 시행한 처치가 <u>아닌</u> 것으로만 연결된 것은?
① 혈액학적 검사, 심전도
② 뇨검사, 위관검사
③ 심전도, 유치카테터 삽입
④ 유치카테터 삽입, 위관검사
⑤ 수술전 투약, 뇨검사

9 수술기록 요청서에 나타난 합병증과 이에 대한 예방대책이 옳게 연결된 것은?
① 감염-항암제 투여
② 유착-운동권장
③ 방광손상-항생제 투여
④ 요관손상-수혈
⑤ 출혈-항생제 소독

10 수술 후 시행된 내용으로 옳지 않은 것은?

① 수술 후 2일째 수술부위의 실밥을 제거하였다.
② 수술 후 8일째 화학요법을 시작하였다.
③ 수술 후 2일째 가스배출이 있었다.
④ 수술 후 1일째 복막 washing, 세포학 및 세포차단 검사물 접수일이었다.
⑤ 수술 후 6일째 유방검사상 덩어리는 촉진되지 않았다.

06 자궁경부암
Cervical cancer

1.1 자궁경부암(Cervical cancer)

특 징: 여성 성기암(24%) 중 85% 차지

원 인: HPV(human papilloma virus, **인유두종 바이러스**), HSV-2**의 감염**

- 사회경제적 수준이 낮은 계층
- 초혼 연령 또는 조기 성경험 여부
- 분만 횟수가 많은 여성, 접대부
- 흡연, 경구피임약 복용 및 남편의 포경여부
- 자궁경부(목)암의 조기진단을 받아 본 적이 없는 여성

증 상: 냉 냄새 심함, 부정출혈, 성교후 출혈, 요통, 하복통, 골반통, 용변장애, 빈혈 및 허약

검 사: 파파니콜라우 도말검사(Papanicolaou smear), 원추조직절제(Conization)

치 료: 초기암: 원추조직절제
진행암: 수술+방사선 요법

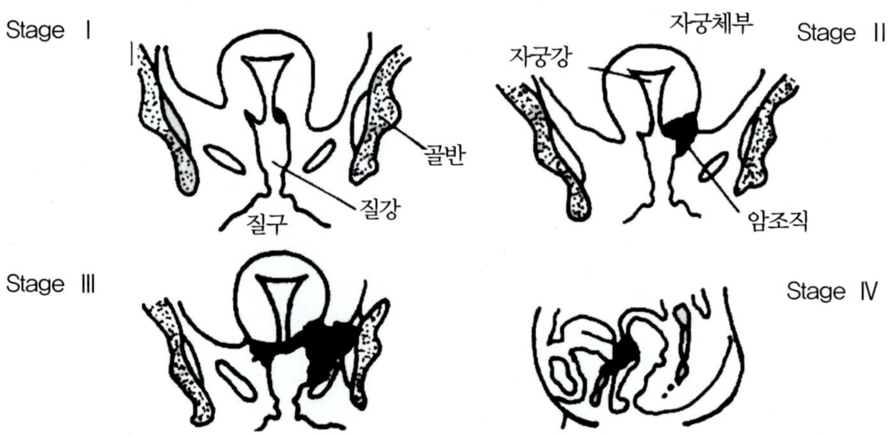

그림 1. 자궁경부암의 국제 임상분류법

1.2 진전도(Stage)

- Stage O: 자궁목의 상피내에 퍼지지 않고 암세포로 변화된 것이 상피내의 암
- Stage I: 암병소가 자궁목에만 국한
- Stage II: 자궁경 밖으로 암이 진행, 골반벽 또는 질하부 1/3까지 침윤 안됨
- Stage III: 암병소가 골반벽 또는 질하부 1/3 이하까지 침윤
- Stage IV: – 골반내 장기 특히 방광 또는 직장까지 침범
  – 복강내 장기(폐, 뼈, 간 등), 골반 밖 임파조직까지 전이

2.1 암 발생의 전형적인 단계

건강세포 → 이형성[dysplasia; 경미(mild)→중등도(moderate)→중증(severe=상피내 암종)] → 국소적으로 진행된 암 → 진행성 암

2.2 상피내 암종(Carcinoma in situ)

- 상피내 암종(CIS) = 중증 이형성(severe dysplasia) = 자궁경부(CIN III)
- 상피내 신생물 = M____/2 = Stage O = 상피내(intraepithelial) = 비침윤성(noninvasive, noninfiltrating)

2.3 암세포 검사(Pap test)

- 질경(vaginal speculum, 질벽을 벌리는 기구)을 삽입
- 암검사를 위해 주걱(spatula)을 이용하여 자궁경관과 질의 내막세포를 긁어냄
- 세포도말(smear)표본을 현미경으로 분석: 자궁암 또는 질암의 조기 진단

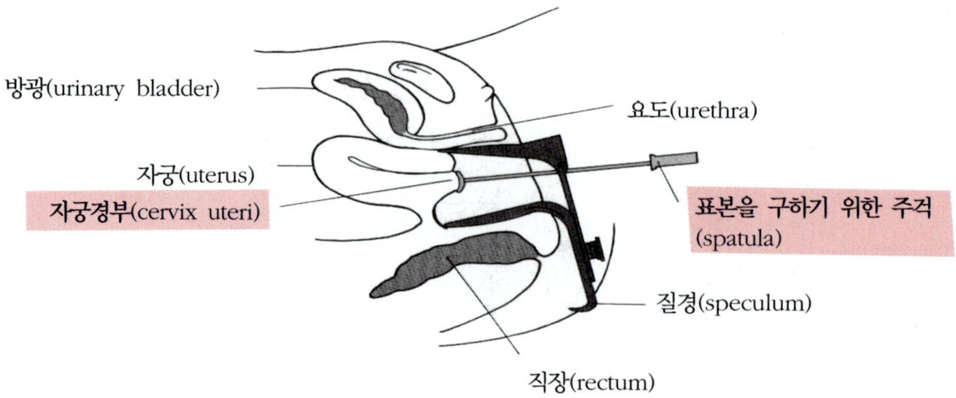

그림 2. 파파니콜라우 도말검사(Papanicolaou smear)

3.1 원추조직절제(Conization)

- ▸ 진단: 자궁경부에서 원추형 조각을 떼어내어 생검(biopsy)
- ▸ 치료: 정상소재암(초기암)인 경우 치료 가능

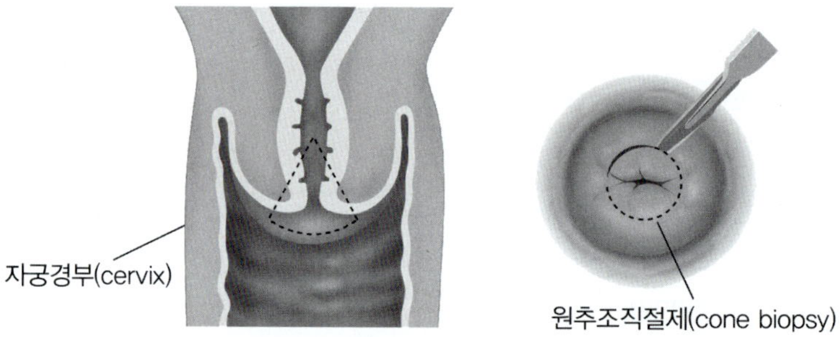

그림 3. 냉동칼 원추절제술(cone biopsy)

3.2 수 술

자궁절제수술(Hysterectomy): 자궁(uterus) 절제

- ▸ 전자궁적출술(total hysterectomy): 자궁과 자궁경부(cervix)의 절제
- ▸ 부분적자궁절제술(subtotal hysterectomy): 자궁경부(cervix)를 남기는 자궁절제술
- ▸ 복식자궁절제술(abdominal hysterectomy): 복부를 통해 자궁(uterus) 적출
- ▸ 자궁근치적출술(radical hysterectomy) = Wertheim's operation
  - 자궁의 침윤 시: 자궁경부, 난소, 난관(자궁관), 질(vagina) 및 주위 임파절의 절제
- ▸ 질식자궁절제술(vaginal hysterectomy): 질을 통해 자궁절제

3.3 불임수술

▶ 난관결찰술(tubal ligation) (여): 불임기법(sterilization) 66.39 (Dx.: Z30.2)
 - 복부를 절개하여 복강경(laparoscope)을 통해 난관 폐쇄
 (남): **정관절제술**(vasectomy) 63.73

4.1 자궁의 해부학적 부위

▶ **자궁경부(목, cervix)** : 한국 여성의 호발암 부위(=trachelo)

▶ **자궁(uterus)** : IUP(intrauterine pregnancy), 정상 임신부위(예: IUP 37~42주 미만)

▶ 난관(**자궁관, uterine tube**) = salpingo = fallopian tube = tubal
 - 불임기법(steralization) : 자궁관 폐쇄
 - 난관임신(tubal pregnancy) : 자궁외 임신 → 유산
 - 난관결찰술(tubal ligation) : 여성 영구피임

▶ **질(vaginal)** : NSVD(normal spontaneous vaginal delivery): 정상 자연분만 부위

▶ **난소(ovary)** : 양쪽에 위치, 난소암은 치사율이 높음(=oophoro)

▶ **외음부(Vulva)** = episio 질(vagina) = colpo 자궁(uterus) = hystero= metro

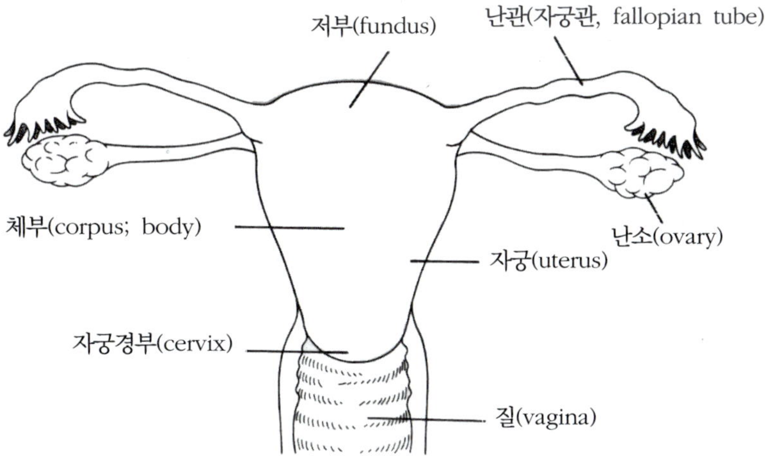

그림 4. 자궁의 해부학적 위치

의무기록 작성 및 서명

- **인 턴** : 신체검진, 병력기록
- **전공의** : 입퇴원기록, 퇴원요약, 경과기록, 수술기록 등
- **전문의** : 입퇴원기록, 수술기록 서명

4.2 차트 용어

▶ 임신검사(pregnancy test)

－HCG(융모성 성선자극호르몬) 유무를 확인하는 혈액 또는 소변검사

▶ 방광경검사(cystoscopy)

－방광경을 이용한 방광의 시각적(visual) 검사 방법

▶ 림프절(lymph node, LN)

－right pelvic(0/6) → 림프조직 6개 떼어낸 것 중 전이 없음

－right pelvic(2/6) → 림프조직 6개 떼어낸 것 중 2개가 전이

▶ 초경(menarche) ↔ 폐경(menopause)

▶ 위축(atrophy) ↔ 비대(trophy)

차트 용어							
· Adequate	적절한	· Antibiotics	항생제	· Cough	기침	· Deep	깊은
· Fever	열	· Hydration	수분	· Inhalation	흡입	· Mild	경미한

약 어	원 어	
AST(SGOT)	Aspartate aminotransferase	간기능 검사
ALT(SGPT)	Alanine aminotransferase	간기능 검사
BPLD	Bilateral pelvic lymph node dissection	양측 골반 림프절 절개술
CBC	Complete blood count	전혈구 조사
CBS	Clear breathing sound	깨끗한 호흡음
CCG	Chromic catgut	크로믹 장선(흡수성 봉합사)
CIN	Cervical intraepithelial neoplasia	자궁경부 상피내 신생물
CIS	Carcinoma in situ	상피내 암종
DUB	Dysfunctional uterine bleeding	기능부전성 자궁출혈
ⓜ	Murmur	잡음
HCG	Human chorionic gonadotropin	융모성 성선자극호르몬
HSO	Half stitch out	실밥 반 제거
IVP	Intravenous pyelogram	정맥내 신우조영술(콩팥깔때기 조영술)
Pap smear	Papanicolau smear · 자궁경부 또는 질의 암검사	파파니콜라우 도말검사
ⓡ	Rale	수포음, 나음
RHB	Regular heart beat	규칙적인 심박동
NC	No complaints	불평없음
NPD	No pathological diagnosis	병리학적 진단없음
RAH	Radical abdominal hysterectomy	근치 복식 자궁절제술
TAH	Total abdominal hysterectomy	전체 복부 자궁절제술
V/Vx	Vulva and vagina	외음부 및 질

등록번호	330 22 66	성별 F
성명	김 말 복	
주민등록	671201-1234567	

입 퇴 원 기 록
Admission and Discharge Record

<table>
<tr><td colspan="3">주 소 : 서울시 송파구 잠실본동 235</td></tr>
<tr><td colspan="3">출신지 : 직 업 : 전 화 :</td></tr>
<tr><td colspan="3">연고자성명 : 관 계 : 주 소 : 전 화 :</td></tr>
<tr><td>입원 : 2017 년 월 일 GY 과 병동 호</td><td rowspan="3">전과</td><td>20 년 월 일 과 병동 호</td></tr>
<tr><td>퇴원 : 2017 년 월 일 과 병동 호</td><td>20 년 월 일 과 병동 호</td></tr>
<tr><td>재원일수 :</td><td>20 년 월 일 과 병동 호</td></tr>
</table>

최종진단명	분 류 번 호
주진단명 : Carcinoma of cervix	
Stage Ib	
기타진단명 :	
수술 및 처치명	
수술명 : RAH	
Bilateral pelvic lymph node dissection	
기타수술 및 주요검사 : Incidental appendectomy	
Baseline study	

<table>
<tr><td colspan="2">치료결과 : 1. 완쾌 2. 경쾌 3. 호전안됨 4. 진단뿐 5. 가망없는 퇴원 6. 48시간내 사망 7. 48시간이후 사망</td></tr>
<tr><td colspan="2">퇴원형태 : 1. 퇴원지시후 2. 자의퇴원 3. 탈원 4. 전원</td></tr>
<tr><td colspan="2">병원감염 : 1. 수술후 2. 기타처치후 3. 비뇨기계 4. 호흡기계 5. 소화기계 6. 기타</td></tr>
<tr><td colspan="2">원사인 : 부검 : 예, 아니오</td></tr>
<tr><td colspan="2">계속적 진료 계획</td></tr>
<tr><td colspan="2">없음·있음 (약속일 20 년 월 일 시)</td></tr>
<tr><td>담당 전공의 서명 : 조용수</td><td>담당 전문의 서명 : 옥돌찬</td></tr>
<tr><td>의무기록 완성 : 2017 년 2 월 9 일</td><td>의무기록사 서명 : 장선화</td></tr>
</table>

등록번호	330 22 66	성별 F
성명	김 말 복	
주민등록	671201-1234567	

퇴 원 요 약
Discharge Summary

1. Final Dx. : Ca of Cx. Stage 1b

2. PAP if class II

3. Hb/Hct: 12.4/36.3 → 10.1/29.8
   VDRL ⊖
   r-HCG ⊖
   HBs Ag: ⊖
   Chest PA: NAD
   OT/PT: 17/11

4. Baseline study
   RAH $\bar{c}$ BPLD, incidental appendectomy

5. 1주일 후 OPD f/u

6. Suprax 2Ⓣ
   Becuse 2Ⓣ
   Lodine 2Ⓣ
   ] #2 bid by p.o x 5days

윤미수

등록번호	330 22 66	성별 F
성명	김 말 복	
주민등록	671201-1234567	

병 력 기 록
History

1. 주소 (C.C.) : Abnormal PAP Smear

2. 개인 및 사회력 : N-C

3. 과거력 : G4 P1 L3 Do A1
: Postmenopausal study
: Menarche : 16-y-o, Marriage : 23-y-o
: Last del : 18년 전
No other M-S illness

4. 가족력 : N-C

5. 현병력 : 본 50세 여환은 local 산부인과 정기 PAP 검사상 Class II 나와 Further eval. & proper Tx. 위해 OPD 경유 adm. 하였다.

6. 문진(ROS)

두경부 : Headache/ dizziness (−/−)
심 폐 : Chest pain / dyspnea (−/−)
소화기 : A/V/N (−/−/−)
C/D (−/−)
비뇨생식기 : dysuria / frequency (−/−)
신경근육 : Myalgia (−)
기 타

지연전

등록번호	330 22 66	성별 F
성명	김 말 복	
주민등록	671201-1234567	

경 과 기 록
Progress Notes

〈 Admission Note 〉

11.2 This 50yrs old $G_4P_3L_3DoA_1$ house wife was admitted to our hospital dept of GYN under the impression of invasive squamous cell carcinoma of uterine cervix

via OPD on 17-11-21

본 50세된 여환은 local OB Gyn에서 정기적으로 검진 받던 중 한달 전 PAP smear상 class II 나와 K대학병원에 transfer되어 punch biopsy 결과 invasive squamous cell ca. 나와서 금일 OPD 통해 Baseline study 및 op. 위해 내원하였습니다.

PHx : G4 P3 L3 Do A1

LMP, PMP] Menopause state

Menarche : 16-y-o

Marriage : 16-y-o

Last Del : 18년 전

No other M-S illness

FHx : N-C

P/Ex : BP 130/90 mmHg PR 83회/분

G/A : Not so ill looking appearance

Skin : Warm $\bar{c}$ dry

HEENT : not pale conjunctivae

not icteric sclera

Neck : Supple

Chest $\bar{c}$ lung : CBS $\bar{s}$ ⓡ

No wheezing

경 과 기 록

일 자	내 용	서 명
11.21	Heart : RHB $\overline{s}$ ⓜ No thrill Abd : soft & flat No tender point B/Ex : No LOM No CVT tenderness Pelvic exam : ext-genitalia v/vx: free Cx : put. punch bx state Ut : Not enlarged Adnexa : free	홍순민
11.28	〈 Operation Note 〉 1. Name of operation Type III extended hysterectomy with bilateral salpingo-oophorectomy Bilateral pelvic lymph node dissection Incidental appendectomy 2. Name of operator Operator : J. W. Kim M.D. U. A. Choi M.D. 1st assistant : U. O Lee M.D. 2nd assistant : Y.P. Kim M.D. 3. Preoperative diagnosis Invasive carcinoma of uterine cervix Stage IB 4. Postoperative diagnosis Same as the above 5. Anesthesia General anesthesia with endotracheal intubation 6. Operative findings and procedures 1) A low midline abdominal skin incision was made. 2) Entering the abdominal cavity, the uterus was normal in size and shape. Bilateral uterine tubes and ovaries were grossly normal in shape and size.	홍순민

경 과 기 록

일 자	내 용	서 명
11.28	3) Radical abdominal hysterectomy with bilateral salpingo-oophorectomy was done. 4) Pelvic lymph node dissection of both sides were done, of which finding were from tumor. Incidental appendectomy was done. 5) Vaginal vault was completely closed. 6) On the manual exploration, the liver, stomach and intestines were grossly normal. 7) Anatomically repaired with CCGs, Vicryl and silks. 8) EBL was about 1500cc 9) Neither gauze nor drain was inserted.	
11.28	〈 Immediate Postop Note 〉 Fully awakening from general anesthesia well running IV fluids Well functing foley catheter CBS $\bar{s}$ ⓡ RHB $\bar{s}$ ⓜ Mild fever Not pale, not conjuntiva Not icteric sclera No active vaginal bleeding Plan) ① enccurye cough $\bar{c}$ deep breathing ② Adequate hydration Antibiotics ③ cold steam inhalation	홍 순민

경 과 기 록

일 자	내 용	서 명
	〈 POD #1 〉	
11.29	High fever No active vag. bleeding Clear wound Hb/Hct 9.8/28.5 Plan) No hydration Antibiotic	
		양경인
	〈 POD #3 〉	
12.2	Afebril state Foley keep state Gas passing status Hb/Hct 10.1/29.8 Plan) foley training conservative management	
		양경인
	〈 Off Service Note 〉	
12.3	본 50세 $G_4P_3L_3DoA_1$ 여환은 Ca. of Cx Ib로 Baseline, study 시행 후 RAH $\bar{c}$ BSD, BPLD 시행 후 POD#5된 환자로서 현재 foley keep 상태에서 foley training $\bar{q}$ 2hr을 하고 있고 내일 foley training $\bar{q}$ 3hr를 하고 foley remove를 계획하세요. wound clear하고 fever 없고 general condition 괜찮습니다. 수고하세요. pathology 나왔습니다.	
		양경인
	〈 On Service Note 〉	
12.4	본 50세 $G_4P_3L_3DoA_1$ 여환은 Ca. of Cx. Ib로 Baseline study 후 RAH $\bar{c}$ BSO, BPLD 시행 후 POD #6입니다. 현재 foley training $\bar{q}$ 3hr 중이며 on call로 foley remove하겠습니다. wound는 midline silk로 비교적 clean합니다. 내일 H.S.O 하겠습니다. Conservative management하겠습니다.	
		윤미수

경 과 기 록

일 자	내 용	서 명
12.5	POD #7 All stitch out was done. Wound is clear Pathology : (S-17-8365) Cx : residural microinvasive sqa. cell ca. invasion depth 3mm Ovary Rt & Lt ⎤ NPD Tube Rt. & tube ⎦ Parametrium : Rt & Lt : free from tumor Vaginal calf : Ac' and ch' Nonspecific inflammation $\bar{s}$ evidence of tumor LNS: 0/16 : free from tumor Appendix : NPD Foley $\bar{q}$ 3hr training에 voiding sensation과 bladder training sensation 있음. 내일 foley $\bar{q}$ 3hr training 하고 remove 예정임	윤미수
12.7	→ appendix에 wound의 edge가 벌어져서(2cm 정도 길이로) wound reopen시켰으며 Nylon 3-0로 2° closure 시행함 Plan) Daily Dressing IM Anti Pontrl 2Ⓛ 'prn'	윤미수
12.9	Discharge	윤미수

등록번호 330 22 66 성별 F
성명 김 말 복
주민등록 671201-1234567

협의진료기록
Consultation Record

Request For Consultation To

Summary of Present Findings GS 과 김송빈 선생님 귀하
Physician of Department

Invasive Ca. of Cx로 입원가료 중인 50세 여자환자입니다. 하기 분야에 대한 선생님의 고진선처를 부탁드립니다.

감사합니다.

For Sigmoidoscopy

2017. 11. 21 a.m.
Date Hour p.m.

Prof. 옥돌찬/R1 지연전 M.D.
Signature of Attending Physician

Report of Consultation

Opinion and Recommendation

〈 Sigmoidoscopy Note 〉

Full examination was performed.(20cm) There was no abnormal mucosal lesion on this study. Bimanual pelvic exam was performed. No abnl findings on Rectovaginal septum.

2017. 11. 22 a.m.
Date Hour p.m.

Prof. 김송빈/황인준 M.D.
Signature of Attending Physician

등록번호	330 22 66	성별 F
성명	김 말 복	
주민등록	671201-1234567	

협의진료기록
Consultation Record

Request For Consultation To

Summary of Present Findings

URO과 이성수 선생님 귀하
Physician of Department

Invasive Ca. of Cx로 입원가료 중인 50세 여자환자입니다. 하기분야에 대한 선생님이 고진선처를 부탁드립니다.

감사합니다.

For Cystoscopy

2017. 11. 21 a.m.
Date Hour p.m.

Prof. 옥돌찬/지연전 M.D.
Signature of Attending Physician

Report of Consultation

Opinion and Recommendation

IVP 및 Cystoscopy의 특이한 이상 소견은 관찰되지 않습니다.

감사합니다.

2017. 11. 23 a.m.
Date Hour p.m.

Prof. 이성수/박사교 M.D.
Signature of Attending Physician

자궁경부암(Carcinoma of Cervix Uteri)

No ______________ Date 20 ____.____.____

Unit No 330 22 66

Name 김 말 복 Age 49 G 4 P 3 L 3 Abort Spont. 0

Induc. 1

Home address 413-2000 Date of birth 1967. 12. 1.

Address 서울시 송파구 잠실동 Citizen No. 671201-1234567

Husband Name ____________ Occupation ____________ Tel. No. 414-5000

Base Line Study ____________

Hb. 12.4 Ht. 36.3 WBC 4,400 (42.8%)

Platelet 294K BUN 8.5 Urinalysis −/−

VDRL (−) A.O. Smear : Class V

Chest P.A NAD EKG : WNL

IVP WNL

Cystoscopy WNL Sigmoidoscopy WNL

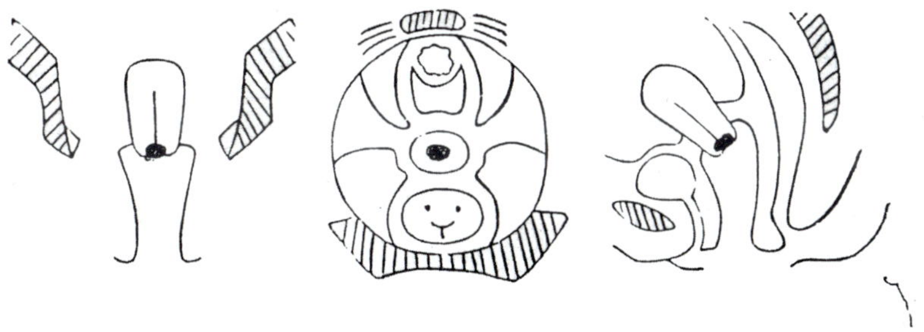

Pathological diagnosis : (외부 punch Bx) : Invasive squamous cell ca. nonkeratinizing

Clinical diagnosis : Ca. of Cx Ib

Therapeutic plans : RAH $\bar{c}$ BPLD

옥돌찬/유미항 M.D.

등록번호	330 22 66	성별 F
성명	김 말 복	
주민등록	671201-1234567	

수술전 체크 리스트
Pre-Operative Check List

		Yes	No
Preparation, for operation, bath, skin, nails 수술전 준비(목욕, 피부준비, 손톱, 발톱)			
Pre-medication given charted	*Pre) Robinul 0.2mg* *Ativan 2.0mg IM* *on call*	V	
Doctor's order sheet on chart special pre-operative order 의무기록에 있는 의사의 지시기록지를 보고 특별한 수술 전 지시를 볼 것		V	
Special medication V blood pints V dextrose CC *F/P/C 3Ⓟ* *HISCL*		V	
Hair prepared, leggings, gown 머리를 갈라 땋고 삼각 끈으로 매고 가운을 입힐 것		V	
Jewellery removed and put in safe care 귀중품 제거와 보관		V	
Artificial teeth removed 의치의 제거, 콘택트렌즈 제거, 보청기 제거		V	
Voided, catheterized, enema 인공 혹은 자연배뇨(시간과 양의 기록) 관장	*H.C.E 6AM* *Lagino/double 6AM*	V	
Has patient fasted? 금식하였는지?	*Foley insert* *MN NPO*	V	
Blood, urine, other report on chart? 혈액, 소변, 기타 검사의 보고지 유무		V	
Identification of child or unconscious patient 혼수상태에 있는 환자나 소아의 이름표(성명, 연령, 주소) 유무		V	
Pre-operative T.P.R., B.P., charted? 수술전 체온, 맥박, 호흡, 혈압측정의 기록	*T P R* *36.3C 78회/miin 20회/min*	V	
Miscellaneous 기 타 *Prep) 복CM x 1*	*B.P. 140/80 mmHg*	V	

Date 11/28 Preparation nurse 양도순 Head nurse 최웅린

등록번호	330 22 66	성별	F
성명	김 말 복		
주민등록	671201-1234567		

수 술 기 록

Operation Record

날짜 : 2017년 11월 28일 집도의 : J. W. Kim M.D
제 1 보조의 : U. O. Lee M.D. 제 2 보조의 : Y.P. Kim M.D.
참여간호사 : 순환간호사

Preoperative diagnosis	:Carcinoma of uterine cervix Fecalith impaction in appendix
Postoperative diagnosis	: Same as the aboves
Name of operation	:Radical abdominal hysterectomy with bilateral salpingo-oophorectomy Bilateral pelvic lymph nodes dissection Incidental appendectomy

Findings & Procedures:

With the patient in supine position and under general anesthesia, the patient's abdomen was prepared, painted and draped in a usual manner after urinary catheterization. A low midline skin incision, extended 5cm above the umbilicus, was made, cutting the subcutaneous tissue, the fascia, and the peritoneum. Entering the abdominal cavity, the uterus was atropied. Bilateral tubes and ovaries were atropied. Adequate exposure of the pelvis was made. The uterus was clamped with two long Kellies, elevated and grasped out of the pelvis. The round ligament on each side was grasped, sutured and ligated with #6 silk, and then divided. The anterior leaf of the broad ligament was separated from the underlying connective tissue and incised in a curved fashion, dividing the peritoneum on the anterior uterine surface above the bladder fold: the bladder and the attached peritoneal flap were then bluntly dissected off the lower uterine segment. The base of the bladder is released from the cervix and upper vagina. The lateral peritoneum on each side was opened and incised along the pelvic brim. Then, the paravesical space was dissected bluntly with index finger. The common iliac artery at the level of its bifurcation internal and external iliac arteries were separated from adjacent tissues. The ureter was identified, left attached to the parietal peritoneum. Then the pararectal space was dissected bluntly with index finger. The posterior leaf of the broad ligament was then divided.

Tissue to path. : ☑Yes, ☐No Drains: ☐Yes ☑No Sponge count correct: ☑Yes ☐No
Dictated/Written by U. O. Lee M.D. Surgeon's Signature J. W. Kim M.D.

수 술 기 록

Operative Procedure

The both infundibulopelvic ligament was grasped, clamped and doubly ligated with #6 silks. The ureter was separated from fascial bundles of broad ligament, dissecting the uterine arteries on each side. The uterine artery was skeletonized, clamped, and doubly ligated with #4 black silks. The parametrial connective tissue on each side was completely divided, sutured and ligated with #6 silk. The parametrium on each side revealed no gross tumor extension. The peritoneum over the posterior aspect of the uterus was incised and prerectal space was bluntly dissected with finger. The uterosacral ligaments were dissected, cut and ligated with #6 silks. The ureter was dissected down along its insertion to the bladder and approximated with interrupted sutures of #2-0 CCG. After dissecting each ureter sufficiently from the cardinal ligaments to about 4cm below the lower cervical limit, two Hiney clamps were placed across the vagina and the vaginal wall. The angles of the vaginal vaults were opened with knife and then sutured to the stump of the cardinal ligaments with #1-0 Vicryl. Resection of the vagina, about 1.0cm below the cervix was achieved. Now the cut edges of the anterior and posterior vaginal wall was sutured involving pubocervical fascia with continous locking sutures of #1-0 Vicryl. Then pelvic lymphadenectomy was performed in the following fashion. The external iliac lymphatic chain was dissected at the level of bifureation of common iliac artery, removing the loose fascial sheath of the external iliac artery, extending to the level of inferior epigastric artery. The psoas muscle and genitofemoral nerve were exposed. Then the hypogastric artery and ligated uterine artery at the level of beginning were identified and adjacent lymphatic chain was dissected, to the level of obturator space, visualizing the obturator nerve, artery and vein. Obturator space was exposed and the soft tissue and lymph nodes in the obturator fossa was dissected. There noted no enlarged lymph nodes. Hemostasis was assured.

Appendectomy was done. The pelvic peritoneum was closed with continuous sutures of #2-0 Vicryl. Hemostasis was reassured. The abdominal wall was closed in layers: a continuous sutures of #1-0 CCG for peritoneum and rectus muscles: interrupted sutures of #4 and #3 silk for the fascia and subcutaneous tissue: the skin was closed with mattress sutures of #3 silks. Estimated blood loss was about 1,500ml. The patient tolerated the entire procedure well and was sent to the recovery room in a stable condition.

Dictacted by U. O. Lee

등록번호	330 22 66	성별 F
성명	김 말 복	
주민등록	671201-1234567	

병리학적 검사 보고서

Pathological Report

병리번호: S-17-8365

검사물 접수일: 17. 02. 02

Organ and tissue received :

1.

2.

3. Sent by ___________

Pathological Findings and Diagnosis

=== continued

Pathological Diagnosis :

Uterus with both adnexae. total abdominal hysterectomy with bilateral salpingo-oophorectomy :

Cervix : Post biopsy state with residual microinvasive squamous cell carcinoma(depth of invasion 3mm)

Endometrium : Post curettage stage

Myometrium : No pathological diagnosis.

Ovary, right and left : No pathological diagnosis.

Fallopian tube, right and left : No pathological diagnosis

Parametrium, right and left : Free from tumor.

Vaginal cuff : Acute and chronic nonspecific inflammation without evidence of tumor.

Lymph nodes, right pelvic (0/6), left pelvic (0/8), right internal iliac (0/2) : total (0/6): Free from tumor.

Appendix, appendectomy : No pathological diagnosis.

Date: 17. 11. 30

Jang Suk, M.D.

Signature of Pathologist

〈김 말 복〉

★ 김말복 차트를 보고 맞는 답에 O표 하시오.

1 인턴 기록을 보고 알 수 없는 것은?

① 자녀가 3명이다.
② 폐경 증후군이 있다.
③ 초경은 16세 때 했다.
④ 유산경험이 있다.
⑤ 가족병력은 없다.

2 환자의 주진단이 맞게 조립된 것은?

① D06.9, M8070/2
② C53.9, M8070/3
③ C53.9, M8070/6
④ C78.09, M8070/3
⑤ C78.01, M8070/6

3 수술기록의 내용과 틀린 것은?

① 절개는 paramidline으로 배꼽에서 5cm 위에서 시작하였다.
② 조직검사를 보냈으며 drainage는 없었다.
③ EBL은 1500ml였다.
④ 암의 진전도는 Ib인 조기암(early cancer)이었다.
⑤ 양쪽 측면 난관(자궁관)과 난소는 모양과 크기가 정상이었다.

4 환자의 통계 중 맞는 것은?

① 재원기간은 19일이다.
② 협의진단 수는 2건이다.
③ 펀치생검 1건, 응급실 통해 내원했다.
④ 전과일은 12월 3일이다.
⑤ 부인과로 전과하였다.

5 주수술명의 분류번호로 짝지어진 것은?

① 47.19, 68.4, 40.21
② 68.4, 65.61, 40.3
③ 68.6, 65.61, 40.3
④ 47.11, 68.6, 40.21
⑤ 68.4, 65.64, 40.3

6 수술직후 상태를 기록한 것 중 맞는 것은?

① 경미한 열이 있었다.
② 약간의 질출혈이 있었다.
③ 수분섭취를 줄이도록 하였다.
④ 심호흡과 목운동을 하도록 하였다.
⑤ 잡음을 동반한 심장박동이 있었다.

7 경과기록지에서 상처가 벌어진 것과 2° closure한 것의 분류번호는?

① T81.0, 47.91
② T81.1, 54.72
③ T88.9, 47.92
④ T88.9, 47.91
⑤ T88.9, 47.09

8 수술 전 준비 상황과 맞지 않는 것은?

① Ativan 2.0mg을 근육내 주사하였다.
② 수혈을 위해 3 pints 준비하였다.
③ Nelaton Catheter를 끼웠다.
④ 혈압은 140/80 mmHg였다.
⑤ 체온은 36.3℃였다.

9 **상기 환자가 시행한 검사의 질병분류는?**

① 48.23, 57.32 ② 42.23, 57.32 ③ 48.23, 44.13

④ 45.23, 68.12 ⑤ 48.25, 57.32

10 **환자의 내용이 맞는 것은?**

① Pap smear를 입원 중에 했으며, 간염 항원이 없다.

② 실밥을 모두 뽑은 날은 12월 4일이다.

③ 방광경 검사는 외과에서 협의진단에 의해 했다.

④ 병리조직검사결과 주위 임파조직에 침윤이 없었다.

⑤ 정맥내 신우조영술 검사상 이상소견이 관찰되었다.

01 쌍둥이 조기진통 분만
Delivery of twin preterm labor

1.1 자궁저부높이(Height of Fundus; HOF)

자궁저부높이 측정

- 자궁저부높이 측정으로 태아 성장과 임신기간 추정
- 줄자를 이용해 치골결합 절흔부터 복부 중앙선을 지나 저궁저부까지의 길이를 측정

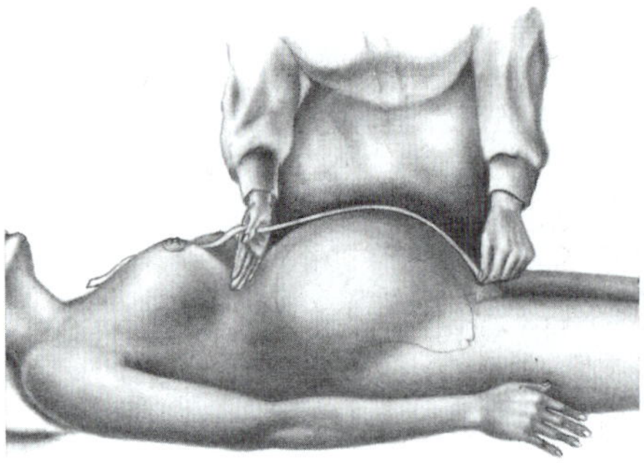

그림 1. 자궁저부높이 측정(HOF)

자궁저부높이 계산

- **자궁저부높이(Height of fundus; HOF)**
  - 자궁저부높이(cm) × 2/7 = 임신월수
  - 자궁저부높이(cm) × 8/7 = 임신주수

자궁저부높이의 임신기간

- 자궁이 커지면서 골반강이 좁아짐에 따라 자궁은 골반 위로 올라감
  - 임신 12~14주: 치골 위에서 촉진 이후 자궁은 상승
  - 임신 22~24주: 제와부 높이에 이르게 되며 말기에는 검상돌기(명치끝)에 근접하게 됨
  - 임신 38~40주: 자궁저부의 높이는 하강하기 시작함에 따라 골반강 내로 진입(출산 준비)

태아의 골반 하강

- ▶ 태아가 골반으로 진입하는 하강감으로 자궁저부로 내려감
- ▶ 초산부: 하강은 분만 시작 약 2주 전에 일어남
- ▶ 경산부: 하강은 분만 시작 시 일어남

출산력의 의미

3	-	1	-	4	-	3
만기분만		조산		유산		생존아

유산 4 ┌ 3 / └ 1 ; 생존아 3 ┌ 1 / └ 2

예) ▶분만: 3회, 조산: 1회, 유산: 4회 (자연유산 3회, 인공유산 1회)

▶생존아: 3명(남아 1명, 여아 2명)

1.2 호흡곤란증후군(Respiratory Distress Syndrome; RDS)

호흡곤란증후군의 의미: 초자막질환

- ▶ 일명 초자막질환(hayline membrane disease)
- ▶ 정상폐포 내면에 존재하는 표면활성물질 결여 때문에 호흡곤란 질환
- ▶ 재태주수 34주 이하의 미숙아, 제왕절개 만출아, 당뇨병 모체의 산아에게 많음

차트 용어

· Adequate	적절한	· Ambulation	보행/외래치료	· Breech	둔위	· Cartilage	연골
· Cephalic	머리/정상분만	· Expelled	만출하다	· Extraction	만출	· Fetal distress	태아곤란증
· Meconium stained	태변착색	· Myometrium	자궁근층	· MTG	자궁수축제	· Placenta	태반
· Pelvis	골반	· Pubic	치골의	· Regular	규칙적	· Transverse	횡의

성별 기호

· 남자: ♂ · 여자: ♀

약 어	원 어	
AC	Abdominal circumference	복부둘레
BM	Body weight	체중
BOW	Bag of water	양수
$\bar{c}$	With	동반
C/S(C/sec)	Cervical section	제왕절개술
DW 5%	Dextrous Water	5% 포도당 용액
EBL	Estimated blood loss ‣ 정상분만 시 과다출혈: 500cc 이상 ‣ 제왕절개 시 과다출혈: 1,000cc 이상	실추정량: 1㎖=1cc 예) EBL 1200cc 제왕절개 시 과다출혈
EDC	Estimated date of confinement	분만예정일
F/C	Foley catheter	폴리카테터, 유치도뇨관
FHT	Fetal heart tone	태아심음(태아 심박동)
F/U	Follow up	추적관리(추적조사)
GD	General diet	일반식
HOF	Height of fundus	자궁저부높이
H/S	Hartman's solution	하트만 용액(1 L=1,000cc)
LLQ	Left lower quadrant	좌하부(좌하복부)
LMP	Last Menstrual period	최종월경주기
MN	Midnight	자정
PL	Preterm labor	조기진통
PP	Presentating part	선진부
PSD	Premature spontaneous delivery	조산
$\bar{q}$	Every	매
req	Request	요청
RLQ	Right lower quadrant	우하부
$\bar{s}$	Without	동반없이
Sx	Symptom	증상
Wks	Weeks	주

신 승 자 요약 차트

등록번호 : 81 56 72　　이름 : 신승자
입원일 : 2017. 5. 1　　퇴원일 : 2017. 5. 8　　퇴원과 : OB

Procedure & Findings

Under the general anesthesia on the supine position, the lower midline skin incision was done. Entering into the abdominal cavity, there was no ascites and no adhesion. Uterine was 8 month size. Both adnexae were free. Lower segmental tansverse c/sec was done. The aliving male baby, weighing 1.85kg, whose Apgar score 1'-2, 5'-3 with no initial crying, no congenital anormaly, transverse lie at 22: 40, no meconium staining was delivered. Breech extraction. Premature sign was seen. For example coarse scalp hair, breast bud (below 2mm), ear cartilage was absence. Placenta was removed by manual, MTG 1A injected into myometrially. Grasping the incised edge of uterus by triangular hemostat, the deep layer of the myometrium was closed by continous locking suture with 1 C.C.G. And the superficial layer of the myometrium were closed by continous suture with 1 C.C.G. *Lee*

5/1　〈 Adm order 〉

1. Check V/S $\bar{q}$ 4hrs & FHT $\bar{q}$ 2hrs
2. GD & NPO from MN
3. Shaving on abd & Pubic area
4. Get op permission op & termination
5. Insert F/C
6. Vag Cleansing before to OR
7. prepare MTG 2Ⓐ
8. req) CBC ABO/Rh, X-matching, Bil, Bun/cr U/A, Na/K/cl
   Bun/cr LFT, Chest, PA, EKG, VDRL, HBsAg/Ab
9. H/S IV $\bar{c}$ 18 G needle
10. Check FHT before T/F to OR
11. Send to OR *Kim*

〈 Postop order 〉

5/3
1. Check V/S $\bar{q}$ 15' x 4 & $\bar{q}$ 30' x 4
   and then $\bar{q}$ 1hr (until stable)
2. NPO
3. EDB & ABR & cough

신 승 자 요약 차트

등록번호 : 81 56 72 이름 : 신승자

입원일 : 2017. 5. 1 퇴원일 : 2017. 5. 8 퇴원과 : OB

4. Watch for Vag. bleeding & P/C
5. Keep F/C & check I/O (If U/O is 30cc/hr. notify)
6. Apply Sand bag on op wd.

5/4 〈 POD #2 〉

1. Check V/S $\bar{q}$ 4hs
2. NPO
3. Ambulation
4. F/I F-5D10 1BT IV
   5DS10
   HS500 IV
   A-SAMP 2Ⓐ IVSS $\bar{q}$ 8hr (AST) *Kim*

5/7 〈 POD #5 〉

1. Check V/S $\bar{q}$ 4hr
2. GD
3. watch for vag bleeding & P/C
4. Check S/V Well
5. Ambulation
6. MED B-DRP 3T #3 1day
   B-MD 3T
   B-KTOR 3T
   B-ERGK 3T

req) CBC, DC, ESR, U/A, GOT/GPT, BUN/Cr *Kim*

5/8 〈 Discharge Order 〉

1. Check V/S $\bar{q}$ 4hr
2. GD
3. Watch for vag bleeding & P/C
4. Check S/V Well
5. breast care
6. Discharge $\bar{c}$ po med for 2day *Kim*

〈신 승 자〉

★ 신승자 차트를 읽고 맞는 것에 O표 하시오.

1 둘째 아기의 수술 내용으로 옳지 않은 것은?

① 자궁의 하위 횡절개를 하였다.
② 하복부 중앙절개를 하였다.
③ 아기는 머리가 먼저 나왔다
④ 아프가 점수는 1분에 2, 5분에 3이었다.
⑤ 자궁수축제를 자궁근육층에 주사하였다

2 태아의 태위가 옳게 연결된 것은?

① 첫째 - 횡위, 둘째 - 두위
② 첫째 - 둔위, 둘째 - 두위
③ 첫째 - 두위, 둘째 - 둔위
④ 첫째 - 횡위, 둘째 - 횡위
⑤ 첫째 - 두위, 둘째 - 횡위

3 산모는 C/S을 하기로 하였다. 그 이유로 옳은 것은?

① O32.2, O69.0
② O36.8, O69.0
③ O32.2, O33.9
④ O33.9, O69.1
⑤ O33.9, O69.8

4 산모에 대한 내용으로 옳지 않은 것은?

① 산모의 골반모양은 출산에 적당하였다.
② 남아 출산 시 실추정량은 과다출혈이었다.
③ 첫째 아기의 출산까지 진통시간은 약 2시간이었다
④ 유산은 3회 있었고 둘째 아기 귀의 연골은 없었다.
⑤ 산모의 자궁저높이는 35cm, 복부둘레는 96cm였다.

5 수술 전 지시내용으로 옳지 않은 것은?

① 모래주머니 부착
② 폴리카테터 삽입
③ 자궁수축제 준비
④ 하트만 용액 주입
⑤ 태아 심박동 체크

6 질병분류로 옳지 않은 것은?

① O60.11
② O30.0
③ O36.8
④ O42.19
⑤ O32.2

04. 기 타 계

Others

MEDICAL RECORD PRACTICE

01 알레르기 중이염 동반 진주종
Cholesteatoma c̄ allergic otitis media

1.1 귀의 구성 및 기능

- 외이(바깥귀)와 중이(가운데귀): 소리의 전도기능
- 내이(속귀): 소리를 받아 뇌의 대뇌피질(cerebral cortex)로 전달

Outer ear 외이		Middle ear 중이		Inner ear 내이(labyrinth)
1. Pinna, auricle(귓바퀴) 2. External auditory canal (외이도/바깥귀길)	➡	3. Tympanic membrane(고막) ‣ 외이와 중이 사이의 막 4. Malleus(추골/망치골) 5. Incus(침골/모루골) 6. Stapes(등골/등자골) 7. Oval window(난원창) ‣ 중이와 내이 사이의 막	➡	8. Cochlea(와우, 달팽이관) 9. Auditory liquid & receptors in the organ of Corti (코르티기관의 청각액과 수용기) 10. Auditory nerve fibers (청각신경섬유) 11. cerebral cortex(대뇌피질)

그림 1. 음진동(sound vibrations)의 경로: 1→10번 순서

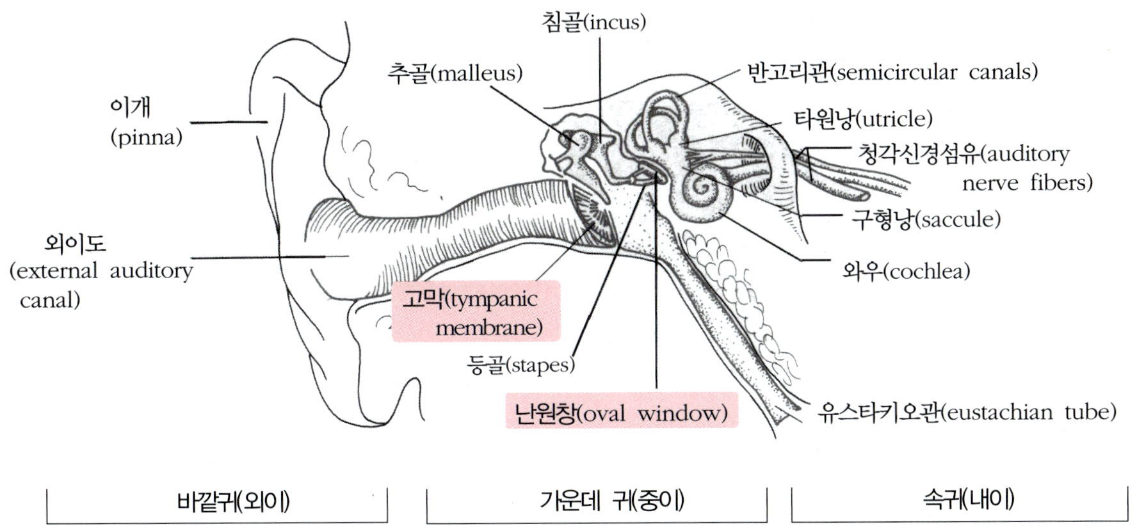

그림 2. 귀(ear)의 구성

1.2 중이(Middle ear) 질환의 종류

화농성 중이염(Suppurative otitis media)

▶ **원인**: 세균에 의한 감염

▶ **치료**: – 항생제(antibiotics) 투여 및 고막절개술(myringotomy)

– 만성 화농성 중이염(Otitis media purulent chronic; OMPC)

– 급성 화농성 중이염(Otitis media purulent acute; OMPA)

장액성(삼출성) 중이염(Serous otitis media)

▶ **원인**: 중이(가운데귀) 내 무균성 장액이 고이는 질환으로 비감염성 염증

▶ **치료**: – 고막절개술(myringotomy)

– 고막천자(장액성 물질을 흡입)

점액성 중이염(Secretory otitis media)

▶ **원인**: 무균성 장액이나 삼출액이 생기는 중이의 염증

2.1 수술 방법

고막절개술(Myringotomy)

▶ 청력상실 또는 꼭지돌기염(mastoiditis) 예방

▶ 화농성 물질 제거

고막성형술(Myringoplasty)

▶ 청력장애가 30dB 이하일 경우에 뚫어진 고막천공만을 재건시켜 주는 수술

유양돌기(꼭지돌기)절제술(Mastoidectomy)

▶ **목적**

– 심한 중이(가운데귀) 질환이 있는 경우 유양동(꼭지돌기굴) 통해 배액(drainage)

– 진주종이 있는 중이염에서 진주종 완전제거(가장 중요한 목적)

고실성형술(Tympanoplasty)

- **목적**: 중이(가운데귀)의 염증병소 제거 및 청력회복
  - 음파의 차폐효과: 고막 형성시켜 줌
  - 음압의 전도: 고막과 가동성이 있는 이소골의 전음연쇄를 형성시켜 음압변환이 되도록 함
  - 전음기구를 새로이 만들어 주는 수술

2.2 난청(Deafness)

- **신경성 난청(nerve deafness)**
  - 와우(cochlea) 및 청신경 장애
- **전음성 난청(conduction deafness)**
  - 음파를 와우에 전달하는 가운데귀의 이소골 및 고막의 장애

2.3 진주종(Cholesteatoma)

- 중이(가운데귀) 내 주머니에 피부세포와 콜레스테롤의 축적
- 이 낭같은 덩어리는 대부분 만성중이염의 결과
- 고막천공(perforation)과 관련

3.1 배액관(Drain)

- **치료목적**: 이미 존재하는 고름, 혈종 또는 장 내용물 등을 외부로 배액
- **예방목적**: 수술 후 출혈 가능성 또는 장 내용물 및 조직액 등이 고여 합병증 유발
- **종류**: Silastic penrose, Close suction drain-Hemovac, Tube drain

3.2 만성부비동염(Chronic sinusitis)

▸ **원인**: 자연개구부의 폐쇄로 인한 환기 및 배설 기능의 장애

- 상기도 감염(URI) 후 이차적 부비동의 세균감염, 치아손상을 통한 세균감염 알레르기성 비염, 심한 안면부 손상 후 후유증
- 체질, 알러지, 세균의 종류, 부비동의 해부학적 구조, 혈관운동신경장애 등
- 소아의 경우 상기도염 및 아데노이드비대증

▸ **증상**: 비폐색, 비루 후각장애, 두통, 주의산만, 피로

▸ **검사**

- 비경검사: 중비갑개 점막의 부종, 중비도의 점액, 농성비루 보임
- 동세척, X-선 검사, PNS CT, 내시경검사

▸ **치료**

- 전신적인 항생제 및 소염제 투여
- 국소적으로 비강내 점막의 종창 제거 → 분비물의 배설/부비동내 통기성 회복

▸ **수술**

- Caldwell-Luc operation
  - 동감염 지속/재발 시, 악성종양 의심, 동이물, 안면골절 시
  - antrochoanal polyp(상악동후비공폴립), oro-antral fistula(구동), 내상악동맥결찰 위한 수술
- 최근에는 내시경적 비내수술(FESS: functional endoscopic surgery) 사용
  : 자연 배설구를 넓혀 주면서 사골동, 상악동 등 부비동 수술을 하는 내시경적 비내수술

3.3 수면무호흡증후군(Sleep Apnea Syndrome)

▸ **증상**: 수면시 심한 코골음 및 주간 과다 졸음

▸ **합병증**: 무호흡에 의한 저산소증은 치명적인 부정맥증

▸ **빈도**: 전 인구의 1%, 40~50대 남성에게 호발

표 1 • 수면 무호흡 증후군의 분류

중추형(Central)		폐쇄형(Obstructive)	
• 정상신체습관	• 불면증	• 대개 비만	• 지적 기능장애
• 수면중 정상행동	• 경미 혹은 간헐적 코골음	• 수면중 비정상적 행동	• 코골음
• 우울증	• 최소한 성적 기능장애	• 야뇨증	• 두통
		• 주간졸음증	

표 2 • 안구진탕 및 금단증후군

▸ Nystagmus(안구진탕)	▸ Withdraw syndrome(금단 증후군)
- 안구운동계 이상 - 무의식적이고 빠른 눈의 리듬감 있는 운동	- 지속적으로 사용하던 물질을 갑자기 중단 - 사용 양을 줄일 경우 발생 - 생리적, 심리적, 행동적 반응 - 불안, 불면증, 두통 등

차트 용어

· Anorexia	식욕부진	· Chill	오한	· Compression	압박	· Destruction	파괴
· Discharge	분비	· Drain	배액관	· Epistaxis	코피	· Headache	두통
· Hyposmia	후각감퇴	· Gait	보행	· Lymphadenitis	림프선염	· Myalgia	근육통
· Mutism	벙어리	· Nausea	오심/구역질	· Otalgia	이통(귀통증)	· Perforation	천공
· Scanty	빈약한	· Sneezing	재채기	· Snoring	코골이	· Sputum	가래/객담
· Temperature	체온	· Tinitus	이명(귀울림증)	· Tympanum	고실	· Wall	벽

약 어	원 어	
AD	Right ear(Latin: auris dextra)	오른쪽 귀
AS	Left ear(Latin: auris sinistra)	왼쪽 귀
AU	Both ear(Latin: auris uterque)	양쪽 귀
BW	Body weight	체중
COM	Chronic otitis media	만성 중이염
EAC	External auditory canal	외이도(바깥귀길)
EEG	Electroencephalogram	뇌파도, 뇌전도
HL	Hearing loss	난청, 귀머거리
I&D	Incision and drainage/skin	절개 및 배농(피부)
MMPI	Minnesota Multiphasic Personality Inventory	미네소타다면성격검사
MN	Midnight	자정
PTA	Pure tone audiogram	순음 청력검사
TM	Tympanic membrane	고막
URI	Upper respiratory infection	상기도감염

등록번호	373 72 68	성별 F
성명	신 완 판	
주민등록	870601-1234567	

입 퇴 원 기 록
Admission and Discharge Record

주 소 : 서울시 서초구 반포동 410

출신지 : 대구시 남구 송현동 253 **직 업** : **전 화** :

연고자성명 : 안주한 **관 계** : 주 소 : 전 화 :

					전과			
입원 : 2017 년 6 월 5 일	과	병동	호		전과	20 년 월 일	과 병동	호
퇴원 : 2017 년 6 월 13 일	과	병동	호			20 년 월 일	과 병동	호
재원일수 :						20 년 월 일	과 병동	호

최종진단명	**분 류 번 호**
주진단명 : Cholesteatoma with allergic otitis media	
기타진단명 : Deaf mutism	
수술 및 처치명	
수술명 : Lt. modified radical mastoidectomy	
with mastoid obliteration	
기타수술 및 주요검사 :	

치료결과 : 1. 완쾌 2. 경쾌 3. 호전안됨 4. 진단뿐 5. 가망없는 퇴원 6. 48시간내 사망 7. 48시간이후 사망

퇴원형태 : 1. 퇴원지시후 2. 자의퇴원 3. 탈원 4. 전원

병원감염 : 1. 수술후 2. 기타처치후 3. 비뇨기계 4. 호흡기계 5. 소화기계 6. 기타

원사인 : 부검 : 예, 아니오

계속적 진료 계획

없음있음 (약속일 2017 년 6 월 20 일 시)

담당 전공의 서명 : 이승길	담당 전문의 서명 : 장민일
의무기록 완성 : 2017 년 7 월 20 일	의무기록사 서명 :

등록번호	373 72 68	성별 F
성명	신 완 판	
주민등록	870601-1234567	

퇴 원 요 약

Discharge Summary

Final diagnosis : Cholesteatoma with chronic allergic OM, both
Deaf mutism
Otorrhea, both

C.C. : Pain c̄ otorrhea from the both ear

P.I : 5살 때 chronic OM 앓은 이후
deafness 상태로 지내왔으며, 1년 전부터 양쪽 귀에 통증을 수반하는
otorrhea가 지속되어 OPD 경유
OP 권유받고 Adm.

P.E : Both tympanic membrane: epithelium c̄ perforation, attic destruction 상태이며
scanty discharge

PTA Rt. - total deafness
Lt - total deafness
mastoid series: both sclerotic c̄ suspecious bony destruction

OP. 2017. 6. 6 Lt. MRM c̄ MO

Hosp. course
Mild otalgia, Lt ⊕
POD #2: Drain removed & compression
그 후 mild nausea, dizziness 발생
POD #6: Stitch out → scanty discharge at drain insertion site

Plan : OPD F/U

Jang

등록번호	373 72 68	성별 F
성명	신 완 판	
주민등록	870601-1234567	

병력 및 신체검진기록
History & Physical Examination

C.C : Otorrhea, both

P.I : 상기 30세된 여자 환자는 5살 때 심한 귀의 염증을 앓은 후 청각 소실이 생기고, mutism으로 지내오던 중, alcoholic인 부친이 심한 우울증 발작 → paranoid로 imp.시 환자를 구타한 사건이 발생 후 양쪽 귀의 통증이 발생함. 일주일부터는 otorrhea 증상으로 본원 ENT OPD visit, op 권유 받고 입원함.

PHx. : Hospitalization : 3년 전, local OB & Gyn에서
Care of uterine scar from C/sec. : delivery ♂ baby

Allergy (+) DM/HTN (-/-)
Cervical Tb. lymphadenitis로 3년 전 medication.
1999년 ♂ 분만 후 또 다시 임신되었으나 자연유산됨.

PEx :V/S : 100/70 - 36 - 80 - 20
G/A : Relatively healthy app.
M/S : alert
HEENT : Rt. TM: nearly total perforated
Discharge (+) but scanty, yellowish color
Lt. TM: Total perforation
Chest : Symmetric expansion
RHB $\bar{s}$ ⓜ
CBS $\bar{s}$ ⓡ
Abd. : Soft and flat
Normoactive bowel sound
Ext. : G-F

Int. 강친절

병력 및 신체 검진기록

일 자	내 용	서 명
	FHx : 어머니가 당뇨병으로 인슐린 치료도중 cataract 발생함. 환자의 부친은 매일 소주 2병 이상을 마시며 최근에는 정신병으로 발전하였으며, 환자는 결혼을 하지 않은 상태에서 ♂ baby를 기르고 있으나 남아가 선천성 viral pneumonia로 local에서 치료를 받고 있다고 함. imp) Cholesteatoma, OM, both deaf-mutism Plan) Lt. TM	
		Int. 강친절

등록번호	373 72 68	성별 F
성명	신 완 판	
주민등록	870601-1234567	

경 과 기 록
Progress Notes

6.5 〈 Admission note 〉

C.C : Otorrhea, both with pain
onset: 8 days ago

P.I : 상기 F/30 환자는 약 2년 전부터 otorrhea가 시작되었으나, 구타당한 후 약 8일 전부터는 통증이 동반되고 심해져서 한약으로 치료하였으나 호전되지 않아 본원 OPD를 방문하여 op 예정으로 adm. recommend 됨.
약 5살 때 귀를 심하게 앓고 난 후 both ear problem이 호전되지 않고 농아가 됨.

PHx : 개인병원에서 C-sec, delivery ♂ baby delivered.
Trauma (−), allergy (+)
current medication (−), Alcohol/smoking (−/−)
major illness: DM (−), HTN (−)
Cervical Tb. lymphadenitis로 medication을 약 2년 전에 먹고 치유됨.
→ left neck scar는 (8세 때, 피부감염으로 I&D한 자국임)

ROS : G/A : relatively healthy looking
Wt : 45kg, wt. loss (−)
fever/chill (−/−), cough/sputum (−/−),
headache (−), anorexia (+), nausea/vomiting (−/−),
myalgia (+), diarrhea (−), constipation (−)

Ear : hearing disturbance (+/+), 5살 이후 농아가 됨.
otalgia (+/+) otorrhea (+/+), fullness (−/−), tinitus (+/+)
dizziness (−/−)

Nose : obstruction (−/−), rhinorrhea (+/+) hyposmia (−/−)
epistaxis (−/−), sneezing (+/+), snoring (−/−)

mouth & throat : Frequent sore throat Hx (−)
sore mouth (−)
mouth breathing (+), swallowing diff (−)

경 과 기 록

일 자	내 용	서 명
	Larynx : dyspnea (−), stridor (−), mutism (+) TM : nearly total perforation, discharge (+) : scanty, yellow hyperemic at anterior superior portion whitish color at posterior, inferior portion maleus의 handle이 보이지 않음 Lt. external auditory canal : clear TM : total perforation, suspeciously suction 시 제거되지 않고 마치 고막이 없이 wall 같이 보임. maleus의 handle이 보이지 않음. discharge (+) : scanty, whitish yellow color Nose : pinkish mucose NSD (−) polyp (−) clear - both Mouth and throat PTH (+/+) $\bar{s}$ injection pharyngeal wall injection (−) postnasal drip (+) Indirect laryngoscopy: free vocal cord movement: hormal mass (−) PTA부터 both ear deafness in AC fistular test : [Rt: negative Lt: positive, objective] Lab : WNL Mastoid series : both sclerotic $\bar{c}$ suspeciously bony destruction Chest PA : [pulm Tb. RUL: activity in uncertain no specific material change since 2017-5-28] (2017-6-5) imp) Chole. OM, both deaf-mutism plan) Lt. TM	R1 *Lee*

경 과 기 록

일 자	내 용	서 명
	〈 Get. op permission 〉	
	Dx. : Choleastoma with chronic allergic OM	
	Op. : Radical	
	Operator : Staff.	
	Complication : recurrence, palsy(입이 돌아감)	
	vomiting, 맛감각 이상	
	General Anes.: lung, kidney, liver 이상 초래	R1 *Lee*
6.6	〈 Brief op note 〉	
	1. Op name : Lt. Modified radical mastoidectomy $\bar{c}$ mastoid obliteration	
	2. Operator : Staff. S.G.Lee	
	3. Assistant : R_3 Y.K.Park	
	4. Preop. Dx. : Chole. OM. Lt.	
	5. Postop. Dx : Chole. OM. Lt.	
	6. Anesthesia : G/A	
	7. Finding : EAC post wall: destruction	
	Mastoid cavity : filled $\bar{c}$ large chole matrix sclerotic	
	TM : total perforation $\bar{c}$ epithelium	
	Ossicle & its joint : all absent	
	Chole capsule 일부는 모두 removal 하지 않고 EAC를 expose시킴	
	8. Procedures	
	1) Supine position $\bar{c}$ Head turn to Rt.	
	2) EAC irrigation	
	3) 1% Lido $\bar{c}$ 1:20만 Epi injection around the Lt ear	
	4) Post auricular incision	
	5) Mastoidectomy $\bar{c}$ open cavity technique	
	6) Removal of chole matrix at mastoid cavity	
	7) Elevation of chole capsule at mastoid cavity	
	8) Mastoid drilling	
	9) Antibiotics solu. irrigation	
	10) Incision at EAC	
	11) F fascia insertion at Mastoid cavity	

경 과 기 록

일 자	내 용	서 명
	12) Mastoid obliteration & Gelform packing at EAC 13) Incision repair c̄ 2-layer 14) Drain insertion 15) Mastoid dressing	*Park*
6.8	POD #2 Drain removal Mastoid dressing apply	*Kim*
	Dressing 후 Headache, Nausea 발생 also Gait nystagmus도 발생하여 Dr. removal 후 Sx. 가라앉음.	*Park*
6.9	POD #3 Good, Clear, wound, but tenderness on the retroauricular incision site. 그러나 discharge는 없음	*Kim*
6.10	POD #4 Dressing, wd: clear	*Kim*
6.11	POD #5 Lt. otalgia: mild하고 욱신거린다고 함. Dr. wd : clear	*Park*
6.12	yesterday psy. consult 결과 : "spont, withdrawl syndrome" Psy. Dr. chai 방문 시 discussion 요함. serous discharge from drain insertion site → Dressing	*Park*
6.13	D r. change Scanty discharge from I&D site rec) Discharge c̄ F/U at OPD	*Kim*

등록번호	373 72 68	성별	F
성명	신 완 판		
주민등록	870601-1234567		

협의진료기록
Consultation Record

Request For Consultation To 정신과 오준철 선생님 귀하

Lt. MRM $\bar{c}$ MO 수술받은 30세 여자 환자는 약 4개월 전 술취한 부친으로부터 구타당한 후 사람을 피하고, 환자 자신의 아기마저 care하려 하지 않는 현상이 있습니다.
귀하께서 내원하시고 정신과적 문제가 있는지를 협의합니다.

2017. 6. 10
Date Hour

이비인후과 장민일/박호민
Signature of Attending Physician

Report of Consultation

환자 면담하였습니다.
수술 후이고 hearing loss인 환자 상태로, oral interview는 하지 못하고 MMPI와 EEG 등을 이용하여 Psy. evaluation하였습니다.
imp) withdrawl syndrome
수술경과를 보아 가면서 다시 한번 방문하겠습니다.
감사합니다.

2017. 6. 11

Signature 오준철

등록번호	373 72 68	성별 F
성명	신 완 판	
주민등록	870601-1234567	

방사선 보고서
X-Ray Report

발 행 처	발 행 일 자	보 고 일 자
	2017. 6. 6	2017

Chest PA, Rt. lat

No significant interval change of
RUL pulm. Tb lesion since 2017-5-28

Reported by Jang M.D.

등록번호	373 72 68	성별 F
성명	신 완 판	
주민등록	870601-1234567	

수 술 청 약 서

성 명: 신 완 판

수술/검사명: Lt. modified radical mastoidectomy

주치의사 :

본인은 본인(또는 상기환자)에 대한 수술 및 마취(또는 검사)의 필요성, 내용, 예상되는 합병증과 후유증에 대하여 자세한 설명을 의사로부터 들었으며, 본 수술 및 마취(또는 검사)로써 불가항력적으로 야기될 수도 있는 합병증 또는 환자의 특이체질로 우발적 사고가 일어날 수도 있다는 것을 충분히 이해하며, 만일 분쟁이 생겼을 때는 의료법 제54조의 2에 의한 의료심사조정위원회에 그 조정을 신청토록 할 것이며, 수술 및 마취(또는 검사)에 협력할 것을 서약하고 다음 사항을 성실, 정확히 고지하며 이에 따른 의학적 처리를 주치의 판단에 위임하여 수술 및 마취(또는 검사)를 하여 줄 것을 청약합니다.

합병증 : 재발, 재수술, 안면신경마비(입이 돌아감), 맛감각 이상, 현훈, 구토

전신마취 : 폐→ 폐결핵 가능성, 간장, 신장에 이상 초래 가능성,

* 기 왕 력 : 결핵성 임파염 완치됨

* 특이체질 :

* 고·저혈압 :

* 심 장 병 :

* 약으로 인한 사고 :

* 알레르기 :

* 당 뇨 병 :

* 출혈소인 :

2017 년 6 월 5 일 7시 분 오전
오후

상기환자 또는 대리인(환자의) 전 환 기 (인)

주 소 공주시 신관동 공주대로

보증인 전진일 (인)

주 소 공주시 신관동 공주대로

* 본 청약서는 본인의 서명이나 날인으로 유효하나 미성년자 및 정신질환자 또는 본인이 서명할 수 없는 상태일 때는 보호자가 이를 대리한다.

신기해 병원장 귀하

등록번호	373 72 68	성별 F
성명	신 완 판	
주민등록	870601-1234567	

수술 전 처치
Pre-Op. Check List

	Yes	NO
1. Pre-medication given charted Atropine (　) mg　Demeroi (　) mg　Valium (　) mg Seconal (　) mg　Morphin (　) mg　Luminal (　) mg robinal (0.2) mg　Midazolam (2.5) mg		
2. Pre-op. T.P. R. B. P Chart B.P (100/70)mmHg　Pulse (66)/min　TEMP (36.5℃)　R.(20)/min		
3. Special medication : H/S L Blood (　) pints　D. W (　)cc　D.S (　)cc.		
4. Operation permission : NPO since (12MN) A.M / P.M　Shaving (V)　Enema (　) Foley-catheter (　)　Levin-tube (　)		
5. Special pre-op order's check	Yes	NO
6. 귀중품 보관 및 제거	V	
7. Blood, urine X-ray 기타 검사 보고지 확인	V	
8. Hair, prepared-legging Gown 머리를 갈라 땋고 삼각끈으로 매고 가운 착용 확인	V	
9. Operative unit preparation 수술부위 준비(목욕, 피부준비, 손톱, 발톱)	V	
10. Miscellaneous(기타)　SA 2Ⓥ Epinephrine 1Ⓐ	V	

Date 2017. 6. 6　　Head Nurse 백두진

Preparation nurse 서동인

등록번호	373 72 68	성별	F
성명	신 완 판		
주민등록	870601-1234567		

수 술 기 록
Operation Record

Date : 2017. 6. 6 Surgeon : N.Y.Park
1st Ass't: J.H.Won 2nd Ass't: Y.O.Lee
Scrub nurse: Circ. nurse:

Preoperative diagnosis : Chole with chronic allergic OM
Postoperative diagnosis : Same as above
Name of operation : Lt. modified radical mastoidectomy $\bar{c}$ mastoid obliteration

Operative findings: Tympanum: attic destruction
Ossicles and its joints: all absent
Mastoid air cell: sclerotic, filled with large chole matrix
Aditus and antrum: filled with chole matrix
Posterior wall of EAC: destruction

Procedure : The patient was prepared and drapped in a routine manner under the general anesthesia. After EAC irrigation with saline 1% lidocaine with 1:100,000 epinephrine was infiltrated around the Lt. ear. The postauricular incision by classic type. Temporalis fascia was obtained and laid aside to dry and mastoid cortex was exposured. Mastoid drilling with inside out technique was started. After complete open cavity mastoidectomy was done, operative field was irrigated with antibiotics soln. Gelfoam was inserted into the external auditory canal. The wound was closed by three layers 3-0 chromic and 4-0 silk sutures. Silastic drain was inserted to the wound site. A standard mastoid dressing was applied.

기록일 : 2017. 6. 6 Written by *Park*

등록번호	373 72 68	성별 F
성명	신 완 판	
주민등록	870601-1234567	

의 사 지 시 기 록
Doctor's Orders

6.5

〈 Admission order 〉

1. Check V/S $\bar{q}$ 6hr
2. BR
3. MN-NPO
4. Check B.W & Temp.
5. Get op. permission
6. Skin prep.
7. Injection: TM 1.0gm subicu.
8. Dalma 2T p.o hrs *Lee*

〈 Pre-op order 〉

1. Check V/S $\bar{q}$ 6hr
2. BR
3. NPO
4. Premed.
5. Injection H/S 1L IV $\bar{c}$
6. Send the pt to OR with chart & x-ray after full voiding at 9 : 00 AM

Lee

〈신 완 판〉

★ 신완판 차트를 읽고 맞는 것에 O표 하시오.

1 최종진단명으로 맞게 분류한 것은?

① H60.4, H65.90 ② H95.0, H65.31 ③ H71, H65.481
④ H71, H65.401 ⑤ H60.4, H65.91

2 입원 시 나타난 증상으로 맞게 기재된 것은?

① 전체적인 모습이 피곤해 보였다. ② 코피는 있었으나 가래는 없었다.
③ 근육통과 이명이 있었다. ④ 오한과 식욕부진이 있었다.
⑤ 코골이와 식욕부진은 없었다.

3 환자에 대한 내용으로 <u>틀리게</u> 기재된 것은?

① 수술 후 2일째 배액관 제거와 드레싱후 두통과 오심이 있었다.
② 방사선검사 결과 폐 우상엽에 결핵성 병변이 보였다.
③ 수술 전 혈압은 100/70이었으며, 6시간마다 활력징후를 체크하였다.
④ 입원 당시 자정에 금식하고 체중 및 체온을 체크하도록 지시하였다.
⑤ 고막은 천공이 되었으며 노란색의 분비물이 약간 있었다.

4 환자의 출산력에 대한 것으로 맞게 분류한 것은?

① O34.09 ② O34.51 ③ O34.49
④ O34.22 ⑤ O34.21

5 협의진단에 나타난 사항으로 맞는 것은?

① 금단증상으로 진단되었고, 그에 대한 분류번호는 F06.2이다.
② 미네소타 다면 성격검사와 뇌파검사를 하였다.
③ 구두면접을 못하여 미네소타다면성격검사만 실시하였다.
④ 환자에게 나타난 질병으로 인해 이비인후과에 의뢰하였다.
⑤ 폐의 우상엽에 결핵에 대한 병변은 없었다.

6 처치명에 대한 분류로 맞는 것은?

① 20.41 ② 20.42 ③ 20.49
④ 20.51 ⑤ 20.21

7 수술에 대한 내용으로 <u>다르게</u> 기재한 것은?

① 외이도에서 절개하였고, 전벽은 파괴되었다. ② 수술부위를 항생제 용액으로 세정하였다.
③ silastic 배액관을 상처부위에 삽입하였다. ④ 고실상와가 파괴되었다.
⑤ 상처는 크로믹과 실크로 봉합했다.

8 환자의 가족력에 대한 분류번호로 맞는 것은?

① J12.0, F10.2 ② P23.0, F10.5 ③ P23.0, F10.2
④ P23.9, F10.3 ⑤ P23.9, F10.5

9 **경과기록지에 기재된 내용으로 틀린 것은?**

① 수술 후 7일째 절개 및 봉합 후 약간의 분비물이 흘렀다.
② 수술 후 2일째 보행 시 안구진탕이 있었으나 배액관 제거 후 증상이 호전되었다.
③ 수술 후 3일째 상처부위에 압통은 있었으나 분비물은 없었다.
④ 수술 후 6일째 수술부위에 삽입한 배액관을 통하여 장액의 분비물이 흘렀다.
⑤ 수술 후 5일째 왼쪽 귀에 통증이 경미하게 있었고 상처는 깨끗하였다.

10 **환자의 과거에 대한 진단명으로 맞게 분류된 것은?**

① I88.9 ② A18.2 ③ L90.5
④ L90.0 ⑤ A18.4

02 욕창 동반 대동맥류

Aneurysm of aorta c̄ bedsore

1.1 욕창(Bedsore): Decubitus ulcer

- 피부 또는 점막의 개방된 미란
- 뼈의 돌출부위에 잘 생김
- 오랜 기간 누워있거나 몸을 움직이지 못하는 환자
- 허리 뒷부분에 척추돌출부의 피부가 압력을 받음
- 조직의 혈액공급 및 영양공급의 장애로 발생
- 피부궤양

피부 병변의 종류

• 반점(macule): 평편 • 구진(papule): 고형 • 궤양(ulcer): 개방미란

1.2 동맥류(Aneurysm)

- 죽상경화증(atherosclerosis)으로 동맥벽이 약해지거나 깨어짐에 따라 동맥이 부분적으로 넓어짐
- 심장, 대동맥 또는 동맥의 벽이 이완되거나 돌출되어 나옴
- 그 안에 혈전이 생겨 깨어지면 색전증(embolism) 초래
- 보통 대동맥에 발생

동맥류파열(Aneurysm rupture)

- 동맥류의 위험성은 동맥벽이 바깥쪽으로 밀려나가, 점차 얇아지고 터질 수 있음

심실동맥류(Ventricular aneurysm)

- 관상죽상경화증(coronary atherosclerosis), 심근경색증(myocardial infaction)의 합병증으로 발생

치 료

- 침범한 환자의 혈관, 부위, 환자건강에 달려 있음
- 뇌의 작은 동맥류: 작은 클립(clip)으로 혈관 폐색
- 큰 동맥의 동맥류(대동맥): 합성이식(synthetic graft)

2.1 류마티스 관절염(Rheumatoid arthritis)

- **정의**: 관절의 통증과 염증이 있는 만성질환
- **원인**: 관절조직에 대한 자가면역 반응
- **특징**: 작은 관절(손, 발) → 큰 관절로 영향
- **발병률**
  - 남성 < 여성
  - 활막(synovial membrane)은 염증이 생기고 두꺼워짐
  - 여러 관절에 침범되어 근위축으로 인한 변형 및 관절강직(ankylosis) 초래
- **증상**: 고열, 관절통, 부종
- **진단**
  - 혈액검사에서 류마티스양 인자(항체)[rheumatoid factor(antibody)] 나타남
  - x-ray 검사상 침범받은 관절 주위의 변화로 판명
- **치료**
  - 열찜질
  - 아스피린, gold compounds, corticosteroid: 염증과 통증을 감소시키는 약

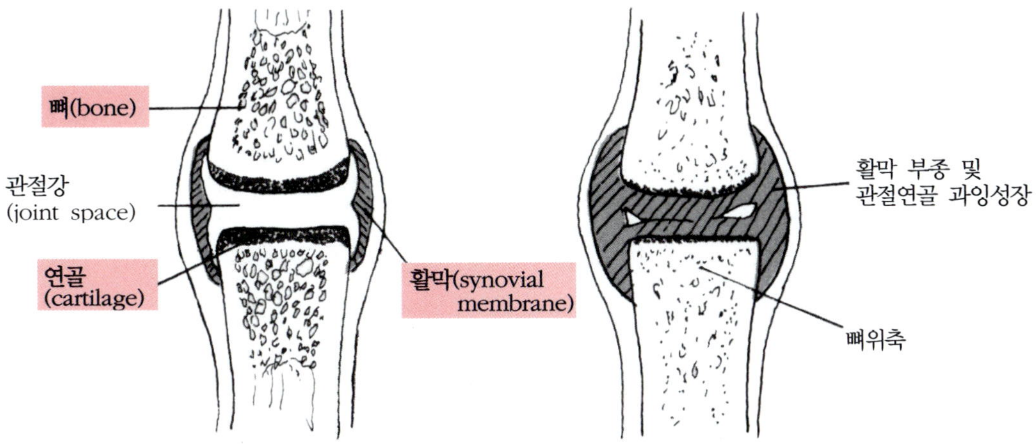

A. 정상 관절(normal joint)　　B. 류마티스 관절염(rheumatoid arthritis)

그림 1. 정상과 류마티스 관절염의 비교

2.2 쿠싱증후군(Cushing's syndrome): 부신피질 과다분비

- **정의**: 부실피질(adrenal cortex)로부터 코티졸을 과잉 생산하게 하는 증상군
- **증상**
  - 비만증, 얼굴(달덩이), 동체(trunk), 목덜미(buffalo hum: 들소목)
  - 골다공증(osteoporosis), 고혈압, 다모증(hirsutism)
  - 고혈당증(hyperglycemia), 고나트륨혈증(hypernatremia), 고칼륨혈증(hyperkalemia)
- **원인**
  - 부신피질자극호르몬(Adrenocorticotropic hormone; ACTH)의 과잉분비
  - 부신피질의 종양

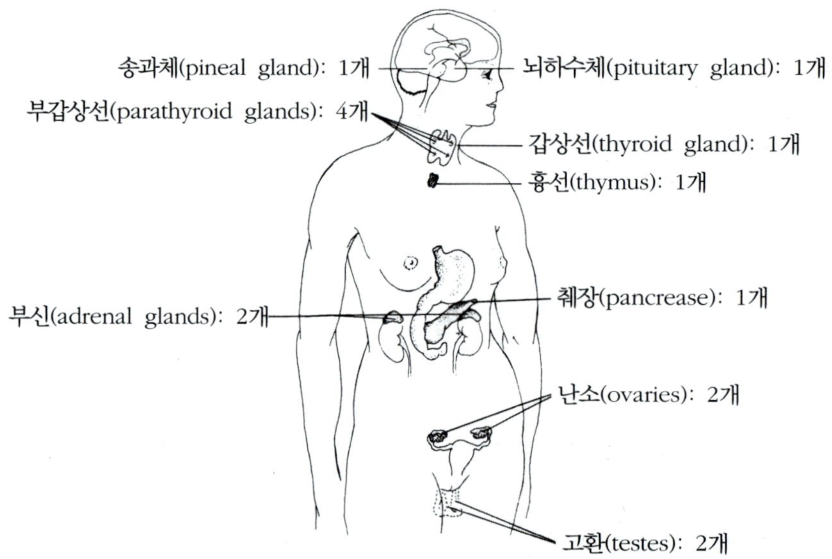

그림 2. 내분비계(endocrine system): 내분비 장기(9개)
분비관 없이 혈액 속으로 분비

3.1 마비(Palsy)

- 운동 기능의 완전 또는 부분적 상실

뇌성마비(Cerebral palsy)

- 임신 또는 주산기(perinatal) 동안의 대뇌 손상이 원인
- 부분적 마비와 근육의 조정 결핍

벨마비(Bell's palsy), 안면신경마비

- 제7번 뇌신경인 안면신경(facial nerve)장애로 인해 안면마비로 입이 비뚤어짐
- 눈을 깜박거릴 때 입술이 당겨 올라가고 말하거나 웃을 때 눈이 감김
  - 얼굴 근육이 독자적으로 움직이지 못하여 얼굴표정이 부자연스러움
- 원인불명
- 완전회복 가능

3.2 질병분류상 주의점

5단위 분류

- 근골격계 및 결합조직의 질환: 해부학적 부위
- 손상, 중독 및 외인에 의한 결과
  - 개방성 또는 폐쇄성 골절여부
  - 두개강내, 흉곽내 및 복강내 손상 시 개방창 동반여부
- 질병이환 및 사망의 외인: 사건발생 시 수행된 행위의 유형

해부학적 부위별 5단위 분류: 진단 및 수술 최대자리(5자리)

- **근골격 침범부위**: KCD-7(1권)

  예) Rheumatoid arthritis, one hand, serology, RA factor, negative M06.04

  (혈청검사 음성인 류마티스 관절염, 한 손)

- **무릎내 이상병태의 국소적 침습부위**

  예) Derangement of MCL meniscus due to old tear M23.25

  (오래된 열상으로 인한 무릎의 내측 곁인대의 반월판 이상)

- **배병증(dorsopathies)의 해부학적 침습부위**

  예) Thoracic spondylolysis M43.04

  [흉추(등뼈)의 척추분리증]

- **생물역학적 병소의 부위**: KCD-7(1권)

  예) Intervertebral disc stenosis of sacral neural canal M99.54

  [천추(엉치)신경관의 추간판협착]

차트 용어

· Constipation	변비	· Deviation	편위	· Dissecting	박리성	· Dizziness	현기증
· Edema	부종	· Hematemesis	토혈	· Hematochezia	혈변	· Hematuria	혈뇨
· Hemoptysis	객혈	· Insomnia	불면증	· Sore throat	인후통/목통증	· Tenderness	압통

약 어	원 어	
ECHO	Echocardiography	초음파 심장조영술
ICU	Intensive care unit	중환자실
LVH	Left ventricular hypertrophy	좌심실비대
MCL	Medial collateral ligament	무릎의 내측결 인대
MI	Myocardial infarction	심근경색증(=heart attack, 심장발작)
OB	Occult blood	잠혈
OD	Once daily	1일 1회
PT	Physical therapy	물리치료
RA	Rheumatoid arthritis	류마티스 관절염
RUQ	Right upper quadrant	우상 1/4
U/O	Urine output	소변배출량

등록번호	210 66 77	성별 F
성명	이 필 승	
주민등록	770503-1234567	

입 퇴 원 기 록
Admission and Discharge Record

주 소 : 서울시 송파구 서울시 송파구 올림픽로4길 15 아시아선수촌 Apt 11-101

출신지 : 직 업 : 전 화 :

연고자성명 : 황주석 관 계 : 주 소 : 전 화 :

	전과	
입원 : 2017년 12 월 15 일 과 병동 호		20 년 월 일 과 병동 호
퇴원 : 2018년 월 일 과 병동 호		20 년 월 일 과 병동 호
재원일수 :		20 년 월 일 과 병동 호

최종진단명	분 류 번 호
주진단명 : Aneurysm of aorta $\bar{c}$ bedsore	
기타진단명 : Rheumatoid arthritis	
Iatrogenic Cushing syndrome	
Bell's palsy	
수술 및 처치명	
수술명 : Conservative management	
Chest C-T	
Abdominal C-T	
Abdominal sonography	
Echocardiography	
기타 수술 및 처치명 : PT	

치료결과 : 1. 완쾌 2. 경쾌 3. 호전안됨 4. 진단뿐 5. 가망없는 퇴원 6. 48시간내 사망 7. 48시간이후 사망

퇴원형태 : 1. 퇴원지시후 2. 자의퇴원 3. 탈원 4. 전원

병원감염 : 1. 수술후 2. 기타처치후 3. 비뇨기계 4. 호흡기계 5. 소화기계 6. 기타

원 사 인: 부검 : 예, 아니오

계속적 진료 계획

없음있음 (약속일 2017 년 1 월 10 일 시)

담당 전공의 서명 : 이수용	담당 전문의 서명 : 정교가
의무기록 완성 : 20 년 월 일	의무기록사 서명 :

등록번호	210 66 77	성별 F
성명	이 필 승	
주민등록	770503-1234567	

퇴 원 요 약
Discharge Summary

Final Dx : 1. Dissecting aneurysm of thoracoabdominal aorta $\bar{c}$ bedsore
2. Rheumatoid arthritis
3. Iatrogenic Cushing syndrome
4. Bell's palsy

C.C : Chest pain and dyspnea

PHx : Arthralgia hx(+) - 계속 진통제(steroid 제제) 복용중

FHx : Her mother - MI로 치료받고 있음

Lab. & X-ray Findings
V/S : BP 220/120 - 105 - 20 LD isoenzymes : WNL
Chest C-T : dissecting aneurysm of aorta
Echo : LVH
Abdominal sonography : fatty liver disease and pleural effusion, Lt.

Hospital Course and Therapeutic Procedures
BP는 medication으로 control, moderate RA는 pain control, Cushing syndrome은 cortisol/ACTH workup 끝난 상태이고 Bell's palsy는 물리치료로써 많이 호전되었으며 '18.1.10 Endocrinology dept. OPD F/U하기로 하고 퇴원

Discharge Medications
1. Inderal 240mg ┐ #3 P.O
Minipress 6mg ┘
Anaprox 3T
Ceclor 3C ┐ #2 P.O
2. Gaster 40mg ┘
Capoten 50mg
(× 4days)
3. Gelfos 4 pks #4 P.O
4. Prednisolone 5mg OD P.O

R_1 *Lee*

등록번호	210 66 77	성별	F
성명	이 필 승		
주민등록	770503-1234567		

병 력 기 록
History

주 소 : Dyspnea, Chest pain

기 간 : 1day

현병력 : 10년 전부터 rheumatoid arthritis가 있어 local hospital에서 처방한 진통제를 복용하시던 분으로 상기 주소로 본원 ER을 경유하여 endocrinology dept로 adm.

과거력 : 약물부작용 ☐Yes ☑No ______ 알레르기 ☐Yes ☑No ______

폐결핵 ☐Yes ☑No ______ 당 뇨 ☐Yes ☑No ______

고혈압 ☑Yes ☐No ______ 간 암 ☐Yes ☑No ______

종 양 ☐Yes ☑No ______ 기 타 ☑Yes ☐No RA

상해 또는 수술력 ☐ Yes ☑ No ______

현재 복용중인 약물 ☑ Yes ☐ No Steroids 제제 복용 for 10 years

흡 연 ☐No ☑ Yes 1 pk/day x 10 yrs.

음 주 ☑No ☐ Yes 주량 및 빈도 ______

월경주기 30일 초경 15세 폐경 ___ 세 최종월경 17년 11월 30일

월경통 ☐Yes ☑ No 임신력 ☐-☐-☐-☐

소아인 경우

출생시 체중___kg 임신기간 ____주 분만방법 ☐자연분만 ☐제왕절개(이유___)

예방접종 ☐완료 ☐안함 ☐진행중 (BCG__ Hepavax__ DPT__ TOPV__ MMR__)

가족력 : 고혈압, 심혈관계 질환: ☑Yes ☐No Her mother: MI로 치료중

악성종양 : ☐ Yes ☑ No (☐간암 ☐유방암 ☐대장암 ☐난소암 ☐기타)

감염성 질환 : ☐ Yes ☑ No (☐간염 ☐결핵 ☐기타____________)

당 뇨 : ☐ Yes ☑ No

기 타 : N-C

계통별 문진 소견

	Yes	No		Yes	No		Yes	No		Yes	No		Yes	No
전신무력감	☐	☑	피로감	☑	☐	발 열	☐	☑	오 한	☐	☑	두통	☐	☑
현 기 증	☑	☐	불면증	☐	☑	목구멍통증	☐	☑	기 침	☐	☑	가래	☐	☑
각 혈	☐	☑	가슴통증	☑	☐	심계항진	☐	☑	오 심	☐	☑	구토	☐	☑
토 혈	☐	☑	복 통	☑	☐	소화불량	☐	☑	식욕부진	☐	☑	혈변	☐	☑
복부팽만감	☐	☑	변 비	☐	☑	설 사	☐	☑	체중변화	☐	☑	부종	☐	☑
배뇨 곤란	☐	☑	혈 뇨	☐	☑	호흡곤란	☑	☐	(NYHA I, II, III, IV)					

기 타____________ *Park*

등록번호	210 66 77	성별 F
성명	이 필 승	
주민등록	770503-1234567	

신 체 검 진 기 록
Physical Examination

전신외관

외관	☐ 병색없음	☐ 만성병색	☑ 급성병색		
의식상태	☐ 정상	☑ 몽롱	☐ 혼미	☐ 반혼수	☐ 혼수
발육 및 영양상태	☑ 정상	☐ 부족	☐ 비만		
피부긴장도	☑ 정상	☐ 빈약			

머리, 눈, 귀, 코 및 목구멍

두개형상	☑ 정상	☐ 이상____________	
결막	☑ 정상	☐ 창백(경함, 심함)	☐충혈(경함, 심함)
공막	☑ 정상	☐ 황달(경함, 심함)	
이루 및 비루	☑ 없음	☐ 있음	
목, 입술 및 혀	☑ 정상	☐ 건조(경함, 심함)	
목 및 편도	☑ 정상	☐ 충혈	☐ 편도비대
기타 ____________			

경부

목	☑ 유연	☐ 경직(경함, 심함)	
경정맥	☑ 정상	☐ 확장	
임파절	☑ 정상	☐ 종대	
갑상샘	☑ 정상	☐ 종대	☐ 종물

가슴 및 폐

시진	☑ 대칭 팽창	☐ 비대칭 팽창
	☐ 흡기시 함몰(늑간, 가슴뼈밑, 늑연하)	
촉진 및 타진	☑ 정상	☐ 이상
청진	☑ 정상	☐ 이상(wheezing, crackle, friction, rub)

심장

최대 박동점	☑ 정상(5th, ICS & H.MCL)	☐ 이상 _______
심박동	☑ 규칙	☐ 불규칙
잡음(murmur)	☑ 없음	☐ 있음(Grade I, II, III, IV, V)
		종류 ___________

신 체 검 진 기 록

복부

시 진 ☑ 편평 ☐ 함몰 ☐ 팽만(경함, 심함)

청 진 ☑ 정상잡음 ☐ 이상잡음(항진, 감소)

촉진 및 타진 ☐ 유연 ☐ 강직 ☐ 종목 ☑ 압통 ☐ 반동압통

☐ 이동탁음(shifting dullness) ☐ 장기촉지 N-C

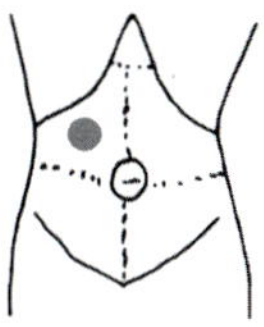

기타 Epigastric tenderness

유방

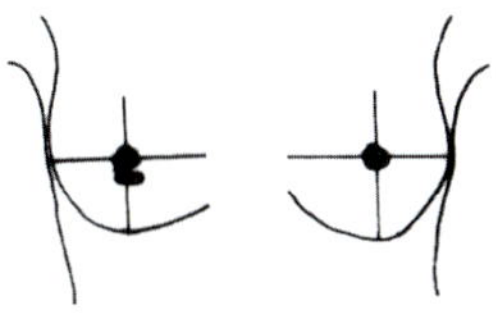

☑정상 ☐ 비정상소견

유 방 통 ☐ 주기성 ☐ 비주기성

유두분비물 ☐ 혈성 ☐ 우유색 ☐ 기타

유방 종괴 (위치____cm 거리 ____cm 크기 ____cm)

등 및 사지

늑골 척추간 압통 ☐ Yes ☑ No

운 동 제 한 ☐ Yes ☑ No

관 절 부 위 압통 ☑ Yes ☐ No

신경계

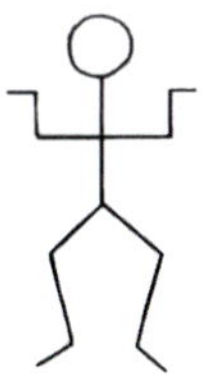

동공 및 대광반사 ☑ 정상 ☐ 이상 __________

운 동 및 감 각 ☑ 정상 ☐ 이상 __________

심 부 건 반 사 기타 N-C

항문

시 진 ☐ 정상 ☐ 치열 ☐ 치핵 ☐ 치루

수 지 검 사 ☐ 전립선 비대(유, 무) ☐ 괄약근 긴장도(감소, 정상, 증가)

☐ 종괴(항문면에서 거리 ___cm, 방향____)

☐ 기타

앞

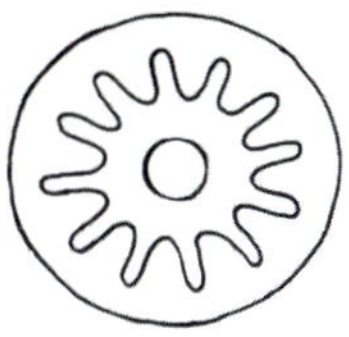

뒤

추정진단 Iatrogenic Cushing Syndrome *Park*

등록번호	210 66 77 성별 F
성명	이 필 승
주민등록	770503-1234567

경 과 기 록
Progress Notes

일 자	내 용	서 명
	〈 ICU Record 〉	
12.15	9: 00 PM S : Mental state is drowsy, poor cooperative	
	O : V/S BP 130/65 mmHg HR 91/min	
	LR (++/++) c̄ isocoria	
	No pathologic reflex	
	Abdominal C-T: dissecting aneurysm of aorta	
	Echodoppler: LVH with LV dysfunction	
	A : Iatrogenic Cushing syndrome	
	Dissecting aneurysm of aorta c̄ bedsore	
	R/O adrenal insufficiency state	
	P : Adrenal function test	
	BP & HR control	*Lee*
12.16	3: 00 PM S : Mental state-drowsy	
	Oral intake - poor	
	O : V/S BP 140/80 → 120/70mmHg HR 90/min	
	U/O : poor	
	BUN/Cr 19/1.1 electrolytes : 133-3.8-98-8.1	
	ESR 36 GOT/GPT 97/32	
	TP/AL 5.4/2.5	
	A : Iatrogenic Cushing syndrome	
	Dissecting aneurysm of thoracoabdominal aorta c̄ bedsore	
	R/O secondary adrenal insufficiency	
	P : Oral prednisolone 10mg # OD maintain	
	BP & HR control	*Lee*
12.17	4 : 00 PM S : Mental state : alert → to drowsy	
	Intermittent irritable state	
	O : V/S BP 128/76mmHg HR 90/min	
	U/O 35-50cc/hr	
	BUN/Cr 16/0.9 Na-K-Cl-Ca : 134-3.2-99-9.1	
	A : Hypokalemia, dehydration	
	P : 1/2 N/S	
	KCL 60meq/supply	*Lee*

경 과 기 록

일 자	내 용	서 명
12.18	S : Mental state: alert to drowsy	
	O : BP 120/80 → 130/70	
	HR 80±10/min	
	U/O 10-50cc/hr	
	PEx: RUQ tenderness (+)	
	A : Dissecting aneurysm of aorta $\bar{c}$ bedsore	
	Iatrogenic Cushing syndrome	
	Adrenal insufficiency	
	P : Inderal dossage ↑	*Lee*
12.19	S : Mental state: alert	
	coorperation: fair	
	O : V/S BP 160/80 → 127/65 HR 80-90/min	
	No fever	
	PEx : trunk & buttock area, Rt. pretibial area : ulceration(+)	
	RUQ tenderness	
	A : Dissecting aneurysm of aorta $\bar{c}$ bedsore	
	Iatrogenic Cushing syndrome	
	Moderate rheumatoid arthritis	
	P : Abdominal sonography for RUQ pain	*Lee*
12.21	Patient was transferred to general ward from ICU	*Lee*
12.26	S : 1) RUQ tenderness 2) Abdominal pain	
	3) Sore at sacral area & Rt pretibial lesion	
	O : V/S stable BP 150/80 → 110/70 HR 90/min → 75/min	
	↑ inderal 0.5mg/IV	
	Hx상 입원전 RUQ trauma (+)	
	A : Dissecting aneurysm of aorta $\bar{c}$ bedsore	
	Iatrogenic Cushing syndrome	
	P : MRI (thoracoabdominal MRI)	*Lee*
12.28	S : RUQ tenderness & abdominal pain is much improved	
	P : conservative treatment	
	cancel MRI	*Lee*
12.30	Neurology consultation for lip deviation	
12.31	PT was done for lip deviation	*Lee*
18.1.5	Discharge $\bar{c}$ medication and OPD F/U '18. 1.10	*Lee*

등록번호	210 66 77	성별	F
성명	이 필 승		
주민등록	770503-1234567		

협의진료기록
Consultation Record

Request For Consultation To 신경과 조준탁 선생님

진단명 및 의뢰사유

상기 40세 여자 환자는 chest pain & dypnea를 주소로 dissecting aneurysm of aorta $\bar{c}$ bedsore의 진단하에 HD #15째인 환자입니다.

Lt. side에 facial palsy가 발견되어 귀과의 고진선처 부탁드립니다.

2017. 12. 30
Date Hour

정교가 / R_1 이수용
Signature of Attending Physician

Report of Consultation

Problem: Lip deviation to Rt. side

Imp) Lt. side Bell's palsy, peripheral type

Tx: 1. Reconsult after control the aneurysm
2. Physical therapy

2017. 12. 30

Signature 조준탁

〈이 필 승〉

★ 이필승 차트를 읽고 맞는 것에 O표 하시오.

1 주진단명의 분류번호가 맞는 것은?

① I71.02 ② I72.1 ③ I72.2
④ I71.9 ⑤ I71.29

2 경과기록지에 대한 내용으로 맞는 것은?

① 입원기간 동안 우상부에 압통과 외상이 있었다.
② 체간, 볼기 및 오른쪽 비골(종아리뼈)에 궤양이 있었다.
③ 자기공명영상을 촬영하였다.
④ 입술편위에 대한 물리치료를 하였다.
⑤ 입원 당시 협조적인 상태였다.

3 신경과 협의진단 후 확인된 진단명과 처치분류번호가 맞는 것은?

① G51.0, 93.39 ② L89, M06.9 ③ G83.9, 93.83
④ G90.2, 73.4 ⑤ G51.0, 93.83

4 의무기록 내용에 대한 설명으로 맞는 것은?

① 입원 시 의식상태는 혼수상태이다
② 초음파 심장촬영술 검사 결과 좌심실 비대 소견이 나타났다.
③ 복부 초음파검사 결과 간경화와 왼쪽에 흉막(가슴막)삼출이 있었다.
④ 환자의 어머니는 협심증을 앓고 있다.
⑤ 입원 다음날 소변배출량은 양호하였다.

5 약물에 의한 부작용으로 생긴 질환과 관련된 진단명의 분류번호는?

① I71.02 ② L89.9 ③ E24.2
④ G51.0 ⑤ E24.4

6 Bedsore에 대한 내용으로 다르게 기재한 것은?

① 피부궤양으로 조직의 혈액공급의 장애로 발생한다.
② 한 자세로 오랫동안 눕는 압력 때문에 생긴다.
③ decubitus ulcer라고도 한다.
④ 면역계이상으로 관절과 내부장기의 만성 염증성 질환이다.
⑤ 피부 또는 점막의 개방된 미란이다.

7 퇴원 시 약 처방의 내용 중 부신피질 호르몬제인 것은?

① Anaprox ② Gelfos ③ Gaster
④ Prednisolone ⑤ Enafon

8 RA에 대한 분류번호가 맞는 것은?

① M05.89 ② M05.31†, I41.8* ③ M06.91
④ I25.2 ⑤ M06.99

9 **진료통계에 대한 내용으로 틀린 것은?**

① 개인의원을 경유하여 본원 응급실을 통해 내원하였다.
② 중환자실의 재원일수는 6일, 일반병동은 15일이다.
③ 입원과는 내분비내과, 퇴원과는 신경과이다.
④ 협의진료는 내분비과에서 신경과로 의뢰하였다.
⑤ 협의진료 건수는 1건이다.

10 **신체검진상 상기 환자에게 나타난 증상인 것은?**

① hematochezia ② dizziness ③ hematemesis
④ sore throat ⑤ constipation

03 백내장 및 녹내장
Cataract and glaucoma

눈(Eye)

1. Cornea	각막(굴절, refraction)
2. Anterior chamber	전안방/앞방(굴절)
Aqueous humor	안방수(굴절)
3. Pupil	동공
4. Crystalline lens	수정체(굴절)
5. Vitreous chamber	초자체방/유리체방
Vitreous humor	초자체/유리체액(굴절)
6. Retina	망막

➡

뇌(Brain)

7. Optic nerve fiber	시신경섬유
8. Optic chiasma	시신경교차
9. Thalamus	시상
10. Cerebral cortex	대뇌피질

그림 1. 빛(light rays)의 경로: 1→10번 순서

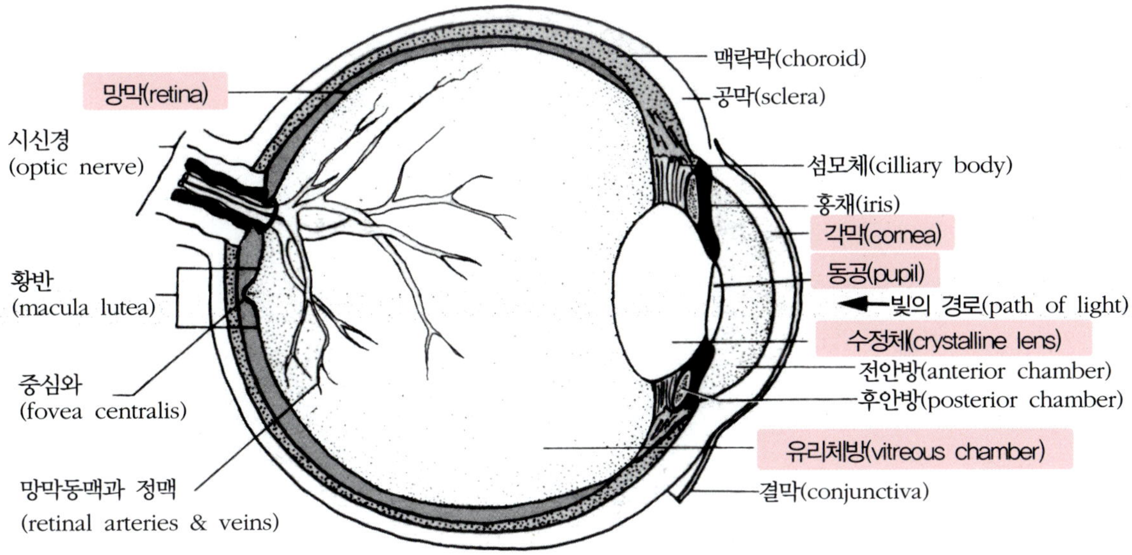

그림 1. 눈(eye)의 구조

표 1 • 백내장 및 녹내장의 비교

백내장(Cataract)	녹내장(Glaucoma)
• 특징: 수정체가 혼탁해져 시력감퇴 진행 • 수술 – 수정체낭내적출(ICCE) – 수정체낭외적출(ECCE) + 인공수정체 삽입술(PCL)	• 특징: 안압의 상승으로 인해 시력상실 초래 • 수술 – 홍채절제술(iridectomy) – 모양체해리술(cyclodialysis)

1.1 백내장의 종류

노인성 백내장(Senile cataract)

- 대개 50세 이후 발생
  - 40대: 초로성 백내장(pre-senile cataract)
  - 40세 미만: 약년성 백내장(juvenile cataract)
- 연령이 증가함에 따라 수정체 섬유단백의 분자량이 증가하면서 투명성을 잃어가는 현상

외상성 백내장(Traumatic cataract)

- 외상으로 수정체가 파열
- 파열되지 않아도 타박으로 수정체 혼탁

합병성 백내장(Complicated cataract)

- 대개 심한 안질환 후 발생
- 심한 만성 각막염, 홍채모양체염, 녹내장, 망막박리, 유리체의 변성 및 출혈 등에 합병되는 수정체 혼탁
- 염증성 독성물질의 직접 작용, 수정체낭의 투과성 변화, 섬모체상피 변화에 의한 방수이상
- 기존의 염증으로 망막의 기능저하 및 조직변성
- 수술 후 시력회복이 되지 않는 경우 빈번

당뇨병성 백내장(Diabetic cataract)

- 연소성 당뇨병 환자에게 발생: 제대로 치료하지 못한 경우
- 당뇨병이 있을 경우: 수술 후 염증 발생, 상처 치유의 지연, 출혈

선천성 백내장(Congenital cataract)

- 원인불명, 유전성
- 태내감염 및 대사이상
  - 풍진백내장: 임신 3개월 때 모체가 풍진에 감염되었을 때 신생아의 양안에 백내장

감염성 질환(infectious diseases)

· rubeola=measles	홍역	· variola=small pox	천연두, 두창
· rubella=german measles	풍진	· varicella=chicken pox	수두

1.2 백내장 검사방법

- 동공산대약 점안
- 작은 손전등, 검안경, 세극등을 검사하여 혼탁의 정도 및 위치 등 확인
- Scheimpflug camera: 수정체의 전후면을 동시에 세극상으로 촬영
  - 자료를 보관 후 그 진행 상태를 계속 관찰(최근)

1.3 백내장 치료방법

수정체낭내적출(Intracapsular cataract extraction; ICCE) → 13.19

- 수정체(lens) 피낭을 포함하여 수정체 전체 적출
- 노인성 백내장에 적용: 최근 사용 저조

수정체낭외적출(Extracapsular cataract extraction; ECCE)+PCL → 13.59, 13.71

- 수정체 피낭을 열고 후낭을 남겨 두고 수정체 내용물만 적출
- 그 자리에 후방 인공수정체 삽입술(PCL)

후방 인공수정체 삽입술(Posterior chamber lens; PCL) → 13.71

- 백내장 적출술 후 거기다 인공물질로 만든 렌즈 삽입
- 수술후 안경 또는 콘택트렌즈 없이도 시력 선명

2.1 수정체수술과 관련된 합병증

▶ 마취 중: 구후출혈(retrobullar hemorrhage), 감염, 안구손상 및 시신경손상

▶ 수술 후: – 인공수정체 탈구(intraocular lens dislocation), 감염, 출혈
– 녹내장, 망막박리 등

표 2 • 점안약

산동제(mydriatics)	축동제(miotics)
• 사용: 부교감신경 마비제 교감신경 흥분제 • 특징: 동공만 산대(조절에 영향없음) • 종류: ·atropine sulfate ·scopolamine hydrobromide, ·homatropine hydrobromide ·cyclogyl ·adrenaline HCI ·ephedrine HCI ·neo-synephrine	• 사용: 부교감신경 흥분제 안압하강 • 종류: ·pilocarpine nitrate ·mecholy ·eserine ·neostigmine bromide ·DFP ·phospholine

* 기타: 항균제(antibacterial agents)

2.2 진단-관련 집단(Diagnosis Related Groups; DRG)

DRG(진단–관련 집단)의 정의

표 3 • 수가제의 비교

DRG(포괄수가제)	행위별 수가제
• 입원환자 분류체계 • 재원기간 유사 • 병원 자원의 소모가 유사한 환자군 • 전향적 산정방법/선불제도 (prospective payment system; PPS) • 건별지불제도(pay-for case system) 예) 충수돌기절제술의 경우 - 충수돌기 환자의 DRG군에 미리 책정 - 일정액의 진료비 지불	• 퇴원환자 분류체계 • 후향적 산정방법/후불제도 (retrospective payment system) 예) 충수돌기절제술 시행 - 진료비는 수술, 처치, 검사 및 약 등의 단가 - 횟수에 따라 지불

DRG 지불제도의 도입 배경

- **행위별 수가제도(Fee-for-service system)의 문제점**
  - 급격한 의료비 상승
  - 진료비 청구심사 업무의 복잡함 및 업무량의 과중
    - 진료비 청구명세서상의 행위, 투약 및 재료 사용 등을 일일이 대조, 심사인력 및 비용, 심사 지불기간 1개월 이상 소요
  - 보험진료비 심사에 따른 의료인 및 보험자 간의 마찰 및 갈등
  - 의료수가관리의 어려움 및 의료서비스 공급 형태의 왜곡현상 유발
    - 각 진료수가 항목간 불균형: 수익성이 높은 수가 항목, 근시교정술 등 비급여 분야에 투자 집중
- **DRG 지불제도의 기대 효과**
  - 의료기관 비용 절감/적정량의 의료서비스 제공
  - 병원경영의 합리화: 의료의 질 향상
    - 재원일수 단축, 병원 생산성 증가 및 전문화
  - 의료기관의 진료청구방법 간편
    - 행정 비용 절감, 진료비 청구 및 심사 조정 마찰 감소
    - 진료비 범위 내에서 의사들의 임상적인 자율권 보장

DRG 대상질환군: 4개 진료과 + 7개 대상질환

- **안과**: 수정체 수술(백내장)
- **이비인후과**: 편도 또는 아데노이드 수술, 기타 다른 수술과 함께 받은 수술
- **외과**: 항문 또는 항문주위 수술, 치질
  - 서혜부(사타구니) 및 대퇴(넙다리) 탈장수술
  - 충수절제술(충수염)
- **산부인과**: 자궁 또는 자궁부속기 수술,악성종양 제외
  - 제왕절개 분만

DRG 번호의 결정

- 주진단과 외과계 시술 등에 의해 결정
- DRG 분류번호는 DRG 본부에서 대상군별로 결정하여 제시
  - 주진단범주(Major Diagnostic Category; MDC)
  - 신체부위 또는 질병특성에 따른 질병군의 23개 대분류
- 연령에 따라 질병군 세분화: 연령구분 필요시
- 기타 진단명(secondary diagnosis)에 따라 합병증 및 동반상병 결정
- 퇴원 시 상태

표 4 • DRG 대분류번호 및 질병군 범주

대분류 번호	질병군 범주
039	· 수정체 수술(vitrectomy)
059	· 편도 및 아데노이드절제술(tonsillectomy & adenoidectomy)
157	· 항문 및 항문주위 수술(anal or stomal procedures)
161	· 서혜(샅) 및 넙다리 탈장 수술(inguinal or femoral hernia procedures)
164	· 복잡한 주진단에 의한 충수절제술(appendectomy)
166	· 복잡한 주진단이 없는 충수절제술(appendectomy)
358	· 자궁 및 자궁부속기 수술(uterine or adnexa procedures)
370	· 제왕절개 분만(cesarean section)

DRG 번호: 6자리

▶ 첫 4자리: 질병군, 5번째 자리: 연령그룹, 6번째 자리: 합병증 및 동반상병 분류

예) 0 5 9 0　0　1

↙ ↘ ↘

질병군 **연령** **합병증 및 동반상병**(수술 후 출혈)

(편도 및 아데노이드) (연령 20세, 연령≥18)

표 5 • 편도 및 아데노이드절제술 DRG 번호

DRG 번호	DRG명칭	입원일수(일) 평균	정상군하한	정상군상한
059001	편도 및 아데노이드절제술, 연령≥18, 합병증 및 동반상병 분류=1	5.51	2	10

진단명 및 수술·처치명 분류번호의 기준

▶ **주진단명**: KCD-7(한국표준질병사인분류)

기타진단명: KCD-7

▶ **수술명**: EDI 코드(의료보험수가 코드)

검사명: EDI 코드 예) 검사코드: E7500-E7750

주진단 및 기타진단의 의미

▶ **주진단(principal diagnosis)**

- 입원하게 된 주원인이 되는 병태
- 입원기간 중의 모든 검사결과를 확인한 후 최종적으로 밝혀진 진단
- 주진단명 선정원칙: U.S. National Committee on Vital and Health Statistics(UHDDS)

▸ **기타 진단(secondary diagnosis): 중증도 결정**

- 합병증(complication): 입원기간중 생긴 이차 질환
- 동반질병(comorbidity)
    - 입원 당시부터 주진단과 함께 가지고 있던 질환
    - 치료 또는 입원기간에 영향을 준 질환

    단, 과거입원과는 관련있지만, 이번 입원과는 무관한 병태(질환)는 제외

합병증 및 동반상병 분류기준

▸ 분류 '2': 기타 진단의 치료에 따른 의료자원의 소모량 증가가 매우 큰 것

▸ 분류 '1': 합병증 및 동반상병 분류 '2'보다 경미한 것

▸ 분류 '0': 기타 진단이 없거나 분류 '1, 2'에 속하지 않는 경우

▸ 합병증과 동반상병에 영향 주지 않는 경우

- 기타 진단이 주진단과 동일하거나 주진단이 속한 질병군과 동일한 질병군에 분류될 경우
- 기타 진단이 의료보험 비급여 대상 진단명

▸ 여러 개의 기타 진단이 있을 경우

- 기타 진단에 의한 합병증 및 동반상병 중 분류단계가 가장 높은 것으로 결정

DRG 환자구분

▸ **정상군**: 입원기간과 행위별 총 진료비가 정상인 환자

▸ **하단열외군**: 입원일수가 정상군의 하한 입원일수보다 짧은 자
(입원일수 < 정상군의 하한 입원일수)

▸ **상단열외군**: 입원일수가 정상군의 상한 입원일수보다 긴 자
(입원일수 > 정상군의 상한 입원일수)

▸ **진료비 열외군**: 총진료비 > 보험자 부담 + 본인부담 진료비

비급여대상

▸ MRI(자기공명전산화 단층 촬영장치), USG(초음파)

▸ 피부질환: 주근깨, 점, 사마귀, 여드름

▸ 포경수술, 보청기, 의수족, 콘택트렌즈의 재료비

▸ 예방접종: 단, 파상풍 혈청주사 중 치료목적으로 사용 시 제외

▸ 보청기, 의수족, 콘택트렌즈의 재료비

열외군(outliers)

▸ 동일한 질병을 가지고도 다른 환자들과 달리 오래 입원(재원기간 길어짐)

▸ 의료이용량이 많은 환자

- 이때 의료기관은 추가지불 신청

▸ **재원일수 열외군(Day-outlier)**

- PPS에 의해 정해진 재원기간을 20일 이상 초과한 경우
- 병원이 추가지불 신청하면 그 이유를 심의하여 타당할 경우

→ DRG 금액에 의한 1일 진료비의 60% 추가 지급

▸ **진료비 열외군(Cost-outlier)**

- 진료비 총액이 DRG 금액의 1.5배 이상이거나 총액이 12,000달러 초과 시

→ 병원이 추가지불 신청하면 심의하여 타당할 경우 차액의 60% 추가 지급

차트 용어

· Aspiration 흡인	· Cortex 피질	· Fundus examination 안저검사	· Hydrodissection 수압박리
· Hyperemic 충혈의	· Irrigation 세척	· Opacity 불투명함	· Rectus 직근
· Superior 상급의	· Trabeculectomy 섬유주절제술	· Viscoelastics 점탄성 물질의	

약 어	원 어	
ABR	Absolute bed rest	절대 안정
AC	Anterior chamber	전안방(앞방)
ECCE	Extracapsular cataract extraction	낭외 백내장 적출술
EOM	Extraocular movement	외안구 운동
HM	Hypermetropia manifast	발현성 원시(hyperopia, hypermetropia)
ICCE	Intracapsular cataract extraction	낭내 백내장 적출술
IOL	Intraocular lens	내안렌즈
IOP	Intraocular pressure	안압
LA	Light and accommodation	빛에 반응하고 조절
LOM	Limitation of motion	운동제한
OD	Right eye(Latin: oculus dexter)	오른쪽 눈
OS	Left eye(Latin: oculus sinister)	왼쪽 눈
OU	Each eye(Latin: oculus uterque)	양안
PCL	Posterior chamber lens(implantation)	수정체 후방(이식술)
PLR	Prompt light reflex	눈이 신속하게 반응
	→ Pupil isocoria $\bar{c}$ PLR(+/+)	동공의 크기 같고 눈이 신속하게 반응
VA	Visual acuity	시력(명료도)
VF	Visual field	시야

등록번호	233 55 77	성별 M
성명	정 대 승	
주민등록	370302-1234567	

입 퇴 원 기 록
Admission and Discharge Record

<table>
<tr><td colspan="4">주 소 : 서울시 성동구 행당동 286-21</td></tr>
<tr><td colspan="4">출신지 : 　　직 업 : 　　전 화 :</td></tr>
<tr><td colspan="4">연고자성명 : 홍주미 　　관 계 : 　　주 소 : 　　전 화 :</td></tr>
<tr><td colspan="4"></td></tr>
<tr><td colspan="2">입원 : 2017년 5 월 6 일 EY 과 8 병동 10 호</td><td rowspan="3">전과</td><td>20 년 월 일 과 병동 호</td></tr>
<tr><td colspan="2">퇴원 : 2017년 5 월 13 일 과 병동 호</td><td>20 년 월 일 과 병동 호</td></tr>
<tr><td colspan="2">재원일수 :</td><td>20 년 월 일 과 병동 호</td></tr>
<tr><td colspan="3">최종진단명</td><td>분 류 번 호</td></tr>
<tr><td colspan="3">주진단명 : Cataract OU</td><td></td></tr>
<tr><td colspan="3">기타진단명 : 2°glaucoma OS</td><td></td></tr>
<tr><td colspan="3">DM</td><td></td></tr>
<tr><td colspan="3"></td><td></td></tr>
<tr><td colspan="3">수술 및 처치명</td><td></td></tr>
<tr><td colspan="3">수술명 : ECCE $\bar{c}$ PCL, implantation, OD</td><td></td></tr>
<tr><td colspan="3">and ant. vitrectomy</td><td></td></tr>
<tr><td colspan="3">기타수술 및 주요검사 :</td><td></td></tr>
<tr><td colspan="3"></td><td></td></tr>
<tr><td colspan="3"></td><td></td></tr>
<tr><td colspan="3"></td><td></td></tr>
<tr><td colspan="4">치료결과 : 1. 완쾌 2. 경쾌 3. 호전안됨 4. 진단뿐 5. 가망없는 퇴원 6. 48시간내 사망 7. 48시간이후 사망</td></tr>
<tr><td colspan="4">퇴원형태 : 1. 퇴원지시후 2. 자의퇴원 3. 탈원 4. 전원</td></tr>
<tr><td colspan="4">병원감염 : 1. 수술후 2. 기타처치후 3. 비뇨기계 4. 호흡기계 5. 소화기계 6. 기타</td></tr>
<tr><td colspan="4">원사인 : 　　부검 : 예, 아니오</td></tr>
<tr><td colspan="4">계속적 진료 계획</td></tr>
<tr><td colspan="4">없음·있음 (약속일 20 년 월 일 시)</td></tr>
<tr><td colspan="2">담당 전공의 서명 : 박동욱</td><td colspan="2">담당 전문의 서명 : 장주호</td></tr>
<tr><td colspan="2">의무기록 완성 : 2017년 6 월 18 일</td><td colspan="2">의무기록사 서명 :</td></tr>
</table>

등록번호	233 55 77	성별	M
성명	정 대 승		
주민등록	370302-1234567		

퇴 원 요 약
Discharge Summary

Final diagnosis : Cataract OU
2°glaucoma OS
D.M.

C.C. : Decreased vision, OU (duration : 5yrs)

P.E : 1. V/A VOD: 0.3
VOS: LP (-)

2. IOP TOD : 14
TOS : 48 AT

3. Ant. seg.

lid & cilia : free OU

conj : hyperemic, swelling — OU

cornea : relative clear OD
mild edematous OS

A.C. : mild shallow OS

Pupil & Iris L/R (+) OD
L/R (−) OS

4. lens

〈OD〉

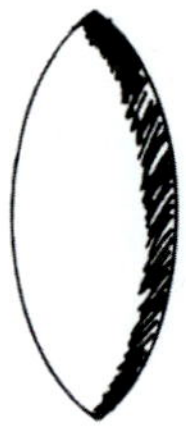

Post subcapsular opacity

〈OS〉

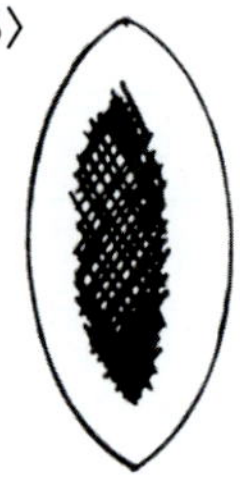

hypernature cataract

5. EOM No LOM
No diplopia

6. Color perception intact OD

퇴 원 요 약

일 자	내 용	서 명

7. lacrimal syringing OU) well passed
8. fundus exam OD) not clearly visible due to lens opcity
   OS) not visible due to lens opcity
9. Gonioscopic exam

OD)

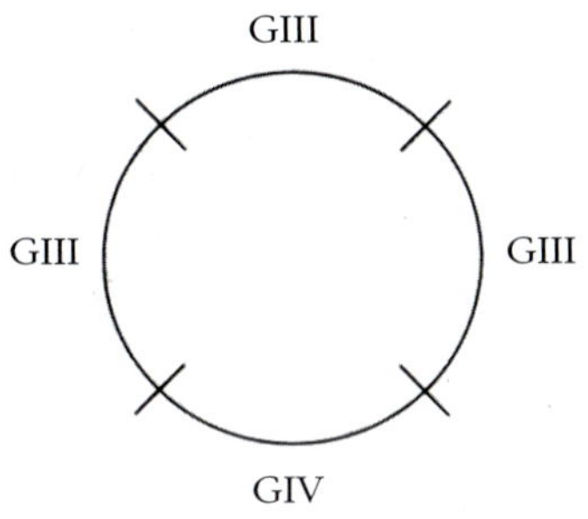

OS)

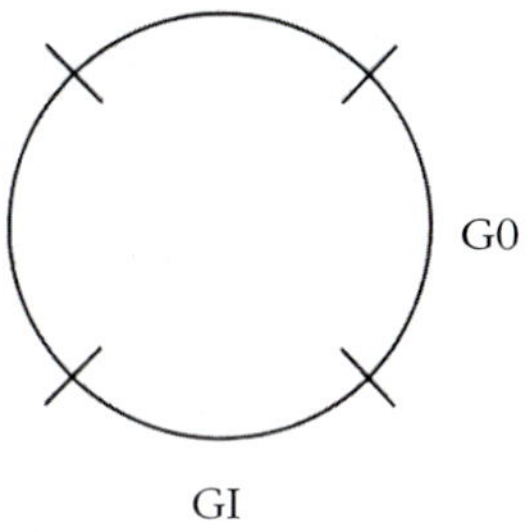

Preop. Dx : Cataract (OU)
2°glaucoma
D.M.

Postop Dx : S/A

Name of operation : ECCE $\bar{c}$ PCL implantation (OD) & ant. vitrectomy

Operator : 고마수

Anesthesia : pinpoint

Discharge medication:
1. EGTV
2. EGFLU 1BT $\bar{q}$ 4 hrs
3. CEFTR 3T, Irritran 3T, MageF 3T — #3 p.o x 7 days
4. MGO25 0.5 3T #3 p.o x 7 days

퇴원계획 : F/U at OPD (2017년 5월 15일)

등록번호	233 55 77	성별 M
성명	정 대 승	
주민등록	370302-1234567	

병력 및 신체검진기록
History & Physical Examination

C.C : Decreased vision (D: 5yrs)

P.I : 상기 80세된 male pt.는 약 5년 전부터 상기 C/C이 develop되었다. 치료받지 않고 지내다가 2016년 12월 local OT에서 cataract(OU), glaucoma(OS), imp.하에 큰 병원을 가도록 권유받고 본원에서 cataract(OU), absolute glaucoma(OS) 진단하에 OP받기 위해 입원하심.

PHx. : N-S except D.M.

P.E : 1. V/A VOD : 0.3
VOS : LP (−)
2. IOP TOD : 14
TOS : 48 AT
3. Ant. seg.

lid & cilia : free OU

conj : hyperemic
swelling OU

cornea: relative clear OD
mild edematous OS

A.C. : mild shallow OS

Pupil & Iris L/R (+) OD
L/R (−) OS

병력 및 신체검진기록

일 자	내 용	서 명

4. Lens

OD)

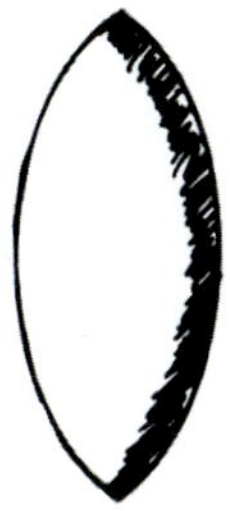

post
supcapsular
opacity

OS)

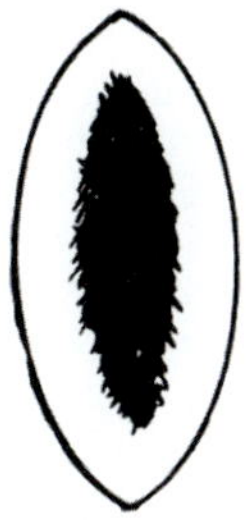

hypernature
cataract

5. EOM — No LOM
No diplopia
6. Color perception — intact OD
7. Lacrimal syringing — OU) well passed
8. Fundus exam — OD) not clearly visible due to lens opcity
but no hemorrhage
9. Gonioscopic exam.

OD)

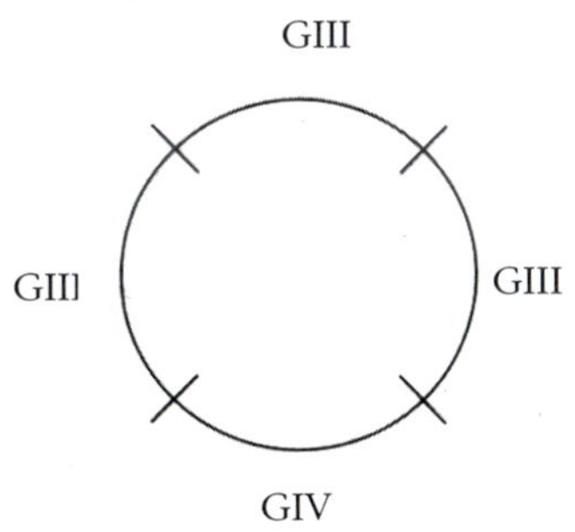

OS)

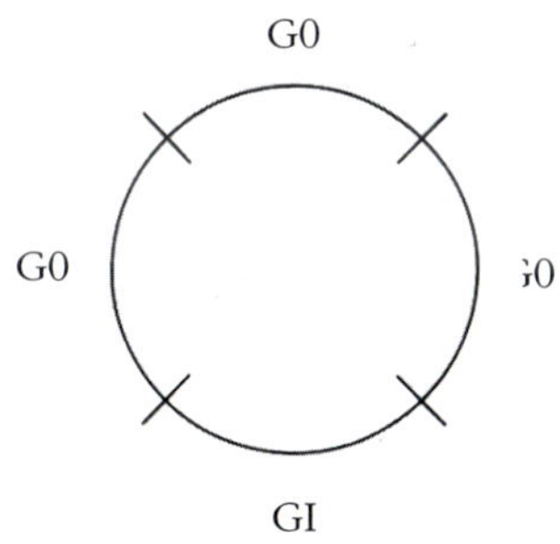

Imp) Cataract OU
2° angle closure glaucoma, OS

등록번호	233 55 77	성별	M
성명	정 대 승		
주민등록	370302-1234567		

경 과 기 록
Progress Notes

5.6 〈 Admission note 〉

C.C : Decreased vision (D: 5yrs)

P. I : 상기 80세된 male pt.는 약 5년 전부터 상기 C/C이 develop되었다. 치료받지 않고 지내다가 16년 12월 local OT에서 cataract(OU), glaucoma(OS) imp하에 큰 병원을 갈 것을 권유받고 본원에서 cataract(OU), absolute glaucoma(OS) 진단하에 OP 받기 위해 입원하심.

P.Hx : N-S except D.M.

P.E. : 1. V/A VOD : 0.3
VOS : LP (−)

2. IOP TOD : 14
TOS : 48 AT

3. Ant. seg.
lid & cilia : free OU
conj : hyperemic
swelling OU
cornea : relative clear OD
mild edematous OS
A.C. : mild shallow OU
Pupil & iris L/R (+) OD
L/R (−) OS

5.6 4. Lens

OD)

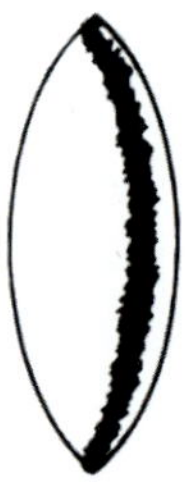

post subcapsular opacity

OS)

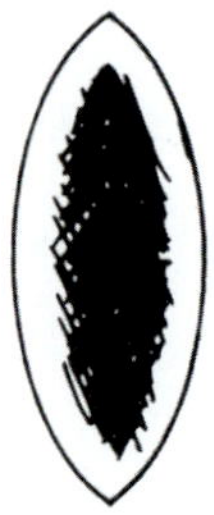

hypernature cataract

경 과 기 록

일 자	내 용	서 명

5.6 5. EOM No LOM

No diplopia

6. Color perception

intact OD

7. Lacrimal syringing OU) well passed

8. Fundus exam OD) not clearly visible due to lens opacity

but no hemorrhage or exudate

9. Gonioscopic exam OS) not visible due to lens opacity.

우각경검사

OD)

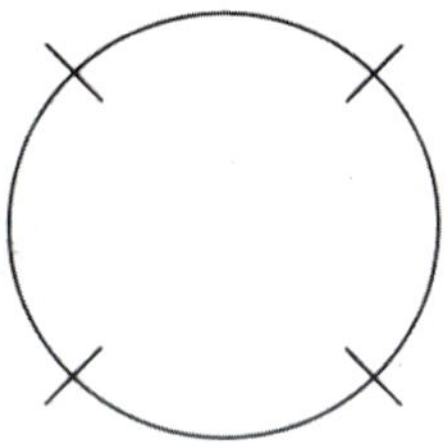

OS)

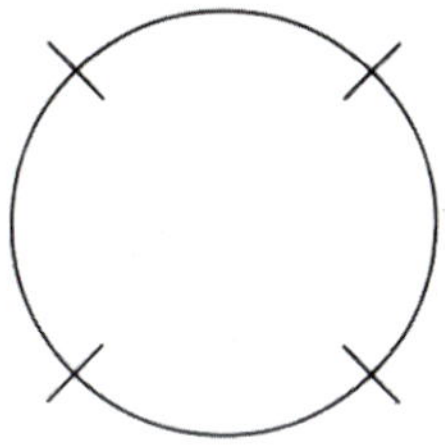

Imp) Cataract(OU)

2° angle closure glaucoma(OS)

Rec) ECCE $\bar{c}$ PCL implantation(OD)

ECCE $\bar{c}$ trabeculectomy (OS)

5.7 〈 Brief Op. note 〉

Surgeon : S.W.Kim M.D. Assistants : G.R.K

Anesthesia : pinpoint

Preoperative diagnosis : Cataract, OU

Postoperative diagnosis : The same as above

Name of operation: ECCE with PCL, implantation, OD

경 과 기 록

일 자	내 용	서 명
5.8	Rayner Model 604 A Power +21.0 D Length 12.50mm LOT 06SC 1398506	
5.8	〈 POD #1 〉 TOD: 10 Cornea: edematous A.C: deep & cells (+ + +) well position IOF Diamox 3T #3 p.o	
5.10	〈 POD #3 〉 Cornea: sl. edematous A.C: deep & cells (+ +) well position IOL	
5.12	〈 POD #5 〉 Cornea: sl. edematous A.C: deep & cells (+ +) well position IOL VOD 0.2 (0.5) x sphtozti cyl-4.0 Ax 20	
5.13	〈 POD #6 〉 Discharge c̄ medication	

등록번호	233 55 77	성별 M
성명	정 대 승	
주민등록	370302-1234567	

수 술 신 청 서

* 환자의 체질상태(환자측으로부터 고지받은 사항)

·기왕력:	·당뇨병: (+)	·약물사고:	·기타사항 :
·특이체질:	·출혈소인:	·알레르기 :	
·심장병:	·고·저혈압: (-)	·마약(알코올)중독	

* 의사로부터 들은 설명의 내용

1) 시술에 대한 필요성: 시력회복, 백내장으로 인한 합병증 예방
2) 예상되는 합병증 및 후유증, 예후: 난시, 염증, 출혈, 각막 및 망막부종, 초자체 출혈, 안내염
3) 시술과 관련한 불가항력적인 사항: 황반부종, 안내염, 망막박리, 후발백내장, 인공수정체 삽입 불가
4) 기왕력이나 특이체질로 인한 우발적 사고: 국소마취제에 의한 합병증 쇼크

* 기타 :

본인(또는 상기환자)은 (수술), 마취, 검사 등의 필요성과 이에 따른 위험성 및 불가항력적인 사항에 대해 주치의사로부터 자세히 설명을 듣고 충분히 이해하여 동의하였으므로 그 결과에 이의 없이 상기와 같은 내용을 확인하고 수술, 마취, 검사 등의 시술을 자유의사에 의거 승낙하므로 이에 따른 의학적 처치를 주치의사의 판단에 의하여 시행하여 줄 것을 청약합니다.

* 만일 의료분쟁 발생 시 의료법 제54조 등 관련 법규에 의뢰하여 처리할 것임.

2017년 5월 6일 7시 분 오전
(오후)

상기환자 또는 대리인(환자의 자) ____________ (인)
주 소 ____________________
증 인 ______________________________ (인)
주 소 ____________________

* 본 청약서는 본인의 서명이나 날인으로 유효하나 미성년자 및 정신질환자 또는 본인이 서명할 수 없는 상태일 때는 보호자가 이를 대리한다.

유주발 병원장 귀하

등록번호	233 55 77	성별 M
성명	정 대 승	
주민등록	370302-1234567	

수 술 전 점 검 표
Pre-operative Check List

Preparation for operation, Bath, Skin, Nails 수술 전 준비(목욕, 피부준비, 손톱, 발톱)		Yes	NO
Pre-medication given charted	VIM 5mg #1 IM Diamox 2T #1 P.O KI		
Doctor's Other sheet on chart, special pre-operative order 의무기록에 있는 의사의 지시기록지를 보고 특별한 수술 전 지시를 볼 것		V	
LVDX $\bar{c}$ celo 2.0g $\bar{c}$ C6 IV(AST) after skin test Special medication Blood Pints Dextrose cc		V	
Hair prepared, Leggings, Gown 머리를 갈라 땋고 삼각끈으로 매고 가운을 입힐 것		V	
Jewellery removed and put in safe care 귀중품 제거와 보관		V	
Denture removed 의치의 제거, 콘택트렌즈 제거, 보청기 제거		V	
Voided, Catheterized, Enema 인공 혹은 자연배뇨(시간과 양의 기록) 관장		V	
Has patient fasted? 금식하였는지		V	
Blood, Urine, Other report on chart? 혈액, 소변, 기타 검사의 보고지 유무		V	
Identification of child or unconscious patient 혼수상태에 있는 환자나 소아의 이름표(성명, 연령, 주소) 유무		V	
Pre-operative T.P.R.B.P charted? 수술 전 체온, 맥박, 혈압, 호흡측정의 기록		V	
Miscellaneous 기타		V	

Date 2017. 5. 7 Preparation nurse___ Head Nurse _______

등록번호	233 55 77	성별 M
성명	정 대 승	
주민등록	370302-1234567	

수 술 기 록

Operation Record

Date : 2017. 5. 7 Surgeon: 홍기술

1st Ass't: 최지구 2nd Ass't: 서만수

Scrub nurse: Circ. nurse:

Preoperative diagnosis: Cataract, OU

Postoperative diagnosis: The same as above

Name of operation: ECCE with PCL implantation, OD

Operation type: Elective (*) Emergency ( )

Position of Pt.: supine position

Skin preparation: 7.5% potadine soap (*) 75% alcohol ( ) 10% potadine ( )
Sterile drap (*) Others ( )

Anesthesia: General endotracheal ( ) Spinal ( ) Epidural ( )
Caudal ( ) Regional (*), Others ( )

Preparation and drapes was done as a usual. Lids speculum was placed. 6-0 nylon bridle suture was done under the superior rectus muscle. Fornix-based conjunctival peritomy was done at the superior lumbus. Hemostasis was with cautery. Partial thickness scleral tunnel incision was performed at the superior post limbus. Entering to anterior chamber was done by the microsurgical knife. Viscoelastics was inserted into anterior chamber. A continous curvilinear capsulorrhexis type anterior capsulotomy was performed with hooked 25 gauge needle. Capsular flap was removed with fine forcep. Wound was extended with corneoscleral scissior from 10 o'clock to 2 o'clock position. Viscoelastics was inserted into anterior chamber repeatedly. Hydrodissection between remaining anterior capsule and cortex was done. Nucleus was expressed with lens spoon and muscle hook saline was irrigated into anterior chamber to reform the anterior chamber. Interrupted replaced sutures were done on incision site. Residual cortex was removed with irrigation and aspiration unit.

Viscoelastics was inserted into anterior chamber. Preplaced suture was removed and IOL was inserted in the bag. forcep and Mcperson forcep. IOL was rotated to horizontal position with Sinskey hook. Miostat was closed with 10-0 nylon interrupted sutures.

Inserted viscoelastics was removed with I & A unit. Suture was tightned and bridge suture was removed. A mixture of gentamycin and dexamethasone was injected subconjunctivally. Dressing and binocular patch were done.

2017. 5. 7 Written by 홍기술

등록번호	233 55 77	성별 M
성명	정 대 승	
주민등록	370302-1234567	

의 사 지 시 기 록
Doctor's Orders

5.6

〈 Admission order 〉

1. Check V/S $\bar{q}$ qid
2. BR
3. FOM diet (Total cal 〈 1600)
4. UST (x4) qid
5. glucopat (x2) qid
6. Aqua 60cc
   KI 0.2] #4 P.O qid
   Codein 0.08
7. EGTV 1BT $\bar{q}$ 2 hrs (OD)

〈 Pre-op order 〉

1. Check V/S $\bar{q}$ qid
2. BR
3. NPO from MN
4. Get op permission sheet
5. LVDX 1BT(500ml)
   Celos 2.0] mix IV (A.S.T) After skin test
   C_6
6. Premed
   VLM 1/2 Ⓐ #1 IM
   Diamox 2T
   KI 2T #1 P.O
7. Prepare
   0.1% epinephrine 1Ⓐ
   GM 80mg 1Ⓐ] to OR $\bar{c}$ chart
   DEXA 1Ⓐ

의 사 지 시 기 록

일 자	내 용	서 명
5.6	8. Miotics를 10분 간격으로 6:00~8:00 AM까지 OD에 점안하시오. 9. Send to Pt. to OR $\bar{c}$ chart & films after full voiding (at 8: 20 AM)	*Park*
5.8	1. Check V/S $\bar{q}$ qid 2. GDM diet 3. BR 4. LVDX 1BT, Celos 2.0g, C_6] mix IV(AST) 5. Astlo 2g #2 IM 6. MGO 25 3T #3 p.o qid 7. EGTV 1BT $\bar{q}$ 2hrs (OS) 〈 Pre-op order 〉 1. Check V/S $\bar{q}$ qid 2. Soft diet & NPO 3. BR 4. Get Op. permission sheet 5. LVDX 1BT, Celoslin 20mg, C_6] mix IV(AST) 6. Pre med Diamox 2T # P.O KI 2T VLM $1\frac{1}{2}$ Ⓐ IM 7. 환자 수술실로 내리면서 Mannitol 300cc IV full dripping $\bar{c}$ 18G needle	
5.8	8. Prepare 0.1% epinephrine 1Ⓐ GM 80mg 1Ⓐ DEXA 1Ⓐ Mitomycin 1Ⓐ] to OR $\bar{c}$ chart	

의 사 지 시 기 록

일 자	내 용	서 명
5.8	9. Insert 18F Foley catheter(silastic) $\bar{c}$ urine reservior bag	
	10. Miotics, Mydriacyl, ocupen을 10분 간격으로 점안하세요.	
	11. Send to Pt. to OR $\bar{c}$ chart & films at "on call"	*Park*
5.9	1. Check V/S $\bar{q}$ qid	
	:	
	생 략	
5.13	1. Check V/S $\bar{q}$ qid	
	2. GDM diet (<1600cal)	
	3. BR	
	4. Astro 1Ⓥ #1 IM	
	5. Discharge $\bar{c}$ med	
	1) EGTV	
	2) EGFLU 1BT $\bar{q}$ 4hrs	
	3) CEFTR 3T, Irritran 3T, MagENF 3T] #3 PO x 7 days	
	4) MGO25 3T #3 PO x 7 days	
	6. OPD Follow-up plan 2001. 5. 15	*Park*

등록번호	233 55 77	성별 M
성명	정 대 승	
주민등록	370302-1234567	

간 호 기 록

Nurses Record

날 짜	시 간	내 용	서 명
5.6	9 AM	Admitted an ambulatory via OPD	
5.7	8 : 30 AM	Send the Pt. to OR with chart $\bar{c}$ X-ray film after voiding	
		Came to ward	
		Rt. eye shield $\bar{c}$ Lt. eye patch	
		ABR adviced	
		:	
		생략	
5.9	1 : 30 PM	Send the Pt. to OR $\bar{c}$ chart & film	
	4 PM	Return to ward	
		V/S checked	
		OP 실패하고 돌아옴	
		No complaints	
	4 : 30 PM	forley catheter removed by Dr xx	
		:	
		생략	
5.13	9 AM	Discharge $\bar{c}$ p.o Med for 7 days	
		OPD F/U teaching	

〈정 대 승〉

★ 정대승 차트를 읽고 맞는 것에 O표 하시오.

1 신체검진상 맞게 기재된 것은?

① 왼쪽 눈의 시력은 0.3이다.
② 오른쪽 눈의 동공 반사가 없었다.
③ 왼쪽 눈의 내압은 48이다.
④ 안구운동은 정상이나 복시가 있다.
⑤ 공막에 충혈이 있었다.

2 진단명에 대한 분류번호로 맞게 짝지어진 것은?

① H26.8, T85.2, E14.9
② H26.91, H40.9, E11.9
③ E11.34+, H28.0*, T85.2, H40.9
④ H26.92, H40.5, E14.9
⑤ E11.34+, H28.0*, T85.2, H26.1

3 상기 환자에 대한 내용으로 틀리게 기재된 것은?

① 입원 당시 환자의 왼쪽 눈 각막은 경미한 부종이 있었다.
② 산동제를 오전 6~8시까지 10분 간격으로 오른쪽 눈에 점안하도록 하였다.
③ 수술 전 피부검사 후 LVDX, celo 2.0g 및 C6을 정맥내 주입하도록 했다.
④ 환자의 질환군은 K-DRG대상 범위에 해당된다.
⑤ 우안은 안저검사상 렌즈의 불투명으로 뚜렷하게 보이지 않았다.

4 상기 환자의 백내장 수술에 대한 마취방법으로 맞는 것은?

① Regional
② IM
③ IV
④ Endotracheal
⑤ Endobroncheal

5 5월 9일 환자가 수술 실패로 병실로 돌아왔는데 이때 시행하려고 했던 수술명은?

① 오른쪽 눈 백내장 낭내적출술
② 홍채절제술
③ 왼쪽 눈 백내장 낭내적출술
④ 왼쪽 눈 백내장 낭외적출술 및 섬유주절제술
⑤ 오른쪽 눈 백내장 낭외적출술 및 홍채절제술

6 수술기록지 내용으로 옳지 않은 것은?

① 점탄물질을 반복적으로 전안방에 삽입
② 잔존 피질은 세정과 흡인기로 제거
③ 7.5% potadine soap로 피부 준비
④ 수압박리는 후방 캡슐과 피질 사이에서 시행
⑤ 나일론 bridle 봉합은 상직근 아래에서 시행

7 상기 환자의 차트는 미비기록이다. 의사에게 보충하도록 요구해야 할 기록은 무엇인가?

① 5월 7일 수술기록
② 5월 9일 경과기록
③ 전과기록
④ Intern note
⑤ 신체검진기록

8 수술명에 대한 분류번호로 맞는 것은?

① 13.19, 13.71
② 13.51, 13.71
③ 13.59, 13.71
④ 13.59, 13.70
⑤ 13.51, 13.70

9 **백내장에 대한 설명 중 틀린 것은?**

① 안압의 상승으로 인해 시력상실을 가져올 수 있는 질환이다.
② 낭내적출술은 수정체 피낭을 포함하여 수정체 전체를 적출하는 것이다.
③ 합병성 백내장은 심한 안질환 후에 초래되는 백내장이다.
④ 수정체가 혼탁해져서 시력감퇴가 서서히 온다.
⑤ 합병성 백내장은 대개 심한 안질환 후에 발생한다.

10 **의무기록에 기재된 약어이다. 정식용어로 틀리게 기재된 것은?**

① lOP: Intraocular pressure
② PCL: posterior cataract lens
③ VA: visual acuity
④ LOM: limitation of motion
⑤ VF: visual field

04 호흡곤란증후군 동반 조산아

Preterm infant c̄ respiratory distress syndrome

1.1 호흡곤란증후군(Respiratory distress syndrome; RDS)

특 징

- 일명 초자막질환(hyaline membrane disease; HMD)
- 미숙아(premature)의 호흡기 문제
- 폐조직 내면의 단백질 결핍은 폐허탈(collaps of lung)의 원인
- 시간경과에 따라 호흡곤란 증가

치 료

- 출생 후 소생술 필요
- 산소공급 및 기타 방법으로 생후 3~4일 무사히 경과 시 회복가능성

발병할 사항

- 모체에 지나친 진정제 사용으로 신생아의 호흡억제
- 호흡중추의 장애를 포함하는 뇌손상
- 폐 및 골격근 발육미숙에 속발되는 호흡운동미약
- 양수, 응혈괴 등의 흡입으로 발생하는 호흡운동장애
- 제대가 목에 걸려 질식
- 당뇨병이 있는 임부의 신생아에서 정상아보다 발병률 6배
- 폐의 활성제 부족

표 1 • 임신기간 및 태아체중

분류번호*		질병명	기준치
O___	정상 임신기간	Term delivery	37주~42주 미만
P___	정상 신생아 체중	Mature infant	2,500g~4,500g 미만 (=2.5~4.5kg 미만)
P07.0	극단적 저체중 출산아	Extremely low birth weight	999g 이하
P07.1	기타 저체중 출산아	Other low birth weight	1,000~2,499g 이하
P07.2	극단적 미숙아	Extreme immaturity	28주미만
P07.3	기타 조산아	Other preterm infant	28주~37주 미만
P05.1	과소체중아	Small for dates	
P08.1	과체중아	Heavy for dates	

*분만 결과: Z37.____: 출생아 또는 사생아
출생아 : Z38.____: 병원내 또는 병원외

황달(Jaundice) = icterus = 과빌리루빈혈증(hyperbilirubinemia)
· 혈류에 빌리루빈(bilirubin)의 과도 축적으로 발생

황달의 세 가지 기전

▸ **폐쇄성 황달(obstructive jaundice)**

– 담즙(bile)의 흐름이 막혀 빌리루빈과 담즙이 장으로 배설되지 못함

예) **담석증**(cholelithiasis)

▸ **간성 황달(hepatic jaundice)**

– 간질환(hepatopathy)으로 인해 간세포의 기능부전 발생

– 간이 빌리루빈과 담즙을 혼합하지 못함

예) **간염**(hepatitis), **간경변**(liver cirrhosis), **간암**(hepatoma)

▸ **용혈성 황달(hemolytic jaundice)**

– 용혈(hemolysis)로 적혈구(erythrocytes)의 과도한 파괴로 혈중 빌리루빈이 상승

예) **태아적아구증**(erythroblastosis), **용혈성 빈혈**(hemolytic anemia)

→ erythroblastosis: 모체와 태아와의 혈액형 부적합으로 인해 생기는 태아의 용혈성 빈혈

질병분류상 주의점: 신생아 황달

▸ **진단명**

– 신생아 황달(neonatal jaundice) 또는 생리적 황달(physiological jaundice) → P59.9

– 조산(preterm, 37주 미만) + 신생아 황달(neonatal jaundice) → P59.0

– 치료: 광선치료(Phototherapy) → 99.83

1.2 아프가 점수(Apgar score)

▸ 영아의 신체상태를 측정하는 점수제도

▸ 출산 후 1분 후 또는 5분 후 측정

▸ 5개 항목

 –심박동률(heart rate), 호흡(respiration), 색깔(color), 근육강도(muscle tone)

 –자극에 대한 반응(response to stimuli)

▸ 점수: 0~10점 부여

 –Apgar 점수가 낮은 신생아: 진료 요함

표 2 • 아프가 채점법(Apgar scoring chart): 총 10점

증후(Sign)	0	1	2
심박동률	없음	100 이하	100 이상
호흡	없음	느림, 불규칙	좋음, 잘 울음
근육강도	약함	사지 약간의 굴절	강한 동작
자극에 대한 반응	무반응	찡그림	기침, 재채기
피부색	푸르고 창백	몸통: 분홍(pink) 사지: 푸른색(blue)	완전 분홍

2.1 출생 후 중요기간

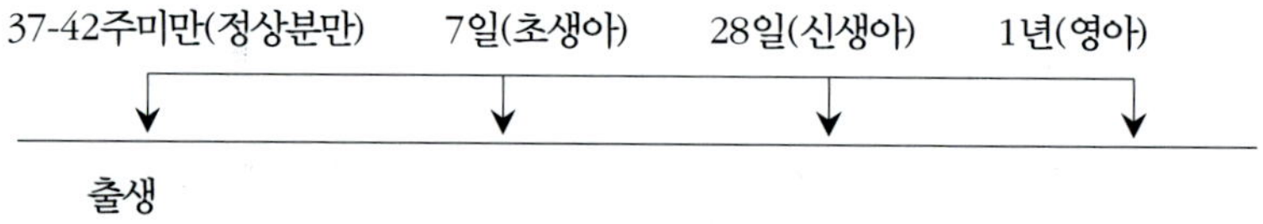

그림 1. 출생 후 기간

▸ 초생아(初生兒): 출생 후 ~ 1주(7일)

▸ 신생아(新生兒): 출생 후 ~ 4주(28일)

▸ 영아(嬰兒, infant): 출생 후 ~ 1년

2.2 사망용어

▸ 선행사인: 사망에 이르게 하는 가장 기본적인 질환 예) 조숙

▸ 중간사인: 사망에 이르게 하는 중간 과정 예) 호흡장애증후군, 위장관 출혈, 파종성 혈관내 응고병증

▸ 직접사인: 직접 사망하는 원인 예) 심폐정지

차트 용어

- 태변(meconium)
  - 만기태아 장내에 있는 암녹색 점액성 물질
- 수분(hydration) ↔ 탈수(dehydration)
- 맥박수(pulse rate; PR)
  - 빈맥(tachycardia): 맥박이 1분에 100회 이상
  - 서맥(bradycardia): 맥박이 1분에 60회 미만

차트 용어

· Caput succedaneum	산류	·Fontanelle	천문/숫구멍	·Grasping reflex	파악반사	·Hazy	흐릿한
· Molding	주형	·Moro reflex	모로반사	·Palate	구개/입천장	·Parity	출산력
· Retraction	함몰/퇴축	·Rhonchus	건성 수포음	·Scaphoid	주상	·Seizure	발작
· Stain	얼룩	·Surfactant	계면활성제	·Ventilator	환기장치		

약 어	원 어	
ABGA	Arterial blood gas analysis	동맥혈 가스분석
AGA	Appropriate for gestational age	임신연령에 적당
ARF	Acute renal failure	급성 신부전
BT	Body temperature	체온
BUN	Blood urea nitrogen	혈액요소질소
CC	Chest circumference	흉위
CPR	Cardiopulmonary resuscitation	심폐소생술
CRP	C-reactive protein	C-반응성 단백질
DIC	Disseminated intravascular coagulation	파종성 혈관내 응고병증
10% DW	10% dextrose (in water) injection	10% 포도당수용액 주입
FFP	Fresh frozen plasma	신선냉동혈장
GA	Gestational age	임신기간
GI	Gastrointestinal	위장의
HC	Head circumference	두위(머리둘레)
HMD	Hyaline membrane disease	초자막질환
ICS	Intercostal space	늑간강
IV	Intravenous	정맥내
IVH	Intraventricular hemorrhage	심실내 출혈
NICU	Neonatal intensive care unit	신생아 중환자실
NPO	Nothing by mouth(Latin: non per os)	금식
NVD	Normal vaginal delivery	정상 질분만
PGE_2	Prostaglandin E_2(유도분만을 위해 1회 1정 복용)	자궁수축제
PCO_2	Carbon dioxide partial pressure	동맥혈의 탄산가스 분압
PO_2	Oxygen partial pressure	동맥혈 산소분압
PR	Pulse rate	맥박수
PROM	Premature rupture of membranes	양막조기파열
RDS	Respiratory distress syndrome ‣ Hyaline membrane disease 초자막질환	호흡장애 증후군
RR	Respiration rate	호흡률
WPW	Wolf-Parkinson-White(syndrome)	볼프-파킨슨-화이트 증후군

등록번호	111 55 77	성별 M
성명	박신통 아기	
주민등록	170108-1234567	

입 퇴 원 기 록
Admission and Discharge Record

주 소 :			
출신지 :	직 업 :	전 화 :	
연고자성명 : 변도철	관 계 :	주 소 :	전 화 :

	전과	
입원 : 2017년 1 월 8 일 PED 과 병동 호		20 년 월 일 과 병동 호
퇴원 : 2017년 1 월 14 일 PED 과 병동 호		20 년 월 일 과 병동 호
중환자실전과일과 2017년 1월 8일 NBICU과 재원일수		20 년 월 일 과 병동 호

최종진단명	분 류 번 호
주진단명 : Prematurity c̄ RDS	
기타진단명 : Pulmonary hemorrhage	
Gastrointestinal hemorrhage	
수술 및 처치명	
수술명 : Supportive care with ventilator care	
기타수술 및 주요검사 : Surfactant	
FFP transfusion	
Photo Tx	

치료결과 : 1. 완쾌 2. 경쾌 3. 호전안됨 4. 진단뿐 5. 가망없는 퇴원 6. 48시간내 사망 7. 48시간이후 사망

퇴원형태 : 1. 퇴원지시후 2. 자의퇴원 3. 탈원 4. 전원

병원감염 : 1. 수술후 2. 기타처치후 3. 비뇨기계 4. 호흡기계 5. 소화기계 6. 기타

원사인 부검 : 예, 아니오

계속적 진료 계획

없음·있음 (약속일 년 월 일 시)

담당 전공의 서명 : 홍준빈	담당 전문의 서명 : 서상훠
의무기록 완성 : 2017 년 2 월 17 일	의무기록사 서명 :

등록번호	111 55 77	성별 M
성명	박신통 아기	
주민등록	170108-1234567	

퇴 원 요 약
Discharge Summary

Final dx : 1. prematurity c̄ RDS　　2. G-I hemorrhage
3. Pulmonary bleeding　　4. DIC
5. IVH

C.C : prematurity & respiratory difficulty
상기 환아는 GA 30^{+5}wks preterm vaginal delivery된 twin중 2nd baby로 initial crying없었으며, Apgar score 0/1min, 2/5min으로 2/10min으로 check 되고 chest retraction 심해지고 morning sing과 O_2 dependency 나타나서 preterm with AGA와 RDS 의심하에 입원 (twin 중 2nd baby)

M.H : 0-0-0-0　PROM (+) : 6일 경과 후 delivery
Meconium stain (+)

P.E : V/S: BT 36.8℃ - PR 180/min - RR 30/min
G/A: Activity, crying → poor
HEENT : Normocephalic
Molding (−), Caput succedaneum (+)
Ches t: Retraction (+) : subcostal, substernal
RHB s̄ ⓜ
Abdomen : soft & scaphoid
No palpable mass
Back & ext : free
Moro & Grasp : Good

Body physiques: B.wt : 1.39kg, Length : 39.5cm　H.C : 30cm　C.C : 23.5cm
ABGA : pH 7.184　PCO_2 : 45.6　PO_2 : 136　HCO_3 : 16.6　O_2 sat 97.9%
CBC : 16.4-50-12800　Plt 19만
Na/K/Cl : 136/5.0/112mEq/L　BUN/Cr : 11/0.8mg/dl
Chest AP : Grade III RDS
HD #1-7 : Supportive care with ventilator care
HD # 3-7 : phototherapy
HD #1 : Surfactant IV 투여
HD #7 : AM 1:00경 PR 200/min 이상의 tachycardia 발생 → AM 3:00경 G-T-C type의 seizure 발생
→ G-tube site로 fresh blood 다량 배출, E-tube site fresh bleeding
→ AM 5:00 bradycardia (PR 50회/min 이하), Hypotension
→ Pupil full dilatation → Cardiac arrest → Expired at 8: 50 AM　*Hong*

등록번호	111 55 77	성별 M
성명	박신통 아기	
주민등록	170108-1234567	

신생아 검진

Examination of Newborn Baby

신생아실 ( ) **NICU (✔)**

재태 주령: **30^{+5} weeks**

분만양식: ☑**NSVD** ☐**Vacuum** ☐**C/S** ☐**Breech Extraction** ☐기타**(forcep delivery)**

산모 병력:

Body physiques

B.Wt : 1.39kg H.C : 30cm Length : 39.5cm C.C : 23.5cm BT : 36.8℃

RR : 30/min PR : 180/min BP : / Average( )

Newborn Examination

General appearance :

Activity - ☐good ☐fair ☑poor Crying - ☐well ☑weak

Others - ☐flaccid ☐motionless ☐pallor

Skin : Color - ☑pinkish ☐cyanotic ☐plethora ☐whitich ☐meconium stained

Others - ☐petechiae ☐rashes ☐desquamation ☐lacerations

HEENT : Anterior fontanel - ☐open ☐closed ☐depressed ☐bulged

Scalp - ☐succedaneum ☐hematoma

Face - ☐symmetry ☐asymmetry ☐cleft lip

Forcep markings - ☐erythema ☐depressed ☐laceration at ( )

Neck : ☑Normal ☐asymmetry ☐palpable mass ☐webbed neck

Lung : Expansion - ☑well ▫ fair ☐poor

Breathing sound - ▫ clear ☑rhonchi ☐rales ☐irregular

Heart : R.S.R - ☐irregular ☐murmur ☐tachycardia ☐bradycardia

Abdomen : ☑soft ☐distended ☐scaphoid

Palpable organ - ☐none ☐liver ☐spleen ☐kidney ☐abnormal mass

Umbilical Cord : Color - ☐normal ☐hemorrhage ☐meconium stained ☐necrotic

Artery - ☐one ☐two ☐absence

Genitalia : Appearance - ☐normal

Testis - ☐one ☐two ☐undescended

Femoral pulse: ☐palpable ☐not palpable

Hip joint movement: ☐full ☐limited on abduction

Extremities : ☑Normal Abnormal-☐polydactylia ☐syndactylia ☐clubfoot ☐symm movement

Reflexes : Moro - ☑good ☐fair ☐poor ☐absence asymmetry

Grasping -☑strong ☐fair ☐poor

Sucking -☐strong ☐fair ☐poor Ventral suspension - ☐increased tone ☐normal ☐decreased tone

Head Lag - ☐good ☐fair ☐poor

Other Congenital or Abnormal Findings : N-C

Kim

등록번호	111 55 77	성별 M
성명	박신통 아기	
주민등록	170108-1234567	

신생아 확인기록

Newborn Identification Form

출생일시 1999년 1월 8일 9 시 35 분 오전 성별 ☑남 □여

신생아 왼쪽 발바닥	신생아 오른쪽 발바닥
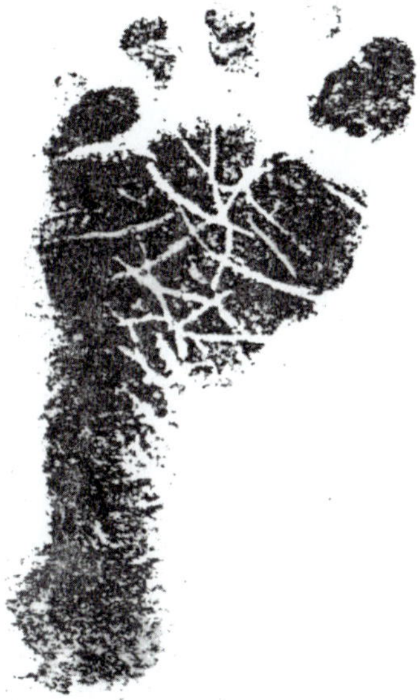	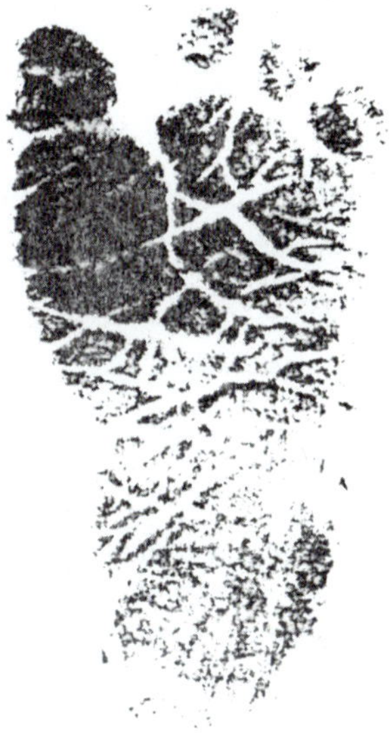

바른손 모지(산모)	확 인 자	비 고
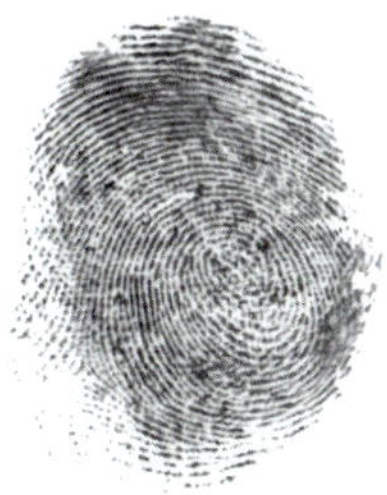	분만 의사 이 승 길 분만개조 간호사	1.39 Kg 30^{+5}주 NSVD 1′- 0 5′- 2 10′- 2

등록번호	111 55 77	성별 M
성명	박신통 아기	
주민등록	170108-1234567	

경 과 기 록
Progress Notes

〈 Admission note 〉

17.1.8 Name : 박신통 아기
Address : 서울시 송파구 잠실동 20-4
Birthday : 17. 1. 8
Adm. date : 17. 1. 8

C.C. Preterm with respiratory difficulty

P.I 상기 baby는 twin중 2nd로 37세 multiparous women으로 GA 30^{+5}wk에 PROM 된지 6일만에 preterm spontaneous vaginal delivery되었으며 initial crying은 없었으며 1분 Apgar Score는 0점, 5분 apgar score는 2점, 10분 2점으로 check 되었으며, 출생 직후 bradycardia 있어 manual cardia massage하였으며 mask로 O_2 (101/min) bagging하고 suction하면서 heart rate, cyanosis는 improve하였으나 chest wall retraction 심하고 morning 심하며 O_2 dependency 보여 intubation 실시하였으며, prematurity와 respiratory difficulty 있어 입원함

BHx : Meconium stain (+)
MHx : 37세
Parity: 0-0-0-0
PROM (+) : 6일 Labor pain

Body physiques
Bwt : 1.39kg
Length : 39.5cm
HC : 30cm
CC : 23.5cm

P/Ex V/S Bt 36.8℃ PR 〈 180/min RR 〈 30/min
G/A Activity
Crying
Skin Whole body cyanosis → Pinkish (after 10 min)

Hong

경 과 기 록

17.1.8 HEENT Normocephalic, soft fontanelle
Caput (+)
Molding (−)
Lip & palate: intact
Eye discharge (−)
Chest Sym exp c̄ subcostal
intercostal
suprasternal
Coarse breathing sound
Rale (−)
RHB c̄ ⓜ
Abd Soft
Liver/spleen: not palpable
Reflex Moro (+) ⎤ good
grasp (+) ⎦

Imp) prematurity c̄ RDS

Hong

〈 Initial lab 〉

CBC : 16.4 - 50 - 12800 - plt 289000
é : 136-5.0-112 BUN/Cr : 11/0.8 Glu : 56
ABGA : pH 7.184 PCO_2 45.6 PO_2 136 HCO_3 16.6 Sat 90.9
CMV : FiO_2 1.0
Chest : Ground glass app.

〈 Problems 〉

1. Respiratory difficulty
2. prematurity

〈 Initial plan 〉

1. Ventilator care
2. Surfactant use

Hong

17.1.10 #1. Prematurity
Bwt : 1.36kg(20gm wt loss)
Intake 84cc
Output 74cc
P : supportive care

경 과 기 록

17.1.10 #2. Respiratory difficulty

CMV : FiO_2 0.5 Pr 18/3 Rate 30/min

pH 7.327 PCO_2 44.5 PO_2 69.1

HCO_3 22.8 O_2 Sat 91.9%

A : RDS

P : Supportive care

Ventilator setting 조절하면서 경과 관찰 *Hong*

17.1.12 #1 : Prematurity

Bwt : 1.3kg (60gm weight loss)

Intake 108cc

Output 140cc

A : Preterm $\bar{c}$ AGA

P : Supportive care

#2 : Respiratory difficulty

CMV : FiO_2 0.33 Rate 20/min

Pr 18/2

pH 7.447 PCO_2 29.8 PO_2 88.4

HCO_3 20.4 O_2 Sat 93%

A : RDS

P : Supportive care

Ventilator setting 낮추어 가면서 경과 관찰 *Hong*

17.1.13 Prematurity

Bwt : 1.24kg (no weight change)

Intake : 120cc

Output : 48cc (urine output 1.6cc/kg/hr)

	Na/K/Cl	BUN/Cr
	144/4.2/111	42/1.6
→	142/4.4/110	44/1.4

A : Dehydration에 의한 prerenal type ARF 의심

P : Supportive care

Hydration 후 urination 증가 *Hong*

경 과 기 록

17.1.14 Tachycardia

O : Heart rate : 190-205/min

EKG : PR interval 0.08 sec

QRS complex : 0.04 sec

QT interval 0.24 sec QTc=0.42

Rhythm : atrial

Axis : +110° Vertical

A : supraventricular tachycardia

WPW syndrome (−)

P: 일단 facial/malar ice wrap 사용하고 계속 진행되면 digoxin 사용 고려

Hong

Tachycardia 지속되고 2-3 AM 사이 generalized tonic clonic type의 seizure 지속되어 intracranial hemorrhage 의심되며 G-tube irrigation에서 fresh(acute) bleeding있고 E-tube suction시 fresh bleeding 있어 disseminated intravascular coagulopathy 의심되며 Hb 10.6, plt 1만 나왔으며 acute bleeding도 계속 진행된다고 생각됨.

17.1.14 → bradycardia (40-50/min=PR) 보여 manual cardiac massage 실시하고 epinephrine IV 하였으며 두 번 사용으로 회복되었고 Vit.K, phenobarbital 사용하였으며, 계속 heart rate 떨어지고 BP 떨어져 Dopamine IV start하였으며, FFP 사용하였고 PR 다시 떨어지고 bradycardia 보여 epinephrine 사용하였으며, 그 당시로 seizure 없고 G-tube irrigation에서 fresh bleeding은 계속되는 상태였음.

A : DIC로 인하여 intracranial hemorrhage와 pulmonary hemorrhage, acute G-I bleeding 있었던 것으로 생각되며 이로 인해 shock 생긴 것으로 생각됨.

Expired at 2 : 10 P.M

·선행사인 : prematurity
·중간사인 : RDS, DIC, GI bleeding, pulmonary hemorrhage
·직접사인 : cardiopulmonary arrest

Hong

등록번호 111 55 77 성별 M
성명 박신통 아기
주민등록 170108-1234567

임상검사결과 경과표
Lab. Findings Flow Sheet

Item/Date	1/8	1/9	1/10	1/11	1/12	1/13	1/14
Hgb.(12-17gm/dl)	16.4						7.8
Hct.(37-53%)	50						23
WBC(5,000-10,000/mm^3)	12800						15700
ESR(M:10mm/h, F:20mm/h)	1						1
Platelets(150,000-350,000/mm^3)	289000						19000
Diff. counts :							
Myelocytes (0%)							
Metamyelo (0-1%)							1
Band (0-5%)							
Seg(60-70%)	29						51
Lympho(20-30%)	70						28
Mono(2-6%)	1						16
Eosino (1-4%)							2
Normoblast (1100WBL)	15						
Na+(136-145mEq/L)	136				144	142	138
K+(3.5-5.5mEq/L)	5.0				4.2	4.4	4.5
CI-(98-110mEq/L)	112				111	110	105
HCO^3 - (24-31mEq/L)							
Ca++ (8.5-10.5mg/dl)	9.9						
P(inorg) (2.5-4.5mEq/L)	8.1						
Mg	2.4						
Protein(6.0-8.0gm/dl)							
Albumin(3.5-5.5gm/dl)							
s-GOT (5-30 I.U.)	74						
s-GPT(5-35 I.U.)	9						
Bilirubin, Total (0.2-1.0mg/dl)		8.1	6.6	7.6		12.8	21.3
Direct(0-0.2mg/dl)							
TTT(5.5U)							
Alk. phosphatase (0.1-1.0U)							
Fibrinogen(150-400mg/dl)							
BUN (7-19mg/dl)	11				4.2	44	42
Creatinine, serum(0.7-1.7mg/dl)	0.8				1.6	1.4	1.6
urine (0.8-2.0gm/24h)						48.0	
Ccr.(75-125ml/min)							
Osmolarity, serum(289-308mosm/L)							
urine(300-900mosm/L)							
CRP	0.5↓	8.1	6.6	7.6	12.8		
Cholesterol(130-250mg/dl)							
Triglyceride (30-190mg/dl)							
Phospholipids(150-250mg/dl)							

임 상 검 사 결 과 경 과 표

Item/Date	1/8	1/9	1/10	1/11	1/12	1/13	1/14
Glucose, FBS(60-100mg/dl)	56						
LDH(50-400U)							
CPK(80 I.U.)							
Bleeding time(1-4min)							
Coagulation time (3-5min)							
aPTT(28-10sec)							
PT(11-13sec)							
RBC(4.2-6.2mil/mm^3)							
Reticulocytes(0.5-2.0%)						3	
Eosino. count(50-500/mm^3)							
Iron(60-175ug/dl)							
TIBC(250-420ug/dl)							
Urinalysis :							
Catheter(Y/N)							
Color(Y.C.)							
S.G.(1.003-1.030)	1: 015						
pH(4.5-8.0)	6.0						
Protein(0-0.1gm/24h)	++						
Glucose(0.3gm/24h)							
Ketone(neg.)							
Urobilinogen(20X)	trace						
Blood(neg.)	+						
Microscope							
Nitrite	+						
Leu	+						
Feces :							
Blood							
Microscope							

Bacteriology			Miscellaneous
Date	Specimen	Organism	
99. 1. 8.	Blood(중간)	No growth	

등록번호	111 55 77	성별 M
성명	박신통 아기	
주민등록	170108-1234567	

방사선소견서
Radiologic Consultation Report

☐ Ambulatory ☑ X-ray ☑ Portable
☐ C-T ☐ Emergnecy ☐ U-S
☐ R-I ☐ Others ☑ New ☐ Old

Part & Type of Examination
Chest AP 'P' 'St'

History & Clinical Findings

Date 2017. 1. 8. Requested by ____________

접 수	촬영실	촬영자	8 × 10	10 × 12	11 × 14	14 × 14	14 × 17	Pol.	Image	정리자
55			1							

Contrast Media or RI agent: Dose :

Findings

Jan. 8. '17
Chest AP :
Total haziness with air bronchogram and obliteration of heart border is noted in both lungs, suggesting hyaline membrane disease, grade 3.

Min O. E./Park S. P.

등록번호	111 55 77	성별 M
성명	박신통 아기	
주민등록	170108-1234567	

방사선소견서
Radiologic Consultation Report

☐ Ambulatory ☑ X-ray ☑ Portable
☐ C-T ☐ Emergnecy ☐ U-S
☐ R-I ☐ Others ☐ New ☑ Old

Part & Type of Examination

Chest AP 'P' 'St'

History & Clinical Findings

Date 2017. 1. 14 Requested by ____________

접 수	촬영실	촬영자	8×10	10×12	11×14	14×14	14×17	Pol.	Image	정리자
88			1							

Contrast Media or RI agent: Dose :

Findings

Jan. 14 '17

Chest AP :

Apparently hazy-looking both lung fields with no visible peripheral air-bronchogram and slightly ill-defined cardiac border seem to be due to underpenetration and under inspiration rather than aggrevation of HMD.

Seo Q. E./Kim P. T.

등록번호 111 55 77 성별 M
성명 박신통 아기
주민등록 170108-1234567

의사지시기록
Doctor's Orders

일 자	내 용	서 명
	〈 Admission Order 〉	
17.1.8	1. Check V/S $\bar{q}$ 2hr	
	2. Check I/O & Bwt.	
	3. NPO	
	4. Ventilator care. ICS care	
	5. Keep U/A line & AP monitoring	
	6. Keep pulse oxymeter	
	7. Keep G-tube	
	8. Req) 1) prn) chest PA, AP, st 'p'	
	2) CBC $\bar{c}$ plt 'st'	
	3) Diff, ESR	
	4) é (Na/K/Cl) BUN/Cr Glu 'st'	
	5) GOT/GPT Ca/P/Mg	
	6) CRP 'quantity'	
	7) Blood culture	
	8) U/A 'st'	
	9) Prn) ABGA 'st'	
	9. Fluid) 10% D/W 500ml IV 3.5ml/hr	
	10. Inj) Vit K 1.0mg IV once	
	11. Fluid) 5% D/W 500ml, heparin 500U] mix for at time	
	12. Med) surfactant 1Ⓐ s.c.	*Hong*
17.1.9	1. Check V/S $\bar{q}$ 2 hr	
	2. Check I/O & Bwt.	
	3. NPO	
	4. Ventilator care, ICS care	
	5. Keep U/A line & AP monitoring	
	6. Keep pulse oxymeter	

의 사 지 시 기 록

일 자	내 용	서 명
17.1.9	7. Keep G-tube 8. Fluid) 10% D/W 500ml IV 3.5ml/hr 9. Anti) 1) Augmentin 45mg IV $\bar{q}$ 12hr 2) Amikin 15mg IV once 10. Req) 1) prn) chest AP 'st' 'p' 2) prn) ABGA 'st' 11. Req) chest AP 'st' 추) 12. Lasix 2mg IV	*Hong*
17.1.10	1. Check V/S $\bar{q}$ 2hr 2. Check I/O & Bwt. 3. NPO (until next order) 4. ICS care 5. Ventilator care 6. Keep U/A line & AP monitoring 7. Keep pulse oxymeter 8. Keep G-tube 9. Fluid) 10% D/W 500ml, Na 40/8ml] mix IV (T1 4ml/hr) 10. Anti) 1) Augmentin 45mg IV $\bar{q}$ 12hr 2) Amikin 15mg IV once 11. Req) 1) chest AP 'P' 'st' 2) prn) chest AP 'p' 'st' 3) prn) ABGA 12. Phototherapy & TSBLD 13. No 9 change to T1 4.5ml/hr	*Hong*
17.1.11	1. Check V/S $\bar{q}$ 2hr 2. Check I/O & Bwt. 3. NPO (until next order) 4. ICS care 5. Ventilator care 6. Keep U/A line & AP monitoring 7. Keep pulse oxymeter 8. Keep G-tube	

의 사 지 시 기 록

<table>
<tr><th>일 자</th><th>내 용</th><th>서 명</th></tr>
<tr><td>17.1.11</td><td>9. Fluid) 10% D/W 500ml, Na-40 8ml, K-40 5ml] mix IV (T1 5ml/hr)
10. Anti) 1) Augmentin 45mg IV $\bar{q}$ 12hr
2) Amikin 1.5mg IV once
11. Phototherapy
12. TSBLD
13. Req) 1) check AP 'P' 'st'
2) prn) ABGA</td><td>Hong</td></tr>
<tr><td>17.1.12</td><td>1. Check V/S $\bar{q}$ 2hr
2. Check I/O & Bwt.
3. NPO (until next order)
4. ICS care
5. Ventilator care
6. Keep U/A line & AP monitoring
7. Keep pulse oxymeter
8. Keep G-tube
9. Fluid) 10% D/W 150ml, Na-40 2ml, K-40 1ml] mix IV (T1 6ml/hr)
6% ped aminosteril 13ml
10. Anti) 1) Augmentin 45mg IV $\bar{q}$ 12hr
2) Amikin 1.5mg IV once
11. TSBLD
12. Req) prn) ABGA</td><td>Hong</td></tr>
<tr><td>17.1.13</td><td>1. Check V/S $\bar{q}$ 2hr
2. Check I/O & Bwt.
3. NPO (until next order)
4. ICS care
5. Ventilator care
6. Keep U/A line & AP monitoring
7. Keep pulse oxymeter
8. Keep G-tube</td><td></td></tr>
</table>

의 사 지 시 기 록

일 자	내 용	서 명
17.1.13	9. Fluid) 10% D/W 150ml Na-40 2ml K-40 1ml 6% ped aminosteril 25ml] mix IV (T1 6.5ml/hr) 10. Anti) 1) Augmentin 45mg IV $\bar{q}$ 12hr 2) Amikin 1.5mg IV once 11. Req) 1) chest AP 'P' 'st' 2) prn) ABGA	*Hong*
	추) 1. Fluid) N/S 10cc for 1hrs 2. ① ele, BUN/Cr 'st' UA 'st' → D/C ② spot urine Na/Cr 'st' 3. Fluid) N/S 12cc for 1hrs IV 4. No. 9 fluid → D/C → T.I. 6.5ml/hr change 5. Fluid) 10% D/W 100ml Na-40 1ml] mix IV (T1 12ml/hr) (8ml/hr) for 4hrs	*Hong*
	추) 1. Req/BUN/Cr ele' 'st' 2. TSBLD 3. Inj) lasix 2.5mg IV 4. Phototherapy	
17.1.14	1. Check V/S $\bar{q}$ 2hr 2. Check I/O & Bwt. 3. NPO (until next order) $\bar{c}$ keep G-tube 4. ICS care 5. Ventilator care 6. Keep U/A line & AP monitoring 7. Keep pulse oxymeter	

의 사 지 시 기 록

일 자	내 용	서 명
17.1.14	8. Fluid) 10% D/W 150ml Na-40 2ml K-40 1ml 6% ped aminostehe 40ml] mix IV (T1 8.5ml/hr)	
	9. Anti) 1) Augmentin 45mg IV c̄ 12hr 2) Amikin 1.5mg IV once	
	10. Req) 1) chest AP 'p' 'st' 2) prn) ABGA 3) Na/K/Cl BUB/Cr 'st'	
	11. Phototherapy & TSBLD	
	추) 12. Req) 1) CBC c̄ plt 'st' 2) diff. ESR. reti 3) GOT/GPT Bil/T/D Ca/P/Mg	*Hong*
	추) 13. Fluid) 30cc/hr → 15cc/hr 1) 15cc/hr (main fluid) 2) FFP 45cc transfusion for 3hr	
	14. Epinephrine 1:10000 1cc x 5	
	15. Vt. K 1.0mg IV	
	16. Luminal 30mg once IV	
	17. Bivon 1.5cc + 증류수 1.5cc x 2	
	18. Dopamin 0.23ml 5% D/W 35ml] mix IV 1.5ml/hr	
	19. Whole blood 1Ⓟ pre → D/C	
	20. Req) 1) KDP 2) CRP] D/C 3) Na/K/Cl BUN/Cr Glu. 4) Blood typing	
	21. Ca gluconate N/S 2cc	
	22. TSBCD → D/C	
	23. Expired at 2: 10 PM 17.1.14	*Hong*

〈박신통 아기〉

★ 박신통 아기 차트를 읽고 맞는 것에 O표 하시오.

1 **의무기록 내용과 일치하지 않는 것은?**

① Apgar score는 1분에 0점, 5분에 2점, 10분에 2점이었다.
② 두번째 방사선검사 결과 양쪽 폐가 희미한 것은 초자막질환보다 흡기 및 투과성하인 것으로 보인다.
③ 청색증은 심해졌으나 흉벽 함몰은 호전되었다.
④ 혈중요소질소의 농도가 증가한 것은 급성 신부전과 관련된다.
⑤ 청색증이었던 환아는 10분 후 분홍색을 띤 피부가 되었다.

2 **박신통 아기 엄마에 대해 맞게 분류된 것은?**

① O42.10 ② O42.91 ③ P01.1
④ O42.00 ⑤ P01.2

3 **입원 시 신체조사 내용과 일치하는 것은?**

① 눈의 분비물이 있었다. ② 수포음이 있었고, 호흡음도 거칠었다.
③ 움켜잡는 반사는 좋지 않은 상태였다. ④ 간과 비장(지라)은 촉진되지 않았다.
⑤ 입술과 구개(입천장)에 염증이 있었다.

4 **상기 출생아에 대한 분류번호로 맞는 것은?**

① Z37.2 ② Z37.3 ③ Z38.3
④ Z38.4 ⑤ Z38.0

5 **신생아의 호흡장애 증후군이 발생하는 경우가 아닌 것은?**

① 폐의 활성제 과다 ② 모체에 지나친 진정제 사용
③ 제대가 목에 걸려서 질식 ④ 당뇨병이 있는 임부
⑤ 호흡중추 장애 포함한 뇌손상

6 **박신통 아기의 주진단명에 대한 분류번호로 맞는 것은?**

① O36.5 ② O60.0 ③ P07.20
④ P07.11 ⑤ P07.13

7 **입원 3일째 의사지시기록에 대한 내용으로 틀리게 기재한 것은?**

① 다음 지시 때까지 유동식을 하도록 지시 ② 10% 포도당 수용액 500ml를 정맥내 주입
③ 늑간강 care와 광선치료 ④ 섭취량과 배설량 체크
⑤ 필요할 때마다 동맥혈가스분석 요구

8 **상기 환아의 출생 시 내용과 맞지 않는 것은?**

① 출생 시 태변 착색이 있었다. ② 출생 시 흉위는 23.5cm였다.
③ 출생 직후 심장마사지를 하였다. ④ 출생 시 키는 30.5cm였다.
⑤ 머리둘레는 30cm였다.

9 진단명에 대한 분류번호로 맞는 것은?

① P01.5, P10.2, P52.3
② P54.3, P22.0, P53
③ P54.3, P60, P52.3
④ P24.0, P60, P53
⑤ P54.3, P60, P53

10 상기 환아가 치료한 처치에 대한 질병분류번호로 맞는 것은?

① P59.9
② P59.0
③ P58.9
④ P59.8
⑤ P58.2

01 만성 화농성 중이염
Chronic suppurative otitis media

1.1 중이염 및 고막성형술의 의미

중이염(Otitis media)

▸ 고막 안쪽 중이 점막에 염증 발생

고실성형술(Tympanoplasty)

▸ 중이의 손상된 고막을 재생시켜 정상적으로 기능하도록 하는 수술

고막, 고실 및 중이의 의미

▸ 고막: 외이도를 통해 전달된 음파를 진동시키는 역할

▸ 고실: 고막의 안쪽에 위치하며 뼈로 둘러싸여 있음

▸ 중이: 외이와 내이 사이에 있는 작은 공간

1.2 지방간(Fatty liver)

지방간의 의미

▸ 정상 간은 지방이 차지하는 비율은 5% 정도, 지방간은 이보다 많은 지방이 축적된 상태

지방간의 분류

▸ 알코올성 지방간

- 알코올을 많이 섭취하게 되면 간에서 지방 합성이 촉진
- 정상적인 에너지 대사가 이루어지지 않아 발생

▸ 비알코올성 지방

- 비만, 당뇨병, 고지혈증, 약물 등이 원인

2.1 팔로4징후(Tetralogy of Fallot; TOF)

팔로4징후(Tetralogy of Fallot; TOF)의 의미

- 4가지(tetra) 결함을 포함하는 선천성 기형
- 선천성 심장질환 중 증상이 가장 심함
- 호흡곤란(dyspnea), 청색증(cyanosis), 실신(syncope) 등이 나타남

팔로4징후(TOF)의 선천성 기형: 대동맥 + 폐동맥

- 대동맥 우측편재(Shift of the aorta to the right)
- 심실중격결손(Ventricular septal defect; VSD)
- 폐동맥협착(Pulmonary artery stenosis; PS)
- 우심실 비대(Hypertrophy of the right ventricle; RVH)

2.2 젤폼(Gelform, 색전물질)

- 외용지혈제의 일종
- 정제젤라틴에 포름알데히드를 더해 열을 가해 중합시키고 기포 불어 넣어 스폰지상으로 한 것
- 절개조직과 창상조직 파열, 모세관과 세정맥 출혈, 실질장기 절제시 출혈 등 지혈 효과

차트 용어

Attic	고실	Disturbance	장애	Chill	오한
Dizziness	현기증	Exposed	노출된	Fascia	근막
Gelfoam	색전물질(젤폼)	Hyperemia	충혈	Mastoidea	유양돌기염
Mastoidectomy	유양돌기절제술	Media	중간	Nasal obstruction	비폐색
Otalgia	이통	Ossicle	이소골(작은뼈)	Orifice	구멍
Otitis	이염	Otorrhea	이루	Performation	수행
Perforation	구멍	Patent	개존(열려있는)	Recommend	권유
Rhinorrhea	비루	Sigmoid sinus	S상 정맥동	Sore throat	인후통
Suppurative = purulent	화농성	Sputum	객담(가래)	Tinnitus	이명

약 어	원 어	
COM	Chronic otitis media	만성 중이염
D/C	Discontinue	중지
EAC	External auditory canal	외이도
E-tube	Endotracheal tube	기관내 삽관
G-F	Grossly free = fee = N-S = intact = N-C = WNL	정상
lA	Impedance Audiometry Impedance	청력검사
lCWA	Intact canal wall mastoidectomy	무손상 판벽 유양돌기 절제술
PTA	Pure Tone Audiometry	순음 청력검사
NSD	Nasal septal deviation	비중격만곡증
OM	Otitis media	중이염
SAA	Same as above	상동
PORP	Partial ossicular replacement prosthesis	부분적 소골치환 보형물 교정
TM	Tympanic membrane	고막
TSP	Tympano sclerosing part	고실경화부위

장 역 전 요약 차트

등록번호 : 68 23 51　　　　　　이름 : 장역전
입원일 : 2017. 12. 11　　　　　퇴원일 : 2017. 12. 28　　　　　퇴원과 : IM

Diagnosis : #1 Chr. supp. OM, Rt.
　　　　　#2 Fatty liver

C.C : Hearing disturbance, Rt.

P.I　중학교 때 귀 앓은 후 Otorrhea 있어 local Tx 받아오다 '08년 Lt. ICW & PORP. attic reconstruction at S ENT (prof C.l. Cho) 받으신 후 청력 호전은 크게 없어 OPD를 통해 Rt. ear의 c.c.에 치료를 위해 op 권유받고 금일 입원

P.Hx : HTN (−) tbc (−)　Drug allergy (−)
　'07. 7.　Total correction of tetralogy of Fallot
　'10. 12.　Lt. ICWA & PORP attic reconstruction

ROS : chill (−), sputum (−), headache (−), hearing disturbance (+) both
　dizziness (+), otorrhea (−), otalgia (−), tinnitus (−), rhinorrhea (−)
　nasal obstruction (−), dyspnea (−), sore throat (−)

P/Ex : Ext deformity (−)
　NSD (+) Lt.
　Ext. deformity (−)
　EAC　Rt : G-F
　　　Lt : free
　TM performation (+) Rt.
　hyperemia (−)

imp) Chr Supp OM Rt.

〈 Op. note 〉

12/13　Preop Dx : Rt. Suppurative COM
　　　Postop Dx : SAA

장 역 전 요약 차트

등록번호 : 68 23 51　　이름 : 장역전
입원일 : 2017. 12. 11　　퇴원일 : 2017. 12. 28　　퇴원과 : IM

Op name : Rt. simple mastoidectomy $\bar{c}$ tympanoplasty type I
Op procedure : under GA
Anesthesia : general
Incision : retroauricular
Graft TM : temporalis muslce fascia
TM findings : large sized central perforation
Tympanomeatal flap was elevated
Fossa mastoidea was exposed and simple mastoidectomy was done
Ossicles : all intact but ossicle was attached to the tympanic membrane
Sigmoid sinus : some exposed during op → covered by fascia
Tympanic orifice of E-tube : patent
Chorda tympani n. : intact
Gelfoam insertion on tympanum
Graft fascia insertion by underlay method
Gelfoam was packed at external auditory canal.
Drain. Subcutaneous and skin suture. Compression dressing　　오기쁨

〈 POD #2 〉
12/15　Outer dressing was changed.
Clean op wound. Gelfoam was intact　　오기쁨

12/16　〈 POD #3 〉
Outer dressing was changed.
Clean op wound　　오기쁨
Gelfoam was intact

12/17　〈 POD #4 〉
Dressing was done　　이행운
Cleaned op wound
Gelfoam was intact

12/18　〈 POD #5 〉
Dressing was done　　오기쁨/
Cleaned op wound　　이행운
Half stitch out was done.

장 역 전 요약 차트

등록번호 : 68 23 51　　이름 : 장역전

입원일 : 2017. 12. 11　　퇴원일 : 2017. 12. 28　　퇴원과 : IM

12/12 〈 Admission Orders 〉

1. Check V/S $\bar{q}$ 6hrs
2. BR
3. GD
4. Get Op. permission from patient and his relative
5. Get pre-anesthetic order from anesthesiologist
6. Req.
   PTA. 1A → D/C

12/13 〈 Pre-Op Order 〉

1. Check V/S $\bar{q}$ 6hrs
2. BR
3. NPO from midnight
4. Follow pre-anesthetic order
5. F/I
   F - SD/S 10 IV
   A - CTZ 2Ⓐ mixed IV with AST
6. Prepare
   F - HS 500mL
   A - N/S 1L, IV set → D/C
   S-S
7. Shave the Rt. temporal area
8. Transfer the Pt. to OR after full voiding with all Labs, X-ray, and Chart
9. Prepare
   F - HS 500mL
   5% Dextrose in Normal Saline
   A - N/S 1L, IV set → D/C
10. Shave the Rt. temporal area
11. Transfer the Pt. to OR after full voiding with all Labs, X-ray, and Chart

12/14 〈 Postop Order 〉

1. Check V/S $\bar{q}$ 30 min x 2
   If stable Check $\bar{q}$ 6hrs

장 역 전 요약 차트

등록번호 : 68 23 51　　　　이름 : 장역전

입원일 : 2017. 12. 11　　　　퇴원일 : 2017. 12. 28　　　　퇴원과 : IM

2. BR
3. SD if gas is out
4. Keep humidification
5. Recommend to avoid nose blowing

II. F/I

F - 5D/S remained

A - CTZ　2 Ⓐ IVSS c̄ AST

A - FOF (CTZ)　2 Ⓐ IVSS

I - PAMBA　2 Ⓐ IM

12/15 〈Repeat〉

1. I - PAMBA ┐
   Fluid ┘ D/C

12/19 Discharge c̄ P.O med ┐

c̄ B - LFX 3T ┘ #3

OPD F/U　12/21

〈장 역 전〉

★ 장역전 차트를 읽고 맞는 것에 O표 하시오.

1 **환자에게 나타난 증상으로 옳은 것은?**

① 비루 ② 호흡곤란 ③ 현기증
④ 인후통 ⑤ 비폐색

2 **환자에 대한 설명으로 옳지 않은 것은?**

① 우측 외이도는 정상이었다. ② 비중격 만곡이 좌측으로 있었다.
③ 좌측은 고실성형술을 시행한 상태이다. ④ 수술 후 5일째 실밥의 반만 제거하였다.
⑤ 수술상처는 깨끗했고 진주종 비대가 있었다.

3 **질병분류번호로 옳은 것은?**

① H65.40 20.41 19.52 ② H66.30 20.41 19.4
③ H66.30 20.42 19.4 ④ H65.20 20.42 19.4
⑤ H66.40 20.49 19.52

4 **수술기록지에 대한 내용으로 옳은 것은?**

① 고막은 인조고막을 사용하였다. ② 고삭 신경이 수술 도중 절단되었다.
③ 기관내 삽관의 고막 구멍은 닫혀 있었다. ④ S상 정맥동의 일부가 노출되어 근막으로 덮었다.
⑤ 고막은 구멍이 크게 났고 분비물이 흐르고 있었다.

5 **환자에게 투여된 수액으로 연결된 것은?**

① 아미노산 용액 - 5% 포도당 용액 ② 염화칼륨 용액 - 5% 포도당 용액
③ 염화칼륨 용액 - 하트만 용액 ④ 아미노산 용액 - 생리식염수
⑤ 하트만 용액 - 생리식염수

6 **환자에 대한 기술로 옳지 않은 것은?**

① 코를 풀도록 하였고 수술 후 6일째 퇴원하였다.
② 환자는 외래를 통하여 수술목적으로 입원하였다.
③ 수술경과는 합병증이나 부작용 없이 좋은 편이었다.
④ 퇴원약은 3일치를 주었고 2일 후 외래로 오도록 하였다.
⑤ 수술 후 활력증후군은 30분마다 2회 점검하도록 하였다.

05. 의무기록 중요 내용

Fundamentals of Medical Record

MEDICAL RECORD PRACTICE

01 진단에 따른 임상처치(질병분류 병행)

Clinical procedures based on diagnosis

1) 진단명:	Obstructive hydrocephalus	폐색성 수두증	G91.1
수술명:	Ventriculoperitoneal shunt	뇌실복강단락	02.34
2) 진단명:	Tuberculous meningitis	결핵성 수막염	A17.0+, G01*
처치명:	Spinal tapping	척추천자	03.31

- spinal tapping = spinal puncture 척추천자

3) 진단명:	Metastatic brain tumor	전이성 뇌종양	C79.3
	Post lung lobectomy status	폐엽 절제 후 상태	Z85.1
	No recurrence of primary site	원발 부위의 재발 없음	
치료명:	Chemotherapy	화학요법	99.25

- lung cancer(폐암) : C34.9 - 진단명
  post lobectomy(폐엽 절제 후) : Z85.1 - 병력(history)/개인력 → 가족력(Z80.___)
- M___/O: 양성 /1: 악·양성 경계 /2: 정상소재암(carcinoma in situ)
  /3: 악성+원발 /6: 악성 + 전이
  /9: 원발·전이 모를 경우

4) 진단명:	Adenoma of thyroid gland, Rt	우측 갑상선 선종	D34, M8140/0
수술명:	Unilateral thyroidectomy	편측 갑상선절제술	06.2

- fibergastroscopy(FGS, 위내시경): 44.13
- fiber gastroscopy(위내시경) + bx(생검): 44.14

5) 진단명:	Adenocarcinoma of early gastric cardia	조기 위 분문의 선암종	C16.00, M8140/3
검사명:	Fibergastroscopy with stomach biopsy	위내시경 및 생검	44.14

Non-surgical biopsy(비수술 생검)		Surgical biopsy(수술생검)	
· by endoscopy	내시경	· by incision	절개
· punch biopsy	천공 생검	· by excision of tissue	조직 절제
· percutaneous needle biopsy	경피 침 생검	· frozen biospy	동결 생검
· aspirational biopsy	흡인 생검	· by open operation	개방성 수술
· superficial smear	표재성 도말		

6) **진단명**: Acute lymphocytic leukemia 급성 림프구성 백혈병 C91.08
검사명: Bone marrow aspiration with biopsy 골수흡인 및 생검 41.31
치료명: Bone marrow transplantation 골수이식 41.00

7) **진단명**: Senile catatract 노인성 백내장 H25.99
수술명: Extracapsular extraction 낭외적출술 13.59
Posterior chamber lens implantation 인공수정체 삽입술 13.71

‣ intracapsular cataract extraction(ICCE)	**낭내적출술**	13.19
‣ extracapsular cataract extraction(ECCE)	**낭외적출술 + PCL**	13.59, 13.71
‣ posterior chamber lens implantation(PCL)	**인공수정체 삽입술**	13.71

8) **진단명**: Glaucoma secondary to keratitis 각막염에 의한 속발성 녹내장 H40.4, H16.9
수술명: Cyclodialysis 섬모체 박리술 12.55

9) **진단명**: Chronic serous otitis media 만성 장액성 중이염 H65.2
수술명: Myringotomy 고막절개술 20.09

10) **진단명**: Ruptured cerebral aneurysm 파열된 뇌동맥류 I60.9
수술명: Aneurysmectomy 동맥류절제술 38.60

11) **진단명**: Chronic cholecystitis with gallstone 담석을 동반한 만성 담낭(쓸개)염 K80.10
수술명: Cholecystectomy 담낭(쓸개)절제술 51.22

· Stone =calculus = litho **결석** · GB=gallbladder=cholecysto **담낭(쓸개)**
· CBD=common bile duct=choledocho **총담관**

12) **진단명**: Pre-eclampsia, severe form 중증 전자간증 O14.1
C/S wound infection 제왕절개 상처의 감염 O86.0
수술명: Lower flap transverse cesarean section 제왕절개 수술 74.1
Secondary closure 수술상처의 재봉합 54.61

12-1) **진단명**: IUP at 6 weeks — 임신 6주
Lt, Salpingitis — 좌측 난관염(자궁관염) O08.0
수술명: D & C — 소파수술 69.01

- Intrauterine pregnancy(IUP) 자궁내 임신: 정상임신
  → tubal pregnancy 난관(자궁관)임신: 비정상임신 → 유산
- Dilatation and curettage(D&C) 확장 및 소파수술 →유산
  - **수술후 감염**: 일반 임상과 → T81.4 + Y62.0
    산과 → O86.0 + Y62.0
  - **산과**: 분만, 미분만(분만 전·후), 유산, 산욕기

12-2) **진단명**: IUP at 37 weeks — 임신 37주
Previous cesarean section state — 이전 제왕절개 상태 O34.22, O99.8
Lt. Parovarion cyst — 좌측 난소방체의 낭종 Q50.5, O82.0
수술명: Repearted C/S — 반복 제왕절개 74.1
Bilateral tubal ligation — 양측 난관(자궁관)결찰술 66.39

- **자궁관**: tubal = salpingo = uterine tube = fallopian tube
- **진단명**: Sterilization — 불임 — Z30.2
  ① Tubal pregnancy — 난관(자궁관)임신 (여성) — O00.1
  ② Vasectomy — 정관절제술 (남성) — 63.73
  ↔ vasovasostomy — 정관정관문합술(복원) — 63.82
- **수술명**: Tubal ligation — 난관(자궁관)결찰술 — 66.39
  (Pomeroy operaion 포메로이수술 66.32)
- Elective C/S (선택적 제왕절개) O82.0
- Emergency C/S(응급 제왕절개) O82.1

12-3) **진단명**: Tubal pregnancy, ruptured — 난관(자궁관)임신, 파열됨 O00.1
수술명: Bilateral salpingectomy — 양측 난관(자궁관)절제술 66.63

13) **진단명**: Herniated lumbar disc — 추간판 전위 M51.2
수술명: Laminectomy — 추궁절제술 80.51

- Dx: herniated lumbar disc(HLD) 추간판 전위: M51.2
- Tx: laminectomy(추궁절제술), diskectomy(원판제거), chemonucleolysis(화학적핵분리술)

14) **진단명**: Single born in hospital — 병원출생 단일아 Z38.0
Living newborn at 35 weeks of gestation — 임신 35주의 병원출생 신생아 P07.31
Hyperbilirubinemia — 고빌리루빈혈증 P59.0

처치명: Phototherapy 광선치료 99.83

- 분만결과(delivery): Z37._: 출생아 또는 사산아 → 단일아(Z37.09), 쌍둥이(Z37.29)
- 출생(born) : Z38._: 병원내 또는 병원외 → 단일아: 병원내(Z38.0), 병원외(Z38.1)
  쌍생아: 병원내(Z38.3), 병원외(Z38.4)
- hyperbilirubinemia(고빌리루빈혈증) = jaundice, icterus(황달)
- 신생아 또는 생리적 황달: P59.9, 조산 + 황달: P59.0

15) **진단명**: Second and third degree burn of chest wall 20% of body involved 흉벽의 2도 및 3도 화상 T21.3 신체표면의 20% 포함 T31.22
수술명: Full thickness skin graft 전층 피부이식 86.63

- second and third degree burn of chest wall: 동일 부위인 경우
  → 화상 정도가 더 높은 것으로 분류(2도<3도)
  예) Corrosion of first degree of finger, 30% of hand surface involved → T23.51, T32.33
  손 면적 30%인 손가락 1도 부식
- full thickness skin graft(FTSG) 전층 피부이식

화상/부식 및 신체표면의 정도	화상(burn)	부식(corrosion)
·1도 화상: 홍반(erythema)	.____1	.____5
·2도 화상: 수포(blister)	.____2	.____6
·3도 화상: 괴사(necrosis)	.____3	.____7
·신체표면의 정도: 10% 미만	T31.0	T32.0
·신체표면의 정도: 10~19%	T31.1	T32.1
·신체표면의 정도: 20~19%	T31.2	T32.2
:	:	:

16) **진단명**: Benign prostatic hypertrophy 양성 전립선(샘) 비대증 N40.0
수술명: Transurethral resection of prostate 경요도 전립선(샘) 절제 60.29

- 진단명: benign prostatic hypertrophy(BPH) 양성 전립샘 비대증 N40
  수술명: transurethral resection of prostate(TURP) 경요도 전립샘 절제 60.29
- 진단명: bladder tumor 방광암 C67.9
  수술명: transurethral resection of bladder(TURB) 경요도 방광 절제 57.49

17) **진단명**: Leiomyoma of uterus, intramural type 자궁의 평활근종, 벽내형 D25.1, M8890/0
수술명: Myomectomy 근종절제술 68.29

- 진단명: myoma(자궁근종) = fibroids(유섬유종)
- 수술명: hysterectomy(자궁절제술) 또는 myomectomy(자궁근종)

18) 진단명: Admitted for displaced IUD　전위된 자궁내 피임장치 제거 위해 입원　T83.3
수술명: Removal of IUD　자궁내 피임기구 제거　97.71

- **피임관리**
  - ·피임장치 삽입을 위해 내원　Z30.1
  - ·피임장치의 기계적 합병증(전위, 돌출 등)　T83.3
  - ·피임장치 조사, 재삽입, 제거　Z30.5
  - ·피임장치 존재　Z97.5
- **불임시술을 위한 입원**　Z30.2

19) 진단명: Postoperative wound disruption　수술부위의 파괴　T81.3, Y65.2
수술명: Secondary suture　재봉합　86.59

20) 진단명: Breast cancer, Rt. upper-outer quadrant　우측 상외사분 유방암　C50.40
수술명: Unilateral radical mastectomy　편측성 근치적 유방절제술　85.45

- radical mastectomy(bilateral)　**근치적 유방절제술(양측)**　85.46
  → 유방+흉근+액와림프절+관련된 피부+피하조직 절제
- simple mastectomy(unilateral)　**단순유방절제술(편측)**　85.43: 유방전체 제거
- modified radical mastectomy(unilateral)　**변형 근치적 유방절제술(편측)**　85.43
  → 유방+임파절+흉벽의 근육절제
- lumpectomy　**덩어리절제술**　85.21: 덩어리 제거

21) 진단명: Rectal cancer　직장암　C20
수술명: Mile's operation　마일즈 수술(직장 복부회음적 절제술)　48.5

22) 진단명: Cevical cancer　자궁경부(목)암　C53.9
수술명: Total abdominal hysterectomy　전체복부 자궁절제술　68.4

- **진단명**: Cervical cancer **자궁경부(목)암**　C53.9
- **수술명**: Conization　**원추조직절제술** → **조기암**(early cancer) 시
  Total abdominal hysterectomy(TAH) **전체복부 자궁절제술**　68.4

23) 진단명: Pyloric stenosis　유문(날문)협착증　K31.1
수술명: Pyloromyotomy　유문(날문)근층 절개술　43.3

- pyloromyotomy(**날문근층 절개술**) = Fredet-Ramstedt operation

24) **진단명**: Appendicitis 급성 충수염 K37
수술명: Incidental appendectomy 부수적 충수절제술 47.1

- incidental appendectomy **충수돌기절제술** → MacBurney's incision(**맥버니절개법**)

25) **진단명**: Phimosis 포경 N47
수술명: Circumcision 포경수술 64.0

26) **진단명**: Cleft lip 구개열 Q35.9
수술명: Cheiloplasty 순성형술 27.59

- cleft lip(**구개열**) = hare lip
- cheilo = lip (**입술**)
- celio = abdomen = laparo (**복부**)
- chiro = hand (**손**)

27) **진단명**: Tongue tie 설소대 Q38.1
수술명: Glossotomy 혀주름띠절개술 25.91

- tongue tie(**설소대**) = frenulum = ankyloglossia

28) **진단명**: Fracture of shaft of tibia 경골(정강뼈)간의 골절 S82.20
수술명: Open reduction c̄ internal fixation 관혈적 정복과 내부 고정술 79.36

- Dx: Fx of humerus **상완골(자뼈) 골절** S42.30
  Op: closed reduction with internal fixation(CR c̄ IF) **비관혈적 정복과 내부고정술** 79.11
- S, M **코드: 진단명(4-5자리)**

29) **진단명**: Otosclerosis 이경 H80.9
수술명: Fenestration 조개창술(속귀 창냄) 20.61

30) **진단명**: Dementia in multiple sclerosis 다발성 경화증에서의 치매 G35⁺, F02.8*
검사명: Electroencephalogram 뇌파검사법 89.14

·EKG(ECG) = Electrocardiogram **심전도** 89.52
·EEG = Electroencephlogram **뇌전도** 89.14

02 주진단의 기준

Criteria of principal diagnosis

주진단	기타진단
· 최종 확진된 진단명 중 입원의 주원인 · 의료자원의 소모가 가장 큰 것 · 병리조직검사, 퇴원요약지 진단명 확인 · 첫번째 자리에 번호 부여 · 주된 병태 표시 참조(1~18번)	· 후유증: late effect =squelelae =~years ago = old · 두 번째 자리부터 번호 부여 · 손상외인: 약물, 수술(처치) 후 병태, 사고, 추락 등 – W(미끄러짐, 추락 등) 예) 계단에서 추락 W10.__ – X(살충제 등 사고, 자살 등) 예) X68.__ – Y(외과적 실패 등) 예) 수술 후 UTI→T81.4+Y62.0

주진단 표시: ___

(1) 검표(†)와 별표(*)의 이원분류: 검표(†)

– Tuberculous meningitis　결핵성 수막염　A17.0†(원인), G01*(장기)

(2) 가장 중요하고 의료자원의 소모가 가장 많은 것

– Fracture of femoral neck, Rt　오른쪽 대퇴골(넙다리뼈목) 골절

– Sprain of ankle, Rt　발목의 염좌

– Open wound of knee, Rt　무릎의 개방성 상처　S72.090, S93.49, S81.0

(3) 다발성 골절, 다발성 머리손상: 다발성

– Open wound of scalp　두피(머리덮개)의 개방성 상처　S01.7(다발성)

– Open wound of lip　입술의 개방성 상처　S01.0, S01.50

(4) 두개골/안면골의 골절과 관련되어 두개내 손상 시: 두개내 손상

– Temporal bone fracture　측두골(관자뼈) 골절

– Intracranial hematoma　두개(머리)내 혈종　S06.80, S02.10

머리뼈(Cranial bone)	얼굴뼈(Facial bone)
·전두골(이마뼈, Frontal bone)	·비골(코뼈, Nasal bone)
·두정골(마루뼈, Parietal bone)	·누골(Lacrimal bone)
·측두골(관자뼈, Temporal bone)	·상악골(위턱뼈, Maxillary bone)
→ 유양돌기(꼭지돌기, Mastoid bone)	·하악골(아래턱뼈, Mandibular bone)
·후두골(뒤통수뼈, Occipital bone)	·관골(광대뼈, Zygomatic bone)
·접형골(나비뼈, Sphenoid bone)	·서골(Vomer)
·사골(벌집뼈, Ethmoid bone)	

* □: 머리뼈(두개골)의 동(굴, sinus of skull)

(5) 관련성이 없고, 한 개의 번호로 연계될 수 없을 경우: 진료받은 임상과

- Cataract 백내장
- Streptococcal meningitis 포도구균(알균) 수막염 G00.3, H26.9
  (Treated in neurology) (신경과에서 치료받음)

(6) 다른 질환 유발시키는 인체면역결핍바이러스(HIV)

- HIV disease and Kaposi's sarcoma 인체면역결핍바이러스 질환과 카포시 육종
  B21.0, C46.9, M9140/3

(7) 치료나 검사를 가장 필요로 했던 사항

- Severe headache 심한 두통
- Suspected brain tumor 뇌종양 의증 R51, C71.9

‣ Suspect=rule out(R/O)=impression 의증

(8) 증상, 징후, 어떤 문제가 혼합된 경우: 주된 치료가 시행된 진단명

- Hematuria 혈뇨
- Varicose veins of legs 다리의 정맥류
- Papilloma of posterior wall of bladder 방광 후벽의 유두종 D41.4
  (Diathermy excision of papilloma was done) 투열요법으로 유두종 제거 R31.8, I83.9

(9) 외인으로 인하여 손상 유발된 경우: 손상내용(골절)

- Fracture of femoral neck caused by fall due to tripping on uneven pavement
  고르지 못한 포장도로에 걸려 넘어져서 발생한 대퇴골경(넙다리뼈목) 골절 S72.090(골절)
  W01.4(손상외인/추락)

(10) 후유증은 추가진단으로만 사용: 현재 잔여 병태

- Contracture of Achilles tendon 아킬레스건(발목 뒤)의 구축
- Late effect of injury to tendon 건(힘줄) 손상의 후유증 M67.17, T93.5(후유증)

(11) 급성과 만성: 급성

- Acute and chronic cholecystitis 급성과 만성 담낭(쓸개)염 K81.0, K81.1

‣ GB=Gallbladder=Cholecysto **담낭(쓸개)** ‣ CBD=Common bile duct=Choledocho **총담관**

(12) 진료의 초점이 된 상황

- Carcinoma of breast 유방암
- S/P mastectomy 2 years ago 2년전 유방절제술 시행상태
- Secondary carcinoma of lung 폐의 속발성 암종
- (Bronchoscopy with biopsy of lung was done) (기관지경 검사와 폐의 생검 실시)

C78.09(전이), Z85.3(병력/개인력)

위암(Stomach cancer): 현재 원발암	위암(Stomach cancer): 과거의 위암 + 현재 완치
· 현재 위암 발생한 상태 · 원발성암(위암) 번호 부여: C____ · 예: 위암이 현재 발생 상태: C16.99 예: 전이된 암(위암), 원발암(폐암) → C34.99(원발성 폐암), C78.8(전이 위암)	· 과거에 위암 발생했으나 현재 완치된 상태 · 위암(원발암)은 완치되었으나 다른 장기에 전이된 경우 · 병력(history): 과거암 번호(Z___) 부여 - 개인력 Z85.___ → 예: 위암의 개인력(Z85.0) - 가족력 Z80.___ → 예: 위암의 가족력(Z80.0)

(13) 2개 이상의 원발성 악성 신생물: 다발성 부위의 악성 신생물

- Multiple myeloma 다발성 골수종 C97(다발성)
- Adenocarcinoma of prostate 전립선(샘)의 선암종 C90.0, C61, M8140/3

(14) 임신의 경우: 합병증 또는 기타 상태(질환, 조숙, 과다체중 등)

- Intrauterine pregnancy at 43 weeks 임신 43주
- Delivered a living normal infant by routine episiotomy O48(과숙), O80.0

정례적 회음 절개술에 의한 정상 신생아 분만

‣ **정상 임신기간: 37~42주 미만** ‣ **정상 신생아 체중: 2.5~4.5kg 미만**

(15) 신생아의 경우: 검사 또는 치료를 필요로 하는 병태

– Term birth, living infant, born in the hospital	병원에서 출생한 정상 신생아	
– Hyperbilirubinemia	고빌리루빈혈증	P59.9, Z38.0
(Phototherapy was done)	광선치료 받음	99.83

- 진단명: · 조산 + 황달(hyperbilirubinemia 고빌리루빈혈증) → P59.0
  · 정상신생아(neonatal), 생리적(physical) → P59.9
- 처치명: 광선치료(Phototherapy) → 99.83
- 황달: jaundice=icterus=hyperbilirubinemia

(16) 수술 또는 처치와 관련된 합병증: 일반 임상과(T81._), 산과(O.__)

– Disruption of operation wound	수술부위의 파열	T81.3(합병증), Y65.2
– Cesarean section wound infection	제왕절개 상처의 감염	O86.0(합병증), Y62.0

(17) 처방대로 사용: 부작용(예: 피부염)

– Contact dermatitis due to properly applied antifungal antibiotics L25.1, Y40.7
처방대로 외용한 항진균성 항생제로 인한 접촉성 피부염

(15) 오용 또는 남용으로 중독된 경우: T___

– Contact dermatitis due to accidental contact of antifungal antibiotics
by a baby at home T36.7(중독), L25.1, X44.0
집에서 아기가 항진균 항생제의 우발적인 접촉으로 접촉성 피부염
- 약물 및 화학물질표: 19장(T__) → 중독(overdose, drug intoxication)

03 의학 약어 및 중요어휘

Medical abbreviation & keywords

약 어	원 어	해 설

A

약 어	원 어	해 설
A	adult	성인
	alive	생존
	anterior	전(前)
	‣ 반대어: Posterior 후(後)	
	assessment(in problem-oriented medical record)	평가(문제지향식 의무기록)
	→ SOAP 형식: 경과기록, 퇴원요약, 협의진료기록 ‣ S(Subjective information) 주관적인 정보 : CC(chief complain, 주소) ‣ O(Objective information) 객관적인 정보 : 임상검사 → GFS(내시경) 등 ‣ A(Assessment) 평가 : 진단명 → CVA(뇌졸중), HTN(고혈압) ‣ P(Plan) 계획 : Op.(수술), RT(방사선치료)	
a	accommodation(eye examination)	조절(시력검사)
	before(Latin: ante)	전(前)
AA	aplastic anemia	무형성 빈혈/골수세포의 형성부전증
	‣ hemolytic anemia(용혈성 빈혈): 과잉파괴로 인한 적혈구의 감소 ‣ pernicious anemia(악성빈혈): 비타민 B12 결핍 ‣ sickle cell anemia(낫적혈구 빈혈): 낫 모양의 적혈구, 흑인 발생	
AAA	abdominal aortic aneurysm	복부 대동맥류
AARF	acute alveolar respiratory failure	급성 폐포 호흡부전
Ab	antibody	항체
Ab.	abortion	유산
abd.	abdomen	복부
	abduction	외전
	‣ 반대어: adduction(내전)	
ABE	actue bacterial endocarditis	급성 박테리아 심내염
ABGA	arterial blood gases analysis(laboratory/blood gas)	동맥혈 가스분석
ABI	atherosclerotic brain infarction	죽상경화 뇌경색

약 어	원 어	해 설
ABO	blood group system	혈액형 시스템(A, AB, B, O)
	‣ erythroblastosis fetalis(태아적아구증) : 모체와 태아와의 혈액형 부적합으로 생기는 태아의 용혈성 빈혈	
ABP	arterial blood pressure	동맥혈압
	‣ 정상혈압(120/80): 120 systolic blood pressure(수축기혈압) 80 diastolic blood pressure(이완기혈압) ‣ 혈압 측정하는 동맥: brachial artery(상완/팔동맥) ‣ 맥박촉지: radial artery(요골/노뼈동맥)	
ABR	absolute bed rest	절대 안정
ABS	acute brain syndrome	급성 뇌증후군
AC	abdominal circumference	복위
	adrenal cortex	부신피질
	air conduction(hearing test)	공기전도(청력검사)
	anterior chamber(eye examination)	전안방(시력검사)
ac.	acid	산
	acute	급성
a.c.	before meals(Latin: ante cibum)	식전
accom.	accommodation(eye examination)	조절(시력검사)
ACA	anterior cerebral artery	전방 뇌동맥
ACBG	aortocoronary bypass graft surgery	대동맥 관상동맥 우회로 이식
ACL	anterior chamber lens	전방 렌즈
	anterior cruciate ligament(of knee/tear)	전방십자형인대(무릎/열상)
ACT	activated clotting time	활동적 응고시간
ACTH	adrenocorticotrophic hormone(medication order)	부신피질자극호르몬(약지시)
	‣ 뇌하수체 전엽: 선하수체(adenohypophysis) – ACTH(부신피질자극호르몬), LH(황체형성호르몬), FSH(난포자극호르몬) – MSH(흑색세포자극 호르몬), GH(성장호르몬), PRL(프로락틴), TSH(갑상선자극호르몬) ‣ 뇌하수체 후엽: 신경하수체(neurohypophysis) – ADH(항이뇨호르몬), oxytocin(옥시토신)	
AD	Alzheimer's disease(dementia)	알쯔하이머병(치매)
	right ear(Latin: *auris dextra*)	오른쪽 귀
	‣ AS(auris sinistra, 왼쪽 귀), AU(auris uterque, 양쪽 귀)	
add.	adduction	내전
	‣ 반대어: abduction(외전)	
ADH	antidiuretic hormone: vasopressin	항이뇨호르몬/내분비계
	‣ 뇌하수체 후엽: ADH(항이뇨호르몬) – 수분재흡수 oxytocin(옥시토신) – 진통자극	
adm.	admission	입원
AE	above elbow	팔꿈치 위
AF	atrial fibrillation	심방 세동
Af	atrial flutter	심방 조동

약 어	원 어	해 설
AFB	acid-fast bacilli(tuberculosis)	항산성 간균(결핵의 원인균)
AFO	ankle-foot orthosis	발목-발 정형술
AFP	alpha-fetoprotein(laboratory/chemistry)	태아성 단백질
	‣ 양수와 산모의 혈중에서 상승 시: 무뇌증(anencephaly), 이분 척추(spinal bifida) 등 ‣ Tumor Marker(종양표지자): 간암 진단에 사용	
AFV	amniotic fluid volume	양수량
AGA	appropriate for gestational age	임신연령에 적당
AGE	acute gastroenteritis	급성 위장염
AGL	acute granulocytic leukemia	급성 과립성 백혈병
AGML	acute gastric mucosal lesion	급성 위점막 병소
AGN	acute glomerulonephritis	급성 사구체신염
AGP	antegrade pyelogram	전위 신우조영상(콩팥깔대기조영술)
AHD	antihypertensive drug	항고혈압제
	arteriosclerotic heart disease	동맥경화성 심장질환
	autoimmune hemolytic disease	자가면역 용혈성질환
AI	aortic insufficiency	대동맥 협착
AID	acute infectious disease	급성 감염성질환
AIDS	acquired immunodeficiency syndrome	후천성 면역결핍증후군
AJ	ankle jerk	발목반사
AK	above knee(operation/amputation)	무릎 위
AKA	above knee amputation	무릎 위 절단
alb.	albumin(laboratory/chemistry)	알부민
ALD	alcoholic liver disease	알코올성 간질환
ALG	antilymphocytic globulin	항림프구 글로블린
alk	alkali	알칼리
alk. phos.	alkaline phosphatase(laboratory/chemistry)	간기능 효소검사
ALL	acute lymphocytic leukemia	급성 림프성 백혈병
ALK	alkaline phosphatase(liver function test/enzyme)	간기능 효소검사
ALS	amyotrophic lateral sclerosis	근위축성 측삭경화증
ALT	alkaline transaminase	간기능 효소검사
A.M.	morning	오전
AMA	against medical advice	자의퇴원
AMI	acute myocardial infarction	급성 심근경색증
AML	acute monocytic leukemia	급성 단구성 백혈병
	acute myelogenous leukemia	급성 골수성 백혈병
AN	anesthesiology	마취과
ANA	antinuclear antibody(laboratory/serology)	항핵 항체

약 어	원 어	해 설
AN	antinuclear factor(laboratory/serology)	항핵 인자
A/N/V/D/C	anorexia, nausea, vomiting, diarrhea, constipation	식욕부진, 오심, 구토 설사, 변비
AOD	arterial occlusive disease	동맥폐쇄성 질환
AOM	acute otitis media	급성 중이염
AOMD	adult onset diabetes mellitus	성인 개시 당뇨병
AP	alkaline phosphatase	간기능 효소검사
	ante partum(obstetrics)	출산(분만) 전
	anterior pituitary(=adenohypophysis)	뇌하수체전엽(선하수체)
	anteroposterior	전후의
	aortic pressure	대동맥압
A-P	abdominal perineal(resection)	복부-회음부(절제)
	anterior-posterior	전후
A & P	ascultation and percussion	청진과 타진
	‣ P/E(신체검진): inspection(시진), palpitation(촉진), ascultation(청진), percussion(타진)	
APB	atrial premature beat(=contractions)	심방성 조기수축
APN	acute pyelonephritis	급성 신우신염
aPTT	activated partial thromboplastin time	활성 피티티
aq. dest	distilled water	증류수
AR	aortic regurgitation	대동맥 역류
ARDS	adult respiratory distress syndrome	성인 호흡곤란증후군
	‣ 빠른 호흡, 호흡곤란, 빈맥, 저산소혈증 및 청색증 등	
ARF	acute renal failure	급성 신부전(콩팥기능상실)
	acute respiratory failure	급성 호흡부전
	acute rheumatic fever	급성 류마티스열
AROM	artificial rupture of membranes	양막 인공파열
AS	aortic stenosis	대동맥 협착
	Apgar score	아프가 점수법
	‣ 영아의 신체상태를 측정하는 점수제도 – 출산 후 1분, 5분 후 측정 – 심박동률, 호흡, 색깔, 근육강도 및 자극에 대한 반응 – 0~10점 부여(Apgar 점수가 낮은 신생아는 진료)	
	arteriosclerosis	동맥경화증
	left ear(Latin: *auris sinistra*)	왼쪽 귀
	‣ AD(auris dextra, 오른쪽 귀), AU(auris unitas, 양쪽 귀)	
A.S.A.	acetylsalicylic acid(aspirin)	아스피린
ASAP	as soon as possible	가능한 빨리
	‣ prn(whenever necessary): 필요할 때마다	

약 어	원 어	해 설
ASD	atrial septal defect	심방중격결손
ASHD	arteriosclerotic heart disease	동맥경화성 심질환
Ass't	assistant	수술보조의사
	‣ surgeon 수술집도의 · 1st Ass't: 제 1 수술보조의사, 2nd ass't: 제 2 수술보조의사 · scrub nurse: 소독간호사, circ. nurse: 순환간호사(circulating nurse)	
AST	aspartic acid transaminase	간기능 효소검사
	‣ 간기능검사 정상치: AST(GOT) – (남) 37 U/L 이하, (여) 31 U/L 이하 ALT(GPT) – (남) 40 U/L 이하, (여) 31 U/L 이하 ↑: 간염, 심근경색, 간암, ↓: 간장괴사	
AU	both ears(Latin: aures unitas)	양쪽 귀
	‣ AS(auris sinistra): 왼쪽 귀, AD(auris dextra): 오른쪽 귀	
AV	aortic valve	대동맥판
	ateriovenous	동정맥 혈관
A-V	atrioventricular	방실의
AVC	acute viral conjunctivitis	급성 바이러스성 결막염
AVH	acute viral hepatitis	급성 바이러스성 간염
AVM	arteriovenous malformation	동정맥기형
AVN	atrioventricular node	방실결절
AVR	aortic valve replacement(operation/cardiac)	대동맥판 치환(수술/심장)
AVS	arteriovenous shunt	동정맥 단락

B

약 어	원 어	해 설
B	basophils	호염기구(백혈구)
	‣ leukocytes(백혈구)의 종류 – granulocyte(과립구): basophil(호염기구), eosinophil(호산구), neutrophil(호중구) – agranulocyte(무과립구): lymphocyte(림프구), monocyte(단핵구)	
BA	brachial artery	상완(팔)동맥
	‣ 혈압을 측정하는 동맥: brachial artery(상완/팔동맥) ‣ 맥박 촉지: radial artery(요골/노뼈동맥)	
	bronchial asthma	기관지 천식
	barium	바륨
	both adnexectomy	양측 부속절제술
bact.	bacteria	세균
Ba. swallow	barium swallow(x-ray/esophagus)	바륨(방사선검사/식도)
baso	basophils(leukocyte)	호염기구(백혈구)
	‣ granulocyte(과립구): basophil(호염기구), eosinophil(호산구), neutrophil(호중구)	

약 어	원 어	해 설
BBB	bundle branch block(ECG=EKG)	차단(심전도)
BBBB	bilateral bundle branch block	양각 차단
B.B.T.	basal body temperature	기초체온
BC	blood chemistry	혈액화학검사
	blood culture	혈액배양
BCC	basal cell carcinoma	기저세포암종
	‣ 악성종양 → 원발장기: 피부(skin)	
BDM	bone densitometry	골밀도 검사
BE	barium enema(x-ray/colon)	바륨관장(x-ray 검사/결장)
	‣ lower GI series: 하부소화장기 x-ray 검사/직장, 결장	
	below elbow(operation/amputation)	팔꿈치 아래(수술/절단)
BCG	Bacille Calmette Gurin Vaccine	BCG 생백신
BG	bone graft(operation/orthopedics)	골이식(수술/정형외과)
bib.	drink(Latin: bibe) (medication order)	마심(약 처방)
b.i.d.	two times a day(Latin: bis in die)	1일 2회
BIH	benign intracranial hypertension	양성 두개내 혈압
Billroth I	stomach + gastroduodenostomy	위절제 시, 남은 위와 십이지장 연결
Billroth II	stomach + gastrojejunostomy	위절제 시, 남은 위를 공장에 연결
	‣ 십이지장 궤양 시 수술방법	
b.i.n.	twice a night	하루밤에 2번
BJ	biceps jerk	이두근반사
BJ protein	Bence-Jones protein(laboratory/urine)	벤스-존스 단백(검사/요)
	‣ 다발성 골수종(multiple myeloma): 뇨에 Bence–Jones 단백뇨가 30~50% 환자에게 발견	
BK	below knee	무릎 아래
BJM	bones, joints, muscles	뼈, 관절, 근육
BM	bone marrow	골수
	bowel movement	장운동
	basal metabolism	기초대사량
BMR	basal metabolic rate	기초대사율
BMT	bone marrow transplant	골수이식
BOW	bag of water	양수낭
BP	blood pressure	혈압
	breech presentation	둔위(볼기태위)
BPD	breech presentation delivery	둔위(볼기태위) 분만
BPH	benign prostatic hypertrophy	양성 전립선 비대증
BPLD	bilateral pelvic lymph node dissection	양측 골반림프절 절개술
BPM	beats per minute	분간 박동

약 어	원 어	해 설
BR	bed rest	안정
	bathroom	욕실
BRBPR	bright red blood through rectum = hematochezia(혈변배설)	직장에서 나온 선홍색 혈액
BS	blood sugar(laboratory/chemistry)	혈당(검사/화학)
	bowel sounds(abdomen)	장음(腸音)(복부)
	breath sounds(chest)	호흡음(흉부)
BSE	breast self examination	유방 자가검진
BSO	bilateral salpingo-oophorectomy ‣ salpingo = tubal = uterine tube = fallopian tube(자궁관) ‣ oophoro = ovary(난소)	양측 난관(자궁관)-난소절제술
BST	bedside testing	침상검사
BT	body temperature	체온
	bedtime	취침시간
	bleeding time(laboratory/coagulation) ‣ 정상: 8분 이하	출혈시간
	body temperature	체온
BUN	blood urea nitrogen(laboratory/chemistry)	혈중뇨질소(검사/화학)
BW	birth weight	출생 체중
	body weight	체중
Bx.	biopsy	생검

C

약 어	원 어	해 설
C1-7	cervical vertebrae	경 /목뼈(7개)
$\bar{c}$	with(*latin: cum*) ‣ $\bar{s}$ without ~이 없이	함께
C	centigrade	섭씨
CA	chronological age	생활연령
	cardiac arrest	심정지
Ca	calcium(laboratory/chemistry)	칼슘(검사/화학)
	carcinoma(cancer)	암
CABG	coronary artery bypass graft	관상동맥우회로 이식술
CAD	coronary artery disease	관상동맥질환
CAG	coronary angiography	관상동맥조영상
CAPD	continual ambulatory peritoneal dialysis	지속성 활동성 복막투석

약 어	원 어	해 설
caps.	capsules(medication orders/prescriptions)	캡슐제(약 지시/처방)
CBC	complete blood count(laboratory/hematology)	전혈구검사(혈액검사)
CBD	common bile duct	총담관
	closed bladder drainage	폐쇄된 방광 배액법
CBR	complete bed rest	완전한 침상안정
CBS	clear breathing sound	깨끗한 호흡음
CC	chest circumference	흉위
	chief complaint	주소
	clinical course	임상경과
	creatinine clearance	크레아티닌 제거
cc	cubic centimeter	cm^2(1/1000 liter)
c.c.	with correction(eye examination)	교정과 함께(시력검사)
CCA	common carotid artery	총경동맥
CCG	chromic catgut	크로믹 장선(흡수성 봉합사)
CCU	coronary care unit	관상동맥질환 집중치료실
CCV	critical care ventilator	중환자 인공호흡기
CEA	carcinoembryonic antigen(laboratory/chemistry)	암태아성 항원(검사/화학)
CFS	colonofiberscopy	결장경 검사
CGL	chronic granulocytic leukemia	만성 과립구성 백혈병
C.gl.	correction with galsses	안경으로 교정
CGN	chronic glomerulonephritis	만성 사구체신염
cGy	centigray(1rad-1/100 gray)	센티그레이
CHB	complete heart block(ECG)	완전 심장차단(심전도)
CHD	congenital heart disease	선천성 심장질환
	coronary heart disease	관상동맥심질환
chemo	chemotherapy	화학요법
CHF	congestive heart failure	울혈성 심부전(심장기능상실)
CHL	conductive hearing loss	전음성 난청
chol.	cholesterol(laboratory/chemistry)	콜레스테롤(검사/화학)
chr.	chronic	만성
CHR	chronic hypertrophic rhinitis	만성 비후성 비염
CI	cerebral infarction	뇌경색
CICU	coronary intensive care unit	관상동맥 중환자실
CIN	cervical intraepithelial neoplasm	자궁경부 상피내 신생물
CIS	carcinoma in situ(=CINⅢ)=M_/2	정상소재암
CK	creatine kinase(same as CPK) (laboratory/chemistry)	크레아티닌 키나제 (검사/화학)

약 어	원 어	해 설
Cl	chloride(laboratory/chemistry) ▸ 콩팥으로 배설되는 전해질	클로라이드, 염소
CLL	chronic lymphocytic leukemia	만성 림프성 백혈병
cm.	centimeter	센티미터(1m의 1/100)
c.m.	tomorrow morning(Latin: *cras mane*)	내일 아침
cm^3	cubic centimeter	큐빅 센티미터
CMF	cytoxan, methotrexate, 5-fluorouracil (cancer chemotherapy)	복합 화학요법 (암)
CMG	cystometrogram	방광내압측정법
CMML	chronic myelomacrocytic leukemia	만성 골수 대적혈구성 백혈병
CML	chronic myelogenous leukemia	만성 골수성 백혈병
CMS	chronic maxillary sinusitis	만성 상악동염
CNS	central nervous system	중추신경계 [뇌(brain)+척수(spinal cord)]
CO	carbon monoxide(laboratory/chemistry)	일산화탄소(검사/화학)
CO_2	carbon dioxide	이산화탄소
COA	coarctation of aorta	대동맥 교착증
COD	cause of death	사망원인
COM	chronic otitis media	만성 중이염
COPD	chronic obstructive pulmonary disease ▸ 기도폐쇄는 기종(emphysema), 만성기관지염과 관련	만성 폐쇄성 폐질환
CP	cerebral palsy	뇌성마비
	chronic pyelonephritis	만성 신우신염
	cor pulmonale	폐성심
	creatine phosphate(laboratory/chemistry)	크레이틴 인
	cleft palate	구개열
	clinical pathology	임상병리과
CPA	cardiopulmonary arrest	심폐정지
CPD	cephalopelvic disproportion	머리(아두)골반 불균형
CPK	creatine phosphokinase(laboratory/chemistry) ▸ 심장이나 골격근 손상의 혈류로 방출	크레아티닌 포스포키나제
CPN	chronic pyelonephritis	만성 신우신염
CPR	cardiopulmonary resuscitation ▸ 3가지 기본 단계 – 머리를 뒤로 제치고 기도를 열어 줌 – mouth to mouth breathing으로 호흡을 회복시켜 줌 – 외부에서 심장을 눌러 혈액순환을 회복시켜 줌	심폐소생술

약 어	원 어	해 설
CPS	chronic paranasal sinusitis	만성 부비동염
Cr	chromium	크롬(원소기호)
CR	complete response	전체 반응
CRF	chronic renal failure	만성 콩팥기능상실
(=ESRD)	(=end-stage renal disease, 말기신질환)	
CR c̄ IF	closed reduction with internal fixation	비관혈적 정복술
	‣ CR c̄ IF 비관혈적 정복 및 내부고정: 절개하지 않고 손으로 복원	
	‣ OR c̄ IF 관혈적 정복 및 내부고정: 골절부위의 절개	
CS	cesarean section(operation/obstetrics)	제왕절개(수술/산과)
CSF	cerebrospinal fluid	뇌척수액
CSM.	cerebrospinal meningitis	뇌척수막염
CST	convulsive shock therapy(procedure/psychiatry)	전기충격치료 (처치/정신과)
CT	computed tomography(procedure/x-ray)	컴퓨터 단층촬영술
	coagulation time(laboratory/coagulation)	응고시간
	clotting time	응고시간
CTD	carpal tunnel decompression(operation/orthopedics)	수근관감압술 (수술/정형외과)
CTS	carpal tunnel syndrome	팔목터널증후군
CUG	cystourethrogram(procedure/urology)	방광요도조영술(처치/비뇨기과)
CV	cardiovascular	심장혈관의
CVA	cerebrovascular accident(=stroke)	뇌혈관 사고, 뇌졸중
	‣ 뇌졸중의 유형: thromotic(혈전성), embolic(색전성), hemorrhagic(출혈성)	
CVAT	costovertebral angle tenderness	늑골척추각 압통
	‣ 신장에 돌과 염증이 있을 때 생길 수 있음	
CVD	cardiovascular disease	심혈관질환
CVP	central venous pressure	중심정맥압 (상대정맥의 도관으로 측정)
CVS	cardiovascular system	심혈관계
CXR	chest x-ray	흉부 방사선 사진
Cx.	cervix(gynecology)	자궁경(목): 부인과
	complication	합병증
cysto	cystoscopy	방광경 검사법

약 어	원 어	해 설

D

약 어	원 어	해 설
D1-D12 (=T1-T12)	dorsal vertebrae (=thoracic vertebrae)	흉추/등뼈(12개)
D5W	5% dextrose in water	5% 포도당 증류수
DAA	discharge against advice	자의퇴원
DAMA	dicharge against medical advice	자의퇴원
D & C	dilatation and curettage(operation/gynecology)	확장과 소파술(유산방법)
D/C	discontinue	중지
D & E	dilatation and evacuation(operation/gynecology) ‣ 유산 방법: 흡입(vacuum aspiration)에 의한 질사출법	확장과 사출(수술/부인과)
Derm.	dermatology	피부과(학)
DES	diethylstilbestrol(합성 estrogen 물질) ‣ 에스트로겐 결핍 등 폐경기 문제 치료에 사용되는 합성 에스트로겐 ‣ 만일 임신 중에 투여되면 딸에게 후속종양을 갖게 할 수 있음.	다이에틸스틸베스롤
Decub	decubitus(lying down)	욕창/누운 상태
DI	diabetes insipidus	요붕증
	diagnostic imaging	진단적 영상
DIC	disseminated intravascular coagulation	파종성 혈관내 응고
dil.	dilute	희석
DIPJ	distal interphalangeal joint	원위 손가락뼈사이 관절
DJD	degenerative joint disease	퇴행성 관절질환
dl.	deciliter	데시리터(=1/10 L)
DLE	discoid lupus erythematosus	원판상 홍반성 루푸스
DM	diabetes mellitus	당뇨병
	dermatology	피부과
DNA	deoxyribonucleic acid	디옥시라이보핵산
DOA	dead on arrival	도착시 사망
	date of admission	입원일
DOE	dyspnea of exertion	노력성 호흡곤란
DPT	diphtheria, pertussis and tetanus(vaccine)	디프테리아, 백일해, 파상풍(백신)
Dr.	doctor	의사
DR	delivery room	분만실
	diagnostic radiology	진단방사선학
DRE	digital rectal examination	직장수지검사
DRG	diagnosis related groups	진단명별 환자군

약 어	원 어	해 설
DSA	digital subtraction angiography	계수 공제 혈관조영술
	‣ 비디오와 컴퓨터를 이용하여 혈관 x-ray 촬영	
DSM Ⅲ	Diagnostic & Statistical Manual, 3rd Edition	진단적 통계용수, 3판
DT	delirium tremens	진전섬망
DTR	deep tendon reflex	심부건반사
DUB	dysfunctional uterine bleeding	기능부전성 자궁출혈
DVT	deep vein thrombosis	심부 정맥 혈전증
D.W.	distilled water	증류수
5DW	5% dextrose(in water) injection 5%	포도당 수용액 주입
Dx.	diagnosis	진단

E

약 어	원 어	해 설
é	electrolyte	전해질
	‣ 131–2.7–100 →131 나트륨(sodium)	
EAC	external auditory canal	외이관
EBL	estimated blood loss(on surgical reports)	혈액손실 추정량/수술기록
	‣ 과다출혈: 정상분만 500cc 이상, 제왕절개 1,000cc 이상	
EBV	Epstein-Barr virus	엡스타인-바르 바이러스
ECC	extracorporeal circulation	체외순환
	endocervical curettage	자궁경(목)내막 소파술
ECCE	extracapular cataract extraction(operation/ophthalmology)	낭외 백내장 적출술
	‣ 백내장(cataract) 제거 방법 – 전체 렌즈조직을 제거하나, 렌즈 capsule의 뒷부분은 자리에 남겨 놓음 ‣ ECCE+PCL(posterior chamber lens, 인공수정체 삽입술) 병행	
ECG(=EKG)	electrocardiogram(procedure/cardiology)	심전도(처치/심장과)
	esophagocologastrostomy	식도결장위 문합술
ECHO	echocardiogram(procedure/cardiology)	초음파 심장조영술
	echoencephalogram(procedure/neurology)	초음파 뇌조영술
E. coli	Escherichia coli(laboratory/bacteriology)	대장균
ECT	electroconvulsive therapy	전기경련요법
EDC	estimated date of confinement	분만 예정일
EDH	epidural hemorrhage	경막외 출혈
EEA	end to end anastomosis	문합술
EEG	electroencephalogram(procedure/neurology)	뇌전도
EENT	eyes, ears, nose, and throat	눈, 귀, 코, 목

약 어	원 어	해 설
EFW	estimated fetal weight	추정 태아 체중
e.g.	for example(*i.e.*: 즉)	예를 들어
EGC	early gastric carcinoma	조기 위암
	esophagogastrocolic anastomosis	식도, 위, 결장문합술
EGD	esophagogastroduodenoscopy	식도, 위, 십이지장경 검사법
EMG	electromyography	근전도검사
ENT	ears, nose and throat(=otorhinolaryngology)	이비인후과(학)
EOM	extraocular movement	외안구 운동
eos.	eosinophil(laboratory/hematology)	호산구(검사/혈액학)
ER	emergency room	응급실
	estrogen receptor	에스트로겐 수용체
ERCP	endoscopic retrograde cholangiopancreatogram	내시경적 역행성 담관췌장조영술
ERT	estrogen replacement therapy(ERT)	에스트로겐 대치요법
ESR	erythrocyte sedimentation rate(hematology)	적혈구 침강속도(혈액학)
ESRD	end-stage renal disease	말기신장질환(콩팥병)
(=CRF)	(=chronic renal failure, 만성신부전)	
EST	electroshock therapy(procedure/psychiatry)	정신쇼크치료(처치/정신과)
	exercise stress test	운동 스트레스 검사
ESWL	extracorporeal shock wave lithotripsy	체외 충격파 쇄석술
et al.	and others(Latin: *et allii*)	기타
ETT	exercise tolerance test	운동부하검사
EVD	external ventricular drainage	외심실 배액
EVL	esophageal varix ligation	식도정맥류 결찰술
exam.	examination	검사

F

약 어	원 어	해 설
F	Fahrenheit	화씨
FB	foreign body	이물질
	finger breadth	손가락 폭
FBS	fasting blood sugar(laboratory/chemistry)	공복 시 혈당
	‣ DM(당뇨병) 유무: glucose → 정상치: 70–120 mg/dl(공복 시 혈당)	
F. cath	Foley catheter	폴리카테터
FCU	flexor carpi ulnaris	척골수근(자뼈손목) 굴근
FDA	Food and Drug Administration	미국식품의약국
FDP	flexor digitorum profundus	심지(깊은 손가락뼈) 굴근
FDS	flexor digitorum superficialis	천지(얕은 손가락뼈) 굴근

약 어	원 어	해 설
Fe	iron(Latin: *ferrum*)	철
FFP	fresh frozen plasma	신선 냉동 혈장
FGS	fiber gastroscopy	위내시경
FH(=FHx)	family history	가족력
FHR	fetal heart rate	태아 심박수
FHS	fetal heart sound	태아 심음
FHT	fetal heart tone	태아 심음
FSH	follicle-stimulating hormone(endocrinology) **‣ 난소자극: 뇌하수체 전엽 → 내분비 장기**	난포자극호르몬/내분비계
FT	full-term(obstetrics)	만기(산과)
FTPC	frontotemporo-parietal craniectomy	전두측두두정(이마관자마루뼈) 두개절제술
FTSG	full thickness skin graft	전층 피부이식
5-FU	5-fluorouracil(cancer chemotherapy)	화학요법(암)
f/u	follow-up	추적조사
FUO	fever of unknown origin	원인불명의 열
FVC	forced vital capacity(PFT)	노력성폐활량(폐기능검사)
Fx.	fracture	골절

G

약 어	원 어	해 설
G	gravida(pregnant)	임부
g	gram	그램
GA	general anesthesia	전신마취
	general appearance	전신외관
	gestational age	임신기간
	gross anormaly	육안이상
	gastric analysis(procedure/gastroenterology)	위액분석
Ga	gallium	갈륨(원소기호)
Garg	gargle	양치질
GB	gallbladder(=cholecyto)	담낭
GCS	Glasgow Coma Scale	글래스고우 무의식척도
GD	general diet	일반식
GDH	gonadotropic hormone	성선자극호르몬
GEA	general endotracheal(intubation) anesthesia	기관내삽관 전신마취
GE	gastroenterostomy(operation/stomach)	위장 문합술
	gastroesophageal	위 식도의

약 어	원 어	해 설
G-F	grossly free (= free = intact = N-S = WNL = N-C)	육안으로 이상 없음
GFS	gastrofiberscopy	위내시경
GH	growth hormone(=somatotropin)	성장호르몬(뇌하수체전엽/내분비계)
GI	gastrointestinal	위장의
GM	glioblastoma multiforme ‣ 악성종양: 원발장기(brain)	다형성 교모세포증
	gastric mucosa	위점막
Gm-	gram stain negative(on bacteriology reports)	음성그람균(박테리아기록지)
Gm+	gram stain positive(on bacteriology reports)	양성그람균(박테리아기록지)
GN	glomerulonephritis	사구체신염
GO	gas out: GO (+)	가스배출
grav	gravida(pregnancy)	임부
GS	general surgery	일반외과
gtts	drops	점적제
GTT	glucose tolerance test ‣ 당뇨병(DM): 다른 날짜에 측정 시(2번) 진단된 경우 ·75g의 포도당(glucose) 이용한 경구 당부하검사 ① 공복 시(8시간 이상 열량섭취 없는 상태에서 측정한 혈당) → 126 mg/dl 이상 ② 2시간째 혈당검사 → 200 mg/dl 이상	포도당부하시험(당뇨병검사)
	gestational trophoblastic neoplasm	임신성 영양배엽 신생물
GU	genitourinary	생식비뇨기의
G.W.	general ward	일반병동
Gyn.	gynecology	부인과

H

약 어	원 어	해 설
h	hour	시간
HA	hospital admission	입원
	hemolytic anemia	용혈성 빈혈
HAV	hepatitis A virus	A형 간염 바이러스
Hb.(Hgb.)	hemoglobin(hematology)[빈혈유무] ‣ 정상수치: (남) 13.0~17.0 g/dL (여) 12.0~16.0 g/dL	헤모글로빈(혈색소/혈액학)
HBAg	hepatitis B antigen(laboratory/virology)	B형 간염 항원(바이러스)
HBP	high blood pressure	고혈압
HBV	hepatitis B virus	B형 간염 바이러스
HC	head circumference	두위(머리둘레)
HCC	hepatocellular carcinoma	간세포성 암종

약 어	원 어	해 설
HCG	human chorionic gonadotropin	융모성 성선자극호르몬/임신검사
HCO3	bicarbonate	중탄산염
	‣ 신장(콩팥)에 의해 보존되는 전해질	
Hct.	hematocrit(laboratory/hematology)	적혈구 용적(검사/혈액학)
HCV	hepatitis C virus	C형 간염 바이러스
HCVD	hypertensive cardiovascular disease	고혈압성 심혈관질환
HD	hemodialysis	혈액투석
	Hodgkin's disease	호지킨스병
HDL	high density lipoproteins(laboratory/chemistry)	고밀도지단백질(검사/화학)
	‣ 혈중에 HDL이 높으면 관상동맥질환 발생률이 낮음	
HEENT	head, eyes, ears, nose, throat	머리, 눈, 귀, 코, 목
Hg.	mercury(Latin: *hydrargyrun*)	수은
HGH	human growth hormone	인간 성장 호르몬
HiBP, HTN	high blood pressure(hypertension)	고혈압
HID, HIVD	herniated intervertebral disc	추간판 탈출
HIV	human immunodeficiency virus	인체면역결핍바이러스 (AIDS의 원인이 되는 바이러스)
HL	hearing loss	난청, 귀머거리
HLD	herniated lumbar disc	추간판 탈출
HM	hypermetropia manifast	발현성 원시(=hyperopia)
	hydatidiform mole(=H-mole)	포상기태
	‣ 양성종양(H-mole, 포상기태) → 악성종양(choriocarcinoma, 융모상피암종) ‣ 원발장기: placenta(태반)	
HMD	hyaline membrane disease	초자막질환
H & N	head and neck	머리 및 목
HNP	herniated nucleus pulposus	수핵탈출증
H_2O	water	수분
HOF	height of fundus	(자궁)저부 높이
HPV	human papilloma virus	인유두종 바이러스
hr.	hour	시간
HR	heart rate	심장박동률
h.s.	hora somni(=at bed time)	취침 시에
	‣ tapering: 약물복용을 점차 줄여 나가는 것	
H/S	Hartman's solution	하트만 용액/의사지시기록
	‣ 1 L = 1,000cc	
HSG	hysterosalpingogram	자궁난관(자궁관)조영술
HSO	half stitch out	반봉합 해체

약 어	원 어	해 설
HSV	herpes simplex virus	단순포진 바이러스
Ht.	height	신장(콩팥)
HTN	hypertension	고혈압
Hx.	history	병력
hypo.	hypodermic injection	피하주사

I

약 어	원 어	해 설
131I	radioactive iodine(nuclear medicine)	방사선 요오드
	‣ 갑상선의 방사선 물질 섭취여부와 간, 신장스캔과 갑상선의 악양성 종양 치료에 사용	
IADH	inappropriate antidiuretic hormone	항이뇨호르몬의 부적합분비
IADHS	inappropriate antidiuretic hormone syndrome	항이뇨호르몬의 부적합분비증후군
IBD	inflammatory bowel disease	염증성 장질환
ICC	intensive coronary care	집중 관상동맥 진료
ICCE	intracapsular cataract extraction(operation/ophthalmology)	낭내 백내장 적출술
	‣ 백내장 제거 방법: 주머니, 낭(capsule)을 포함하여 전체 렌즈를 제거	
ICH	intracerebral hemorrhage	뇌내 출혈
ICP	intracranial pressure	두개내압
ICS	intercostal space	늑간강
	irritable colon syndrome	과민성 대장증후군
ICSH	interstitial cell-stimulating hormone(laboratory/endocrinology)	간질세포자극호르몬
ICU	intensive care unit	중환자실
I & D	incision and drainage(operation/skin)	절개와 배액
IDA	iron deficiency anemia	철결핍성 빈혈
IDDM	insulin dependent diabetes mellitus(Type I)	인슐린의존성 당뇨병(I형/연소성)
Ig	Immunoglobulin(laboratory/serology)	면역글로블린
	‣ 5가지 유형: IgA, IgD, IgE, IgG, IgM	
IHSS	idiopathic hypertrophic subaortic stenosis	특발성 비후성 대동맥판하 협착
IIOC	incompetent internal os of cervix	자궁경(목)관 무력증
IM	internal medicine	내과
	intramuscular(injection site)	근육내의(주사 부위)
Imp.	impression	의증
	‣ Rule out(R/O)=suspect 의증	
IMV	inferior mesenteric vein	하부 장간막(창자사이막) 정맥
	intermittent mechanical ventilation	간헐적 기계 환기
INA	intranasal antrotomy	비내 상악동 절개
INE	intranasal ethmoidectomy	비내 사골(벌집뼈)절제

약 어	원 어	해 설
Inj	injection	주사
IO	internal os(cervix)	내경구(자궁경부/목)
	intraocular	안(眼)구내의
I & O	intake and output	섭취량 및 배설량
IOL	intraocular lens(implantation)	내안 렌즈(이식)
IOP	intraocular pressure	안압
IPH	intraperitoneal hypothermochemotherapy	복막내 저온열화학요법
IPPB	intermittent positive pressure breathing	간헐적 양압 호흡
I.Q.	intelligence quotient	지능지수
	▸ 평균: 90~100, 정신지체: 70 이하	
IUD	intrauterine device(=contraceptive)	자궁내 기구(피임기구)
	intrauterine death	자궁내 사망
IUP	intrauterine pregnancy	자궁내 임신
IUFD	intrauterine fetal death	자궁내 태아사망
IUP	intrauterine pregnancy	자궁내 임신(정상임신)
	▸ 자궁관임신(tubal pregnancy) = 자궁외 임신(ectopic pregnancy) = 유산	
IV	intravenous	정맥내의
	intravascular	혈관내의
IVC	inferior vena cava	하대정맥
	intravenous cholangiogram(x-ray/gallbladder)	정맥내 담낭조영술
IVD	intervertebral disc	추간원판
IVF	in vitro fertilization	시험관내 수정
IVH	intraventricular hemorrhage	심실내 출혈
IVP	intravenous pyelogram(x-ray/kidneys)	정맥내 콩팥깔때기 조영술 (x-ray/콩팥)

K

약 어	원 어	해 설
K	potassium(laboratory/chemistry)	칼륨, 포타슘(전해질의 종류)
kg.	kilogram	킬로그램(=1,000g)
KJ	knee jerk(neurologic examination)	무릎반사(신경과 검진)
KS	Kaposi's sarcoma	카포시육종
KUB	kidney, ureter and bladder(x-ray/urology)	신장(콩팥), 요관, 방광
	▸ 조영제 없는 x-선 촬영	(x-ray 검사/비뇨기과)

약 어	원 어	해 설
L		
L1-L5	lumbar vertebrae	요추/허리뼈(5개)
LA	light accommodation	빛 조절
	left atrium	좌심방
L/A	local anesthesia	국소마취
lab.	laboratory	검사실
LAT	lateral	측면
LAUP	laser assistant uvuloplasty	레이저 구개수 성형술
LBBB	left bundle branch block(ECG)	좌각 차단(심전도)
LBP	low blood pressure	저혈압
L/C	liver cirrhosis	간경변
LD	lethal dose	치사량
	liquid diet	유동식
LD_{50}	median lethal dose	50%의 치사량
LDH	lactic dehydrogenase	유산탈수소 효소
LDL	low-density lipoproteins(laboratory/chemistry)	저밀도지단백
LE	Lower extremity	다리뼈
	lupus erythematosus	홍반성 낭창(루프스)
LE cell	lupus erythematosus cell	홍반성 낭창(루프스) 세포
LFT	liver function test	간기능검사
	‣ **간기능검사의 종류: ALK, bilirubin, ASR(SGOT), ALT(SGPT)**	
LFT c/s	low flap transverse cesarean section	저피판 횡의 제왕절개
LGA	large for gestational age	임신기간에 비하여 과다체중아
LH	lutenizing hormone/endocrine gland ‣ **난소자극 및 배란(뇌하수체 전엽)**	황체형성호르몬/내분비계
LIH	left inguinal hernia	좌서혜(샅)부 탈장
LLL	left lower lobe(lung) ‣ **폐: RUL(우상엽), RLL(우하엽), LUL(좌상엽), LLL(좌하엽)**	좌하엽(폐)
LLQ	left lower quadrant	왼쪽 하부 1/4
LLSB	left lower sternal border	흉골(복장뼈) 하부 가장자리
LMCL	left midclavicular line	좌중간 쇄골선
LML	left medial lateral(episiotomy)	좌측 안쪽의(회음절개술)
LMP	last menstrual period	최종월경주기
LN	lymph nodes	림프절
LOC	loss of consciousness	의식상실
LOM	limitation of motion	운동 제한
LOS	length of stay(단입법 계산: 퇴원일-입원일)	재원일수

약 어	원 어	해 설
Lot	lotion	로션
LOT	left occiput transverse(position of fetus)	좌후두 횡위(태아위치)
LP	lumbar puncture	요추(허리뼈)천자
LROM	limited range of motion	운동범위 제한
LRT	lower respiratory tract	하호흡기
LS	lumbosacral	요천골(허리엉치뼈)의
LSK	liver, spleen, kidney	간, 비장(지라), 신장(콩팥)
LSO	left salpingo-oophorectomy(operation/gynecology)	좌측 난관(자궁관)-난소절제술
LUL	left upper lobe(lung)	좌상엽(폐)
LUQ	left upper quadrant	왼쪽 상부 1/4
LV	left ventricle	좌심실
LVH	left ventricular hypertrophy	좌심실비대
lymphs	lymphocytes	림프구

M

약 어	원 어	해 설
M	male	남 성
ⓜ	murmur	잡음(심장)
M.A.	mental age	정신연령(심리검사)
MAO	monoamine oxidase	모노아민 산화효소
max.	maximum	최대
mcg.	microgram(ug)	마이크로그램(10^{-6}g)
MCH	mean corpuscular hemoglobin	평균 적혈구 색소량
mCi	millicurie	밀리퀴리(방사선 측정 단위)
MCL	modified chest lead(ECG)	변형 흉부유도(심전도)
	medial collateral ligament	내측부 인대(무릎)
	midclavicular line	중쇄골선
MCLNS	mucocutaneous lymph node syndrome	피부점막 림프절 증후군
MCV	mean corpuscular volume ‣ MCV가 높으면 세포는 macrocytic(대구성) ‣ MCV가 낮으면 microcytic(소구성)	평균 적혈구 용적
MD	mid-day	정오
M/D	moderate development	발육 적절
M/D/N	moderate development nurishment	발육 및 영양상태 적절
Mg	magnesium	마그네슘
mg	microgram	마이크로그램
MI	myocardial infarction	심근경색

약 어	원 어	해 설
	mitral insufficiency(incompetence)	승모판부전증
MICU	medical intensive care unit	내과계 집중치료실
MIH	multiple internal hemorrhoid	다발성 내치질
ml.	milliliter	밀리리터(10^{-3} L)
mm^3	cubic millimeter	입방 밀리미터
MM	multiple myeloma	다발성골수종
	[=plasma cell myeloma: 형질세포골수종 → 원발장기: 골수(bone marrow)]	
MMPI	Minnesota Multiphasic Personality Inventory (psychological test)	미네소타 다면적 성격검사
MN	midnight	자정
M/N	moderate nutrition	영양상태 적절
Mn.	manganese(laboratory/chemistry)	망간
mo.	month	월(月)
mono	monocyte	단구(백혈구)
MOPP	mechlorethamine, oncovin, procarbazine and prednisone (cancer chemotherapy)	화학요법(암)
MP	metacarpal phalangeal(joint)	중수지절의(관절)
	metatarsal phalangeal(joint)	중족지절의(관절)
MR	mitral regurgitation	승모판 역류
	mental retardation(mentally retarded)	정신지체
MRF	mitral regurgitant flow	승모판 역류성 유량
MRI	magnetic resonance imaging	자기공명영상
MRM	modified radical mastectomy	변형근치유방절제술
MS	mental status	정신상태
	‣ G/A: alert MS → 전신외관: 명료한 정신상태	
	mitral stenosis	승모판협착증
	multiple sclerosis	다발성 경화증
MSH	melanocyte-stimulating hormone	멜라닌세포자극호르몬
	‣ 피부색소증가(과잉분비): 뇌하수체 전엽 → 내분비계	
MTD	right ear drum	오른쪽 고막
MVP	mitral valve prolapse(syndrome)	승모판 탈출증
MVR	mitral valve replacement(operation/cardiac)	승모판 대치(수술/심장)

약 어	원 어	해 설
N		
Na	sodium(laboratory/chemistry)	나트륨, 소디움: 전해질
N&	normal and active	정상활동
NABS	normoactive bowel sounds	정상활동성 장음
NaCl	sodium chloride(intravenous solution)	염화나트륨(정맥내 용액)
NB	newborn	신생아
	neurogenic bladder	신경원성 방광
NBS	normal breathing sound	정상 호흡음
NC	no complaints	불평없음
NCP	normocephaly	정상두부
NCU	neurological care unit	신경외과 중환자실
NCV	nerve conduction velocity	신경전도속도
N/E	neurological examination	신경계 검사
NEC	not elsewhere classified	달리 분류되지 않음
NED	no evidence of disease	질병의 증거가 없음
NFD	normal forcep delivery	정상 겸자분만
ng.	nanogram(=millimicrogram)	나노그램(10^{-9}g)
NG tube	nasogastric tube	비위튜브
NGU	nongonococcal urethritis	비임균성 요도염
NH_3	ammonia	암모니아
NHL	non-Hodgkin's lymphoma	비호지킨 림프종
NICU	neonatal intensive care unit	신생아 중환자실
NIDDM	non-insulin-dependent diabetes mellitus(Type II)	비인슐린 의존성 당뇨병(II형, 성인)
NM	nuclear medicine	핵의학과
no.	number(#)	번호
NOS	not otherwise specified	상세불명(달리 명시되지 않음)
NP	neuropsychiatric	신경정신과
NPD	no pathological diagnosis	병리학적 진단없음
NPO	nothing by mouth(Latin: *non per os*)	금식
NR	neonate room	신생아실
NS	nervous system	신경계
	neurosurgery	신경외과
N/S	normal saline	생리식염수
NSAID	non-steroidal anti-infammatory drug	비스테로이성 항염증성 약물
NSFTD	normal spontaneous full-term delivery ‣ 정상: 임신기간 37~42주 미만, 신생아 체중 2.5~4.5kg 미만	정상만기의 자연분만

약 어	원 어	해 설
NST	non-stress test(fetal monitoring)	비부하 검사(태아감시)
NSVD	normal spontaneous vaginal delivery	정상 자연 질분만
N/V/D	nausea, vomiting and diarrhea	오심, 구토 및 설사

O

약 어	원 어	해 설
O_2	oxygen	산소
OB	obstetrics	산과
	occult blood	잠혈
OB & GY	obstetrics and gynecology	산부인과
OBS	organic brain syndrome/dementia	기질성 뇌증후군(치매)
OCP	oral contraceptive pills	경구 피임제
OD	right eye(Latin: oculus dexter)	오른쪽 눈
	‣ OS(oculus sinister, 왼쪽 눈), OU(oculus uterque, 양안)	
	once daily	1일 1회
	on duty	근무일
oint.	ointment(medication orders/prescriptions)	연고(약지시/처방)
o.m.	every morning(Latin: omni mane)	매일 아침
OME	otitis media with effusion	삼출성 중이염
OMPA	otitis media purulent acute	급성 화농성 중이염
op.	operation	수술
OPD	out-patient department	외래
	‣ IPD(inpatient departmet): 입원	
OR	operating room	수술실
OR $\bar{c}$ EF	open reduction and external fixation	관혈적 정복 및 외부고정
OR $\bar{c}$ IF	open reduction and internal fixation	관혈적 정복 및 내부고정
	‣ 골절부위를 절개(incision), 나사(screw), 핀(pin), 못(nail)으로 고정	
os	by mouth	구강
	left eye(Latin: *oculus sinister*)	왼쪽 눈
	‣ OD: 오른쪽 눈, OU: 양쪽 눈	
OS	orthopedic surgery	정형외과
OSAS	obstructive sleep apnea syndrome	폐쇄성 수면성 무호흡증후군
OT	occupational therapy	작업치료
OU	both eyes(Latin: *oculus uterque*)	양쪽 눈
oz	ounce	온스

약 어	원 어	해 설

P

약 어	원 어	해 설
P	pulse	맥박
	phosphorus	인
PA	posterior-anterior(chest x-ray)	후전방의(흉부 x-ray)
	pathology	병리학
PAC	premature atrial contracton	조기 심방수축
$PaCO_2$	arterial carbon dioxide tension	동맥 이산화탄소 분압
PaO_2	arterial oxygen pressure tension	동맥혈 산소분압
Pap. smear (test)	Papanicolaou smear(procedure/gynecology) ‣ 자궁경부 또는 질의 암검사(처치/부인과)	파파니콜라우 도말검사
para 2-0-1-2	woman's reproductive history ‣ 예) 2–0–1–2 → 2: 분만(2번), 조산(없음), 유산(1번), 생존아(2명) 임신력(3번)=유산(1번)+생존아(2명)	출산력
PAS	pulmonary artery stenosis	폐동맥협착증
Path.	pathology	병리학
Pb	lead(Latin: *plumbum*)	납
PBI	protein-bound iodine	단백-결합성 요오드
p.c.	after meals(Latin: post cibum)	식후에
PCA	posterior cerebral artery	후방 대뇌 동맥
PCDS	para cul-de-sac	막힌 주머니 주위
PCG	phonocardiogram	심음도
PCL	posterior cruciate ligament of knee	무릎의 후방십자 인대
	posterior chamber lens(implantation)	수정체 후방 이식술
PCM	plasma cell myeloma(bone marrow) (=multiple myeloma: 다발성 골수종)	형질세포골수종(골수)
PCN	penicillin(medication order)	페니실린(약지시)
PCNA	percutaneous needle aspiration	경피적 침흡인
PCP	pneumocystis carinii pneumonia	AIDS 환자의 폐렴유형 (에이즈 관련성 기회감염)
p/d	packs per day(cigarettes)	1일 흡연량
PDA	patent ductus arteriosus	동맥관 개방
PDR	physician's desk reference	약물목록집
PE	physical examination	신체검진
PED	pediatric	소아과
PEEP	positive end-expiratory pressure	호기종말 양압(호흡치료)

약 어	원 어	해 설
per	by, for each	-에, 의해
PET	positron emission tomography	양전자 방출 단층촬영술
PFO	patent foramen ovale	난원공 개방
PFT	pulmonary function test	폐기능검사
PGE_2	prostaglandin E_2	자궁수축제
	‣ 유도분만을 위해 1회 1정 복용	
PH	past history	과거력
(=PHx)	personal history	개인력
pH	symbol for degree of acid or alkalinity	산성, 알칼리성의 정도 (수소이온농도지수)
phos.	phosphorus(laboratory/chemistry)	인
PI	present illness	현재 질병상태
PID	pelvic inflammatory disease	골반내 염증성 질환
PIH	pregnancy induced hypertension	임신성 고혈압
pil.	pill	환제
PKU	phenylketonuria	페닐케톤뇨증
PLR	prompt light reflex	눈이 신속하게 반응
	‣ pupil isocoria c̄ PLR(+/+): 동공의 크기가 같고 눈이 신속하게 반응	
PLT	platelet (laboratory/hematology)	혈소판(검사/혈액학)
	‣ 정상치: 15만~40만/mm^3	
	‣ 혈액: 구성요소(적혈구, 백혈구, 혈소판)+혈장(plasma: 비타민, 호르몬, 단백질 등)	
PM	after noon(Latin: post meridian)	오후
PMH(=PH)	past medical history	과거력
PMN	polymorphonuclear leukocyte	다형핵백혈구
PMP	past menstrual period	전 월경기
PMS	premenstrual syndrome	월경전 증후군
PND	paroxysmal(sudden) nocturnal dyspnea	발작성 야간 호흡곤란 (울혈성 심부전의 증상)
PNET	primitive neuroectodermal tumor	원시성 신경외배엽 종양
PNS	peripheral nervous system	말초신경계
	‣ 뇌신경(cranial nerve) 12쌍+척수신경(spinal nerve) 31쌍 = 말초신경	
	parasympathetic nervous system	부교감신경계
P/O	phone order	전화지시
p.o.	by mouth(Latin: *per os*)	경구로
PO_2	oxygen partial pressure	동맥혈 산소분압
POD	postoperative day	수술 후
poly	polymorphonuclear leukocyte	다형핵 백혈구

약 어	원 어	해 설
PORP	partial ossicular replacement prosthesis	부분소골대치 인공삽입물
Powd.	powder	가루약, 산제
PP	postpartum	분만 후
	postprandial	식후의
	presenting part	현위
PPD	purified protein derivative(procedure/tuberculin skin test)	정제단백질유도체(결핵검사)
PR	pulse rate	맥박수
	‣ 정상 맥박: 1분에 60~80회	
	‣ 빈맥(tachycardia): 1분에 100회 이상, 서맥(bradycardia): 1분에 60회 미만	
	partial responses	부분적 반응
P.R.	per rectal	경직장
PRBC	packed red blood cells(blood transfusion)	농축적혈구(수혈)
PRC	plasma renin concentration	혈장 레닌 농도
PRCA	pure red cell aplasia	적혈구계 무형성증
preg.	pregnant	임신한
preop.	preoperative	수술 전
prep.	prepare for surgery	수술준비
primip	primipara: primiparous	초산부: 초산의
PRL	prolactin	프로락틴
	‣ 모유분비 자극: 뇌하수체 전엽 → 내분비계	
p.r.n.	as occasion requires(Latin: pro re nata)(medication order)	필요한 경우
prof.	profession	직업의
PROM	premature rupture of membranes	양막 조기파열
prot.	protocol	원부
PS	plastic surgery	성형외과
	pulmonary artery stenosis	폐동맥협착
PSA	prostate-specific antigen	전립선(샘) 특이 항원
PSGN	poststreptococcal glomerulonephritis	사슬알균 후 사구체신염
PSVT	paroxysmal supraventricular tachycardia	발작성 심실상 빈맥
pt.	patient	환자
	pint	파인트
PT	parathyroid	부갑상선
	paroxysmal tachycardia	발작적 빈맥
	physical therapy	물리치료
	prothrombin time(laboratory/coagulation)	프로트롬빈시간
	‣ 정상치: 12~15 sec, 70% 이상	

약 어	원 어	해 설
PTA	prior to admission(arrival)	입원 전
	pure tone audiometry	순음 청력검사
PTBD	percutaneous transhepatic biliary drainage	경피경간 담즙배액법
PTCA	percutaneous transluminal coronary angioplasty	경피적 경혈관 관상동맥 확장술
PTC	percutaneous transhepatic cholangiography	경피경간 담관조영술
PTCD	percutaneous transhepatic cholangiographic drainage	경피경간 담관조영배액법
PTH	parathyroid hormone	부갑상선 호르몬
PTT	partial thromboplastin time(laboratory/coagulation) ‣ 정상치: 27~43 sec	부분트롬보플래스틴시간
PU	pulmonary medicine	호흡기 내과
PUD	peptic ulcer disease	소화성 궤양 질환
pulv.	powder	분제, 가루약
PUVA	psoralen-ultraviolet-light(treatment)	소랄렌-자외선-광선(치료)
PVB	premature ventricular beat	심실성 조기수축
PVC	premature ventricular contraction	심실성 조기수축
PVM	paravertebral muscle	척추 방외근후

Q

약 어	원 어	해 설
Q(q)	every	매
qam	every morning	매일 아침
q.d.	every day(Latin: quaque die)	매일
q.h.	every hour	매시간
q.2h	every two hour	매 2시간마다
q.h.s.	at bedtime	취침 시
q.i.d.	four times a day(Latin: quater in die)	1일 4회
q.n.	every night	매일 밤
q.n.s.	quantity not sufficient	충분하지 않은 양
q.o.d.	every other day	2일 1회, 격일로
q.o.h.	every other hour	격일 시간
q.p.m.	every evening	매일 저녁
q.q.h.	every four hours	매 4시간마다
q.s.	sufficient quantity	적량
QSE	quadriceps setting exercise	사두정착운동

약 어	원 어	해 설

R

약 어	원 어	해 설
ⓡ	rales	수포음
r	roentgen(x-ray/measurement)	뢴트겐
R	respiration	호흡
R-	Rinne's test negative(hearing test)	린네 시험음성(청력검사)
R+	Rinne's test positive(hearing test)	린네 시험양성(청력검사)
RA	right atrium	우심방
	rheumatoid arthritis	류마티스 관절염
Ra	radium(nuclear medicine)	라듐(핵의학)
rad	radiation absorbed dose	방사선 흡수선량
RA factor	rheumatoid arthritis factor(laboratory/serology)	류마티스 관절염 인자
RAH	radical abdominal hysterectomy	근치 복식 자궁절제술
RBBB	right bundle branch block(ECG)	우각 각 차단(심전도)
RBC	red blood cells(laboratory/hematology)	적혈구(검사/혈액학)
	‣ 정상수치: (남) 20만~630만/mm^3, (여) 400만~540만/mm^3	
RCA	right coronary artery	우관상 동맥
RCU	respiratory care unit	호흡기 집중 치료실
RD	regular diet	정상 식이
RDS	respiratory distress syndrome	호흡장애증후군
	(=hyaline membrane disease, HMD)	(=초자막질환)
	‣ 폐가 정상적으로 확장하는 데 필요한 계면활성제(surfactant)가 없어 생기는 신생아질환 → 호흡곤란과 청색증	
Rec	Recommendation	권고
recur.	recurrence	재발
RF	rheumatoid factor	류마티스 인자
RGP	retrograde pyelogram	역행성 신우(콩팥깔대기) 조영술
RH	radial hemolysis	요골(노뼈) 출혈
Rh+	Rhesus positive(blood)(laboratory/blood bank)	Rh 양성(검사/혈액은행)
Rh-	Rhesus negative(blood)(laboratory/blood bank)	Rh 음성(검사/혈액은행)
RHB	regular heart beat	정상 심박동
RHD	rheumatic heart disease	류마티스 심장질환
Rh factor	Rhesus factor(laboratory/blood bank)	Rh 인자(검사/혈액은행)
	‣ Rh+인 사람의 적혈구에 정상적으로 나타나는 항원(antigen)	
RIA	radioimmunoassay (laboratory method)	방사선면역측정법
RIH	right inguinal hernia	오른쪽 서혜(샅) 탈장

약 어	원 어	해 설
RIND	reversible ischemic neurological deficit	가역성 허혈성 신경학적 결손
R→L	right to left	오른쪽에서 왼쪽으로
RLL	right lower lobe(lung)	우하엽
RLQ	right lower quadrant	우하복부 1/4
RML	right mediolateral(episiotomy)	우측 중외측의(회음절개술)
	right middle lobe(lung)	우중엽(폐)
RN	registered nurse	등록(면허) 간호사
RNA	ribonucleic acid	리보 핵산
RO	routine order	일상적 기본지시
R/O	rule out	의증
ROM	range of motion	운동범위
	rupture of membranes(obstetrics)	양막 파열(산과)
ROS	review of system[=SR(systems review)]	계통별 문진 소견
RPR	rapid plasma reagin(test for syphilis)	급속 혈장(매독검사) (=VDRL)
RR	recovery room	회복실
	respiratory rate	호흡률
RSO	right salpingo-oophorectomy(operation/gynecology)	우측 자궁관-난소절제술
RSR	regular sinus rhythm(heart)	정상 동(굴)리듬(심장)
RT	radiation therapy	방사선요법
	renal transplant	신장이식
	rebound tenderness	반사통
rt.	right	오른쪽
RTC	return to clinic	진료소 회송
RTO	return to office	사무실로 돌아감
RU	residual urine	잔여뇨
RUL	right upper lobe(lung)	우상엽 1/4(폐)
RUQ	right upper quadrant	우상 1/4
RV	right ventricle	우심실
Rx	take(prescription)	처방전

S

약 어	원 어	해 설
SB	serum bilirubin	혈청 빌리루빈
	small bowel	소장(작은 창자)
S1-S5	sacral vertebrae	천추(엉치뼈): 5개
$\bar{s}$	without(Latin: sine)	없이

약 어	원 어	해 설
S/A	same as	~와 같은
SA, S-A	sinoatrial(node)	동방결절
	‣ 심장의 박동이 처음 발생하는 위치/pacemaker 삽입 부위	
SAA	same as above	상동
SAD	seasonal affective disorder	계절성 감정장애
SAH	subarachnoid hemorrhage	거미막하(밑) 출혈
sal.	saline	식염수
SAS	sleep apnea syndrome	수면무호흡증후군
SBE	subacute bacterial endocarditis	아급성 세균성 심내막염
SBP	systolic blood pressure	수축기 혈압
SBS	smooth breathing sound	원활한 호흡음
sc.	subcutaneous(injection site)	피하주사
	without correction(eye examination)	교정없이(시력검사)
SCC	squamous cell carcinoma(=sq. cell ca.)	편평세포암종
SCU	surgical care unit	외과계 중환자실
SD	soft diet	연식
SDH	subdural hematoma	경막하(밑) 혈종
sed. rate (S.R.)	erythrocyte sedimentation rate	적혈구 침강속도
S-F position	semi-Fowler's position	반좌위 자세
SG	specific gravity	비중
SGA	small for gestational age	과소체중아
S.gl.	without correction(without glasses)	교정 없이(안경 없이)
SGOT	serum glutamic oxaloacetic transaminase (laboratory/chemistry)	간기능 효소검사
SGPT	serum glutamic pyruvic transaminase	간기능 효소검사
SH	social history	사회력
	somatotrophic(growth) hormone	성장호르몬/뇌하수체전엽
	serum hepatitis	혈청 간염
Si	silicon	실리콘, 규소
SIADH	syndrome of inappropriate secretion of antidiuretic hormone	항이뇨호르몬 부적합 분비증후군
	‣ 항이뇨호르몬(ADH)의 과잉분비: 뇌하수체 후엽	
sig.	let it be labeled	용법
S.L.	sublingual	설하/혀밑
	‣ salivary glands(타액선/침샘) – sublingual gland(설하선/혀밑샘) – parotid gland(이하선/귀밑샘) – submandibular gland(악하선/턱밑샘)	

약 어	원 어	해 설
SLE	systemic lupus erythematosus	전신성 홍반성 루프스
SLR	straight leg rasing	직하지 거상
SO	salpingo-oophorectomy(operation/gynecology) • 난관/자궁관(salpingo=tubal=uterine tube=fallopian tube), 난소(ovary=oophoro) • 질(vagina=colpo), 자궁(uterus=metro=hystero), 자궁경부(trachelo=cervix), 외음(episio=vulva)	자궁관-난소절제술(수술/부인과)
SO_4	sulfate	황산
SOAP	subjective, objective, assessment, plan (problem-oriented medical records) • 경과기록, 퇴원요약, 협의진단기록 – subjective information, S 주관적 정보(=C.C 주소): 환자 또는 가족이 제공 예) 증상, 병력 등 – headache(두통), abdominal pain(복통) – objective information, O 객관적 정보: 신체검진, 임상검사 예) CT, MRI, 초음파, 위내시경 – assessment, A 평가: S, O의 정보에서 진단 – 질병분류함 예) GFS(위내시경)상 stomach cancer(위암) C16.9 – plan, P 계획: 진단 및 치료 계획 예) chemotherapy(화학요법), RT(방사선 요법)	주관적, 객관적, 평가, 계획 (문제지향식 의무기록)
SOB	shortness of breath	숨이 참
	stool occult blood	대변 잠혈
sol	solution	용액
sos	one dose if necessary(Latin: *si opus sit*) (medication order)	필요시 한 번 용량
SOW	sips of water	물 한 모금
S/P	status post(no change-as before)	지속상태 후
sp.gr.	specific gravity(urine)	비중
SPECT	single-photon emission computed tomography	단일 광전자방출 전산화 단층촬영술
SPRM	spontaneous premature rupture of membrane	자연적 조기 양막 파열
SQ	subcutaneous(injection site)	피하의(주사부위)
SR	systems review(patient's history)	각계조사(환자병력)
	sedimentation rate	침강률
SSA	side-to-side anastomosis	측과 측 문합술
ss	one-half(Latin: semissen)	1/2, 절반(약 지시/처방)
SSE	saline solution enema	식염수 관장
	soap solution enema	비눗물 관장
	soapsuds enema	비누액 관장
ST	slight trace	극미량
Staph.	staphylococcus(laboratory/bacteriology)	포도구균(알균): 검사/세균학

약 어	원 어	해 설
STD	sexually transmitted disease	성병(=VDRL)
STS	split thickness skin graft(operation/plastic surgery)	중간층 피부이식 (수술/성형외과)
stat.	immediately	즉시
Strep.	streptococcus(laboratory/bacteriology)	연쇄상구균(사슬알균/검사/세균학)
S.T.S.	serological test for syphilis	매독 혈청검사
SUN	serum urea nitrogen(laboratory/chemistry)	혈청요질산(검사/화학)
Supp	suppository	좌약
SVC	superior vena cava	상대정맥
SVD	spontaneous vaginal delivery	자연 질분만
Sx.	symptoms	증상
S & W Enema	soap and water enema(procedure/enema)	비누물 관장
syr.	syrup	시럽

T

약 어	원 어	해 설
T1-T12	thoracic vertebrae	흉추/등뼈(12개)
T_3	triiodothyronine(laboratory/endocrinology)	삼요도타이로닌(검사/내분비학)
T_4	thyroxine(=tetraiodothyronine)	티록신(=사요드타이로닌)
T8	T cell lymphocyte(cytoxic or killer cell)	T세포림프구(세포독성, 살세포)
T	temperature(on temperature charts)	체온(T.P.R.)
	tenderness	압통
TA	traffic accident	교통사고
T&A	tonsillectomy and adenoidectomy (operation/nose and throat)	편도절제술과 아데노이드 절제술(수술/코 및 목)
tab.	tablet(medication orders/prescriptions)	정제
TAH	total abdominal hysterectomy(operation/gynecology) ‣ 복부절개 → 전체 자궁[fundus(저)+corpus(자궁체)+cervix(자궁경부)] 제거 수술	전체복부 자궁절제술
TAT	toxin-antitoxin	독소 항독소
TB	tuberculosis	결핵
	total bilirubin	총빌리루빈
TFT	thyroid function test	갑상선기능검사
T/H	total hysterectomy	전 자궁절제술
THR	total hip replacement	전 고관절 치환
TIA	transient ischemic attack ‣ 뇌의 혈액공급이 일시적으로 간섭받음	일과성 허혈성 발작
t.i.d.	three times daily(Latin: ter in die)	1일 3회

약 어	원 어	해 설
tinct.	tincture	팅크제
TJ	triceps jerk	삼두근반사
TKR	total knee replacement	전 슬관절 치환
TLSO	thoracic lumbar sacral orthosis	흉요천골(등허리엉치뼈)의 정형술
TM	tympanic membrane	고막
TMJ	temporomandibular joint	악관절(관자아래턱관절)
	‣ mandibular bone(하악골)은 측두골 부위에서 두개골과 만나 양쪽에 악관절 형성	
TNM	tumor, nodes, metastases	종양, 림프절, 전이
T/O	telephone order	전화지시
TOF	tetralogy of Fallot	팔로사징
	‣ 4가지 결함/선천성 기형: 폐동맥+대동맥 – pulmonary artery atenosis(PS, 폐동맥협착) – ventricular septal defect(VSD, 심실중격결손) – shift of the aorta to the right(대동맥 우측편재) – hypertrophy of the right ventricle(RVH, 우심실 비대)	
TP	total protein(laboratory/chemistry)	총단백질(검사/화학)
T-P	temporoparietal	측두 두정골(관자마루뼈)의
TPN	total parenteral nutrition(intravenous therapy)	전비경구적 영양
	‣ 정맥으로 투여되는 영양 수액제	
TPR	temperature, pulse, respirations	체온, 맥박, 호흡
TRUS	transrectal ultrasound (prostate gland)	경직장 초음파 (전립선 검사)
TS	thoracic surgery	흉부외과
TSH	thyroid stimulating hormone	갑상선자극호르몬
	‣ 갑상선자극: 뇌하수체 전엽 → 내분비계	
TSICU	thoracic surgery intensive care unit	흉부외과 중환자실
TSP	total serum protein	총혈청단백질
TT	thrombin time	트롬빈시간
	‣ 정상치 < 22 sec	
TUR	transurethral resection	경요도 절제술
TURB	transurethral resection of bladder	경요도 방광절제술
TURP	transurethral resection of prostate	경요도 전립샘절제술
TVH	total vaginal hysterectomy(operation/gynecology)	전 질식 자궁절제술
Tx.	therapy, treatment	치료

약 어	원 어	해 설
U		
U	unit(on laboratory reports)	단위(검사기록지)
UA	urine analysis(laboratory/urine)	소변검사(검사)
	uric acid(laboratory/chemistry)	요산(검사/화학)
UC	uterine contractions	자궁수축
UGI	upper gastrointestinal series (x-ray/esophagus, stomach, and duodenum)	상부 위장관 조영술 (x-ray 검사/식도, 위 및 십이지장)
	upper respiratory infection	상기도 감염
UIQ	upper inner quadrant	상내부 1/4
ung.	ointment(Latin: *unguentum*) (prescriptions)	연고(처방)
U/O	urine output	요배출량
UOQ	upper outer quadrant	상외부 1/4
UPJ	ureteropelvic junction	요관 신우 이행부
UR	urology	비뇨기과
URI	upper respiratory infection	상기도 감염
URQ	upper right quadrant	우상부 1/4
URS	ureteroscopic removal of stone	요관경적 결석제거
	ureteroendoscope	요관경
US, U/S	ultrasound	초음파
USO	unilateral salpingo-oophorectomy	편측 자궁관-난소절제술
USP	United States Pharmacopeia	미국 약전
UTI	urinary tract infection ‣ 소변 균배양검사 결과: 박테리아가 100,000/ml 이상 검출 – E-coli(대장균), staphylococcus(포도상구균/포도알균), streptococcus(연쇄상구균/사슬알균), pus(농) ‣ N39.0 → 수술 후 UTI: T81.4, Y62.0 산과 시 UTI: O___, Y62.0	요로감염
UVJ	ureterovesical junction	요관방광이행부
V		
V_1, V_2 …	chest lead 1, chest lead 2, … (ECG)	흉부유도 1, 2, … (심전도)
VA	visual acuity(eye examination)	시력(명료도/시력검사)
VCUG	voiding cystourethrogram(procedure/urology)	배뇨성 방광 조영술
VD	venereal disease	성병
	vaginal delivery	질분만

약 어	원 어	해 설
VDRL	Venereal Disease Research Laboratory (test for syphilis)	성병검사(매독검사)
VF	visual field(eye examination)	시야
	ventricular fibrillation	심실 세동
VH	vaginal hysterectomy(operation/gynecology)	질식 자궁절제술(수술/부인과)
VIN	vulvar intraepithelial neoplasia	외음부 상피내 신생물
Vit.	vitamin	비타민
VLBW	very low birth weight	극소 저체중 출생
VLDL	very low density lipoproteins(laboratory/chemistry)	초저밀도 지방단백질
V/O	verbal order	구두지시
VPB	ventricular premature beat	심실성 조기수축
VPC	ventricular premature contractions	심실성 조기수축
V/S	vital signs ‣ V/S $\bar{q}$ tid: 3시간마다 활력징후 체크할 것	활력징후
VSD	ventricular septal defect(heart)	심실중격결손(심장)
VT	ventricular tachycardia ‣ bradycardia(서맥)	심실성 빈맥
VTH	vaginal total hysterectomy	질식 전자궁 절제술

W

약 어	원 어	해 설
Ⓦ	wheeze	씩씩거리는 호흡
WA	ward ambulation	병동보행
WAIS	Wechsler Adult Intelligence Scale (psychological test)	웨크슬러의 성인지능테스트
WB	whole blood	전혈
WBBS	whole body bone scan	전신골주사
WBC	white blood cell(laboratory/hematology) ‣ 정상치: 4천~1만/mm3	백혈구(수)(검사/혈액학)
wd.	ward	병실
wds.	wounds	상처
WISC	Wechsler Intelligence Scale for Children	웨크슬러의 아동용 지능테스트
wk.	week	주
WN	well nourished	영양이 좋은
WNL	within normal limit	정상범위내
W/O	written order	서면 지시
WPW	Wolff-Parkinson-White(syndrome)	볼프-파킨슨-화이트 증후군

약 어	원 어	해 설
wt.	weight	무게

X

약 어	원 어	해 설
x3, x4	3 times, 4 times	3배, 4배
x2d, x3d,…	for 2 days, for 3 days, …	2일 동안, 3일 동안 …

Y

약 어	원 어	해 설
YAG	yttrium, aluminum, garmet(laser)	이트륨, 알루미늄, 가멧(레이저)
yr.	year	년

Z

약 어	원 어	해 설
ZES	Zollinger-Ellison syndrome	졸링거-엘리슨 증후군
Zn	zinc	아연

1.3 상 징 Symbols

기호	원 어	해 설
+ or ⊕	positive, present	양성, 증상있음
− or ⊖	negative, absent	음성, 증상없음
↑	increase	증가
↓	decrease	감소
>	greater than	보다 큼
<	less than	보다 작음
≤	less than or equal to	~이하
≥	greater than or equal to	~이상
≅	approximately	대략
=	equals	동등
△	change	변화
±	either positive or negative	양성 또는 음성
+	slight reaction	경미한 반응
++	noticeable reaction	눈에 띄는 반응
+++	moderate reaction	적당한 반응
++++	large amount(or pronounced reaction)	현저한 반응
+ reaction	acid reaction	산성 반응
− reaction	alkaline reaction	알카리성 반응
→	to the right, results in, transfer to	오른쪽으로, 결과, 전환
←	to the left	왼쪽으로
↑↑	extensor respone, Babinski sign (neurological examination)	신근반응, 바빈스키 징후 (신경학적 검사)
↓↓	planter response, Babinski sign	족저반응, 바빈스키 징후 (신경학적 검사)
ⓜ	murmur	심장 잡음
1x	once	한 번
2x	twice	두 차례
1°	first degree	1도
2°	second degree	2도
#	number, no.	예) POD #1: 수술 후 1일째
/	per 예) smoking(흡연): 1pack/day 하루에 1갑	~에 대해
♂	male, M	남성
♀	female, F	여성

기호	원어	해설
†	death	사망
*	birth	출산
◉	start of operation(on anesthesia records)	수술개시(마취기록지)
X	start of anesthesia(on anesthesia records)	마취개시(마취기록지)
ⓧ	end of anesthesia(on anesthesia records)	마취종료(마취기록지)
V	systolic blood pressure(on anesthesia records)	수축기 혈압(마취기록지)
∧	diastolic blood pressure(on anesthesia records)	이완기 혈압(마취기록지)
O	respirations(on anesthesia records)	호흡(마취기록지)
-●	pulse rate(on anesthesia records)	맥박수(마취기록지)
△	temperature(on anesthesia records)	체온(마취기록지)
S	suction(on anesthesia records)	흡입력
λ	wave length	파장
μc	microcurie	마이크로퀴리
μEq	microequivalent	마이크로당량
μf	microfarad	마이크로패럿
μg	microgram(1/1000 of milligram)	마이크로그램
μμg	micromicrogram(picogram)	마이크로미크로그램
μμ	micromicron	마이크로미크론
μ	micron	마이크론
μsec	microsecond	100만분의 1초
μv	microvolt	마이크로 볼트
μw	microwatt	마이크로 와트
mμc	millimicrogram(nanocurie)	밀리마이크로그램
mμ	millimicron	밀리마이크론

04 임상과 약어

Abbreviation used in clinical department

표 5-1 • 제1진료부서

약 어	원 어	해 설
IM	Internal medicine	내과
	‣ Pulmonology: 호흡기내과 ‣ Gastroenterology: 소화기내과 ‣ Endocrinology: 내분비내과 ‣ Nephrology: 신장내과	‣ Cardiology: 순환기내과 ‣ Hemato-oncology: 혈액종양내과 ‣ Allergology: 알레르기내과
PED	Pediatrics	소아과
GS	General Surgery	일반외과
TS, CS	Thoracic and Cardiovascular Surgery	흉부외과
NS	Neurosurgery	신경외과
OS	Orthopedic Surgery	정형외과
PS	Plastic & Reconstructive Surgery	성형외과
OB & GY	Obstetrics and Gynecology	산부인과
DM	Dermatology	피부과
UR	Urology	비뇨기과
OT	Ophthalmology	안과
OL	Otorhinolaryngology	이비인후과
NP	Psychiatry	신경정신과
NR	Neurology	신경과
AN	Anesthesiology	마취과
FM	Family Medicine	가정의학과
DT	Dentistry	치과
RH	Rehabilitaion	재활의학과
ER	Emergency Room	응급실
OR	Operating Room	수술실
ICU	Intensive Care Unit	중환자실
	‣ MICU(Medical Intensive Care Unit)	내과계 중환자실
	- CCU(Coronary Care Unit)	심혈관내과 중환자실
	- RCU(Respiratory Care Unit)	호흡기내과 중환자실
	‣ SCU(Surgical Care Unit)	외과계 중환자실
	- NCU(Neurological Care Unit)	신경외과 중환자실
	‣ NICU(Neonatal Intensive Care Unit)	신생아 중환자실

표 5-2 • 제2진료부서

약 어	원 어	해 설
DR	Diagnostic Radiology	진단방사선과
TR	Therapeutic Radiology	치료방사선과
NM	Nuclear Medicine	핵의학
CP	Clinical Pathology	임상병리과
PA	Pathology	병리과
RH	Rehabilitation	재활의학과
MR	Department of Medical Records	의무기록과
PH	Division of Pharmacy	약제부
NU	Division of Nursing	간호부
BE	Biomedical Engineering	의공학과
SL	Special Laboratories	특수검사부
CS	Office of Central Supply	중앙공급실

표 5-3 • 기타 부서 및 직위

직 명	해 설
Office of Planning and Budget	기획조정실
Offices of Education and Research	교육연구부
Offices of Hospital Information Systems	의료정보실
Division of General Affairs	총무부
Division of Patient Affairs	원무부
Division of Finance	경리부
Division of Construction and Engineering	시설부
General Director	원장
Vice General Director for Clinical Services	진료부원장
Vice General Director for Administrative Service	행정부원장
Assistant Director, Division of General Affairs	총무부장
Manager, Department of Medical Records	의무기록과장
Assistant Manager, Department of Patient Affairs	원무과계장
Chief Technologist	기사장

05 차트의 기본용어
Terminology of basic chart

표 5-4 • 차트 기본 용어

용어 해설					
Abortion	유 산	Enlargement	확 대	Onset	시 작
Afebrile	열이 없음	Epigastric	상복부	Operation	수 술
Alert	명료한	Epistaxis	코 피	Organ	장 기
Amenorrhea	무월경	Eruption	발 진	Pain	통 증
Anemia	빈 혈	Extremity	사 지	Palpation	촉 진
Anorexia	식욕부진	Fatigue	피로감	Palpitation	심계항진
Ascites	복 수	Fever	열	Papule	구 진
Asthma	천 식	Findings	발견사항	Parity	출산력
Back	등	Flat	편평함	Pathologist	병리의사
Bearing down sensation	중압감	Gas passing	가스방출	Procedure	처 치
Biopsy	생 검	Gross	육 안	Profuse	아주 많음
Bowel	장	Headache	두 통	Pyroxia	발 열
(=intestine=entero)		Hematochezia	혈변배설	Pyuria	농 뇨
Chill	오 한	Hematemesis	토 혈	Rebound tenderness	반사통
Clear	깨끗함	Hematouria	혈 뇨	Recent	최 근
Conjunctiva	결 막	Hemoptysis	객 혈	Retraction	함 몰
Constipation	변 비	Hemorrhage	출 혈	Remove	제 거
Contraceptive pills	피임약	Icteric	황달의	Routine check	기본검사
Convulsion	경 련	Indigestion	소화불량	Scar	흉 터
Cough	기 침	Inflammation	염 증	Sclera	공 막
Cyanosis	청색증	Insomnia	불면증	Severe	심 한
Dehiscence	열 개	Isocoria	동공등대	Slight	경미한
Delivery	분 만	Jaundice	황 달	Soft	부드러움
(=para)		Labor	진 통	Sore throat	목통증
Diagnosis	진단명	Layer	층	Specimen	검체, 표본
Diarrhea	설 사	Macule	반 점	Sponge count	거즈세기
Dictated	전 사	Mass	(암)덩어리	Squeeze	짜 다
Discomfort	불편감	Meconium	태 변	Stable	안정됨
Dizziness	현기증	Melena	혈 변	Stich-out	실밥뽑음
Drain	배액관	Menarche	초 경	Surgeon	수술집도의
Drainage	배 액	Menstruation	월 경	Suture	봉 합
Dyscharge	분비물, 퇴원	Menorrhagia	월경과다	Tenderness	압 통
Dysmenorrhea	월경곤란	Mild	경미한	Ulcer	궤 양
Dyspnea	호흡곤란	Moderate	적당, 중등도	Vertigo	현기증
Dysuria	배뇨곤란	Menopause	폐 경	Vomiting	구 토
Edema	부 종	Nausea	오 심	Weak	약 함
Embedding	포 매	Nocturia	야뇨증	Wound	상 처
Engorgement	충 혈	Occupation	직 업		

06 의사지시기록의 중요어휘

Keywords of doctor's order

표 5-5 • 의사지시기록 및 기타기록(경과·수술·병리기록)의 중요어휘

약 어	원 어	해 설
ABGA	Arterial blood gases analysis	동맥혈 가스분석
ABO	Blood group system(A, AB, B, and O)	ABO식 혈액형
ABR	Absolute bed rest	절대안정
BR	Bed rest	안정
CTD	Closed thoracotomy drainage	폐쇄적 개흉술 배액
EBL	Estimated blood loss	추정된 실혈량
EKG(=ECG)	Electrocardiogram	심전도
EMG	Electromyography	근전도
FBS	Fasting blood sugar	공복 시 혈당
FFP	Fresh frozen plasma	신선 냉동 혈장
GD	General diet	일반식(정상식이)
GO	Gas out	가스배출
H/S	Hartman's solution	하트만용액(1 L =1,000cc)
ICP	Intracranial pressure	두개내압
I/O	Intake and output	섭취량 및 배설량
IM	Intramuscle	근육내
IVS	Intravenous	정맥내
LD	Liquid diet	유동식이
MN	Midnight	자정
MRI	Magnetic resonance imaging	자기공명영상촬영
NPO	Nothing per os	금식
OR	Operating room	수술실
ⓟ	Pint	파인트/5pints(수혈)
PA	Posterior anterior	후-전방의
po	by mouth	경구로
POD #2	Postoperative day two	수술 후 2일째
PR	Per rectum	직장을 통해
PRBC	Packed red blood cells	농축 적혈구
PRN	Whenever necessary	필요할 때마다
q	Every	마다
qd	Every day	매일
qid	Four times daily	하루에 4번
qod	Every other day	이틀에 한번
RD	Regular diet	일반식
SD	Soft diet	연식
SF position	Semi-fowler's position	반좌위 취하기
SOW	Sips of water	물 한모금 마시도록 함
SSE	Soapsuds enema(=soap solution enema)	비눗물 관장
S-S enema	Saline solution enema	식염수 관장
tid	Three times a day	1일 3회
U/A	Urin analysis	소변검사
U/O	Urine output	요 배설량
USG	Ultrasonography	초음파검사
VDRL	Venereal Disease Research Laboratory	매독검사
V/S	Vital sign	활력징후
W/B	Whole blood	전혈

표 5-6 • 의사지시기록지(Doctor's order)의 중요어휘

출제빈도 높은 내용	
1. Check V/S $\bar{q}$ 6hr	→ 6시간마다 활력징후 체크
2. Get op. permission	→ 수술승낙서 받아 놓기
3. Send the patient to OR with chart and X-ray film	→ 환자를 수술실로 보낼 때는 기록과 방사선 필름을 함께 보낼 것을 지시
4. Preparation of blood(PRBC 5 Ⓟ) X-Matching	→ 농축적혈구 5pints를 교차시험해 둘 것
4-1. Prepare W/B 4pints after ABO Rh & cross matching	→ 혈액검사 후 전혈 4파인트 준비
4-2. req) Pack cell 2pint, FFP 2pint prepare	→ 수술 시 필요한 혈액농축적혈구 2pint와 신선동결혈장 2pint를 준비하라고 지시
5. X-ray 검사(chest PA, skull series)	→ 흉부 방사선 촬영
6. H/S 1L IV(OR용)	→ 정맥주사용 하트만 1,000cc를 수술실용으로 준비할 것
7. ABR c change position $\bar{q}$ 3 hrs	→ 절대 안정시키고 매 3시간 간격으로 체위를 변경해 줄 것
7-1. BR with SF	→ 침상휴식 및 반좌위 취함
8. NPO from M/N	→ 밤 12시 이후부터 금식시킬 것
9. S-S enema 500cc P.R. bid	→ 직장을 통한 비눗물 관장 500cc
9-1. Glycerine enema 70cc	→ 글리세린 70cc 관장할 것
10. Humidification	→ 가습기를 사용하라고 지시/습도유지
11. Skin preparation	→ 피부 준비시킴
12. Check I/O daily(hourly)	→ 섭취배설량 매일(매시간) 측정
13. Full stitch out	→ 실밥 완전 제거
14. Sand bag apply	→ 모래주머니 부착
15. Whole shaving aseptic dressing on the scalp	→ 털을 깎고 무균 드레싱을 할 것
16. Electrolyte check after enema	→ 관장 후 전해질 체크할 것
17. Rt. short leg splint	→ 다리에 부목을 댐
18. Urine bag change qod	→ 소변주머니를 매일 교체
19. Insert F-catheter	→ 유치카테터 삽입
20. Antibiotic Tx.	→ 항생제 치료
21. Abd-US " Dr-on call"	→ 복부 초음파 시행하려면 의사를 호출하라고 지시
22. Mevacor 1T po qd	→ Mevacor를 매일 한 정씩 복용할 것
23. PRN) Lorazepam 0.6mg po(if insomnia)	→ 불면증이 있으면 lorazepam 0.6mg을 복용할 것
23-1 PRN if) headache, ocular pain ⇒ notify to Dr. Yoon	→ 두통이나 눈의 통증이 있으면 의사에게 연락하도록 지시
24. Emazon 3.0mg IVS $\bar{q}$ 6hr	→ emazon이라는 해열제 3.0mg을 6시간마다 정맥내 주사
24-1. Maltos spp. 2pill P.R. bid	→ 직장을 통한 maltos 2pill 좌약주입
25. Humidification	→ 가습기 사용 지시
26. NPO except medication	→ 내복약을 제외하고 금식할 것
27. Electrolyte check after enema	→ 관장 후 전해질 체크할 것
28. Mannitol 400cc O.R.	→ 만니톨 400cc를 수술방으로 보냄
29. U/A with micro(=ⓜ)	→ 소변 검사(소변 세균검사)
30. HBs Ag/Ab	→ 간염 항원·항체 검사

표 5-7 • 의사지시기록 및 기타기록(경과·수술·병리기록)의 중요어휘

의무기록지(Doctor's order)	
31. Prepare ICP sensor & monitor	→ 내뇌압 측정준비
32. Tumor marker (CEA)	→ 종양표지자 검사할 것
33. CTD count $\bar{q}$ 1hr. if 〉 50cc	→ 개흉배액량이 50cc 이상이면 1시간마다 측정
34. O_2 4L/min	→ 산소를 1분 4L씩 준다.
35. Frozen section slip 접수	→ 동결절편 검사지 접수
36. hyperalimentation	→ 정맥영양공급
37. ABR $\bar{c}$ head elevation 20°	→ 수술 후 20° 정도 머리를 올려서 안정하도록 함
경과기록지(Progress notes)	
1. H-vac와 foley remove	→ H-vac과 폴리카테터 제거
2. Serous discharge on back wound	→ 수술상처에 장액성 액이 흐름
3. Gas out(G/O)	→ 가스 배출
4. Self voiding	→ 자가배뇨
5. POD #2 wound: complete cure	→ 수술 후 2일째 상처는 완전 치유
6. POD #3 removed rubber drain	→ 배농관은 수술 후 3일째 되는 날 제거
7. uroflowmetry/residual urine ≒ 50cc	→ 요유량계 검사상 잔료는 50cc
수술기록지(Operation record)	
1. EBL: 800cc	→ 혈액 손실 추정량은 800cc(수술기록지)
병리보고서(Pathological report)	
1. Metastases to 4 lymph nodes(4/56)	→ 림프절은 56개 중 4개가 전이(병리조직학적 보고서)

07 임상검사
Laboratory tests

임상검사 단위

- mg: milligram (one thousand of a gram)
- dl: deciliter (one tenth of a liter of 100ml)
- mEq: milliequivalent
- thou: thousand
- cu mm: cubic millimeter(mm^3)
- ⬆: 검사항목 증가
- ⬇: 검사항목 감소
- ml: milliliter
- U: unit
- I: liter
- g: gram
- mill: million
- μ: micro
- ng: nanogram
- pg: picogram
- IU: international unit
- sec: second

표 5-8 • 주요 임상검사

분 류	검사항목	정상치	임상적 의미
혈액학적 검사 (hematology)	혈색소 (hemoglobin; Hb)	남: 13.0～17.0 g/dl 여: 12.0～16.0 g/dl	↑: 적혈구증다증 ↓: 빈혈
	혈구 용적 (hematocrit; Hct)	남: 36～54 g/dl 여: 36～47 g/dl	↑: 구토, 하리, 선천성심질환 ↓: 빈혈, 부종
	혈소판수 검사 (platelet count)	10～40x104/mm^3	↑: 만성백혈병, 진성다혈증, 출혈, 원발성 혈소판증다증, 골절 ↓: 급성백혈병, 재생불량성빈혈, 쇼크 방사선장해
	적혈구(RBC)	남: 20만～630만/mm^3 여: 400만～540만/mm^3	↑: 진성다혈증, 탈수, 부신부전증, 심폐질환 ↓: 각종빈혈, 수혈증
	백혈구(WBC)	4천～1만/mm^3	↑: 만성백혈병, 급성감염증 ↓: 재생불량성 및 악성빈혈, 과립수감소증
바이러스 검사 (virous test)	HBs Ag HBs Ab	+ ┐ B형 간염 − ┘ 보균자	− ┐ 항체 − ┐ 간염 예방주사 + ┘ − ┘
생화학검사 (biochemical tests) ① 효소(enzymes)	AST(GOT)	남: 37 U/L 이하 여: 31 U/L 이하	↑: 급성간염, 심근경색(GOT〉GPT) 근질환(GOT〉GPT), 악성종양 폐쇄성 황달, 알코올성 간염 ↓: 간장괴사
	ALT(GPT)	남: 40 U/L 이하 여: 31 U/L 이하	
② 지질(lipids) = 고지혈증	콜레스테롤 (Cholesterol)	230 mg/dl 이하	↑: 고혈압, 동맥경화, 심근경색, 협심증, 뇌졸중, 심장마비

표 5-8 • 주요 임상검사(계속)

분 류	검사항목	정상치	임상적 의미
③ 포도당(glucose) (GTT: 당부하검사) = 혈당검사	공복 시 식후 2시간째	·126 mg/dl 이하 ·200 mg/dl 이하	↑: 당뇨병
④ 혈압	수축기/이완기	120/80 mmHg 이상	↑: 고혈압, 140/90 mmHg 이상 ↓: 저혈압, 100/60 mmHg 이하
⑤ 전해질 (electrolytes; e′)	나트륨 (sodium; Na)	135～145 mEq/L 소변: 40～220 mEq/day	↑: 수분결핍, 염분과잉, 신질환, 원발성 aldosteron증 ↓: 하리, 구토, 만성신부전, Addison씨병, 당뇨병성 산증
	칼륨 (potassium; K)	3.5～5.3 mEq/L 소변: 25～125 mEq/day	↑: 요독증, 부신부정증, 신장염, 백혈병 ↓: 구토, 만성신부전, 당뇨병성 산증
	칼슘 (calcium; Ca)	8.1～10.5 mg/dl	↑: 비타민D 과잉증, 부갑상선 기능항진증, 악성종양 ↓: 부갑상선 기능저하증, VitD 결핍증, 골연화증, 신부전증
	염소 (chlorine; CI)	98～110 mEq/L 소변: 110～250 mEq/day	↑: 탈수증, 만성신장염, 염분과잉, 화상 ↓: Addison씨병, 구토, 신우신염, 하리
	마그네슘 (magnesium; MG)	1.8～2.4 mg/dl	↑: 근무력증, 전신마취 ↓: 과도한 신경흥분, 경련증상
⑥ 단백질-질소 화합물 (protein nitrogen)	총빌리루빈 (total bilirubin)	0.2～1.2 mg/dl	↑: 간질환, 급만성 간염, 간경변, 폐쇄성 황달
	크레아틴 (creatinine)	혈청: (남)0.6～1.1 mg/dl (여)0.5～0.9 mg/dl 소변: 1～1.5g/day	(혈청) ↑: 신기능장해 ↓: 근위축, 임신 (소변) ↑: 간질환, 근육질환, 갑상선중독증
	혈액뇨질소 (blood urea nitrogen)	혈청: 4.5～23.5 mg/dl 소변: 9.3～16.3 g/day	↑: 신부전, 간경변, 요독증, 악성종양 ↓: 임신, 저단백식, 간부전, 요붕증
	글루코스 (glucose)	70～110 mg/dl	↑: 당뇨병, 요독증, 갑상선기능항진증,간질환 ↓: 간장해, 인슐린 과잉증
특수생화학검사 (special biochemical tests)	수은 (mercury; Hg)	혈청: 0.5 μg/dl 이하 소변: 20 μg/dl 이하 (독성: 50 μg/day 이상)	↑: 수은중독
	납, 연 (lead; Pb)	혈액: 0.5 μg/dl 이하 소변: 80 μg/dl 이하	↑: 연중독

표 5-8 • 주요 임상 검사 (계속)

분 류	검사항목	정상치	임상적 의미
뇨검사 (urine tests)	벤스-존스 단백 (Bence-Jones protein)	Negative(−)	골수종
면역혈청검사 (immuno-serology)	매독검사 (VDRL)	Non-reactive	감염 3~6주 후에 항체 생성 2차 매독기에 역가 최고치
내분비검사 (endocrinology) ⑦ 성선 (sexual gland)	에스트로겐(estrogen) =estradiol(여성호르몬) : 여성의 2차 성징 (체모 및 유방발육 등) ※ estrogen receptor(+) progesterone receptor(+) → 유방암	(여) 소아:40pg/ml 이하 (주기) 1-10일: 61~394pg/ml 11-20일: 122~437pg/ml 21-30일: 156~350pg/ml 폐경후: 40pg/ml 이하	↑: 난소암 ↓: 난소 발육부전, 뇌하수체 기능 저하증
	프로게스테론 (progesterone) 여성호르몬/황체호르몬 (자궁의 준비 및 유지)	여: 난포(follicular): 0.1~0.5 황체(luteal): 2.5~28.0 midluteal: 3.8~28.0	60세 이상: 0~0.2ng/ml 피임제복용: 0.1~0.3ng/ml 임신: 1st trimester(9.0~47.0ng/ml) 2nd trimester(17.0~146ng/ml) 3rd trimester(55.0~225ng/ml)
	테스토스테론 (testosterone) =androgen(남성호르몬) : 남성의 2차 성징(수염, 체모, 목소리 등)	남: 2.7~10.7ng/ml	
⑧ 태반 (placenta)	β-HCG	남: 2ng/ml 이하 여: 5ng/ml 이하 분만 후 72시간 이후는 정상	단위: mIU/ml 임신 6주: 8천-3만, 임신 10주: 5만-10만 임신 20주: 1만-5만 임신 40주: 2천-5만 자궁외 임신: 150-800mIU/ml ↑: 임신, 융모성 종양
혈액응고검사 (blood coagu-lation test)	부분트롬빈 시간 (partial thrombin time ; PTT) 프로트롬빈 시간 (prothrombin time; PT)	27~43 Sec 12~15 Sec	· 응고 경로에서 초기에 작용하는 인자의 존재 측정 · 혈액의 응고능력을 측정 · 혈장표본에 칼슘 추가, 혈괴(clot)가 생긴 것이 보이는 데 걸린 시간 측정 · 항응고제를 사용한 환자에게 추적검사로 사용

표 5-8 • 주요 임상 검사 (계속)

분 류	검사항목	정상치	임상적 의미
혈액응고검사 (blood coagulation test)	부분트롬빈 시간 (partial thrombin time ; PTT)	27～43 Sec	· 응고 경로에서 초기에 작용하는 인자의 존재 측정
	프로트롬빈 시간 (prothrombin time; PT)	12～15 Sec	· 혈액의 응고능력을 측정 · 혈장표본에 칼슘 추가, 혈괴(clot)가 생긴 것이 보이는 데 걸린 시간 측정 · 항응고제를 사용한 환자에게 추적검사로 사용
	ABO typing Rh typing	Negative	수혈, 장기이식, 수혈부작용, 신생아용혈성 빈혈, 친자감별 ※ erythroblastosis fetalis 태아적아구증 → 모체와 태아와의 혈액형 부적합으로 발생하는 태아의 용혈성 빈혈
	Crossmatching	Compatible	· 수혈혈액의 적합성 여부 검사
종양표지검사 (Tumor Markers)	CEA AFP	5.0ng/ml 이하 20.0ng/ml 이하	· 대장암, 암의 전이, 알코올중독, 흡연 · 급·만성간염, 간경변, 간세포암, 임신, 태아기형
	β2-microglobulin	60세 이하: 2.4mg/L 이하 60세 이상: 3.0mg/L 이하 300μg/L 이하	· 림프종, 간담도계질환, 신장질환 면역결핍증, 중금속중독, 염증성질환
	Ferritin	남: 20～400ng/ml 여: 10～130ng/ml	· 폐암, 림프종, 췌장암, 유방암, 간장질환,
	PAP	3.2ng/ml 이하	· 전립선(샘)암, 골전이
	CA-125	35U/ml 이하	난소암, 자궁내막염, 자궁경부암
	CA-19, 9	37U/ml 이하	위암, 췌장암, 직장암, 담도암
	TA-4 (SCC)	2.0ng/ml 이하	폐암, 폐질환 SCC ↑ : 편평세포자궁암, 폐암, 식도암
	CA 15-3	13±5.2U/ml 이하	전이성유방암진단
	TATI (tumor associated trypsin inhibitor)	혈청: 3～31 μg/ml 소변: 7～50 μg/g·Cr	↑: 췌장암, 위장암, 난소암(특히 점액성), 자궁목암, 자궁내막암, 폐암

08 의약품 종류

Classes of drugs

표 5-9 • 의약품 종류

약품명	성분명	의약품 분류
Acertil	Perindopril tert-butylamine	혈압강화제
Acetic acid		방역용 살균소독제
Acetic acid 3%		방역용 살균소독제
Actilyse inj	TPA	기타의 순환계용약
Activated charcoal		해독제
Adalat-A	Nifedipine	혈관확장제
Adcal		칼슘제
Adchon	Adenochrome monoamino	지혈제
	guanidine methanesulfonate	
Adelavin 9 inj		이담제
Adenocor inj	Adenosine	부정맥용제
Adriamycin RDF, PFS inj	Doxorubicin HCl	주로 악성종양에 작용
Advantan 0.1% oint	Methylprednisolone aceponate	기타의 외피용약
Afloxan	Proglumetacin dimaleate	해열, 진통, 소염제
Aipron	Ipriflavone	대사성 의약품
Airtal	Aceclofenac	해열, 진통, 소염제
Alavac-s		기타의 생물학적 제제
Alaxyl granule		하제, 완장제
Albumin inj 20%, 5%	Human Serum Albumin	혈액제제류
Alcaine oph. sol	Propracaine HCl	안과용제
Aldactazide		혈압강화제
Aldactone	Verapamil	부정맥용제
Aldactone	Spironolactone	이뇨제
Alkyloxan tab, inj	Cyclophosphamide	항악성종양제
Almagel-F susp	Almagate	제산제
Alocin inj	Azlocillin Na	주로 그람양성, 음성균에 작용
Alphaferon inj	Interferon α 2a	항악성종양제
Alum hexa sol 20%(원)	Aluminum chloride hexahydrate	발한제, 지한제
Amikin inj	Amikacin	주로 항산성균에 작용

약품명	성분명	의약품 분류
Amilo	Amiloride	이뇨제
Aminofusin TPN		단백 아미노산제제
Aminoleban EN pow		단백 아미노산제제
Aminophylline pow, inj	Aminophylline	강심제
Aminosteril KE nephro		단백 아미노산제제
Aminosteril Ped		아미노산제제
Amphojel	Aluminum hydroxide	제산제
Andilase		정장제
Androderm	Testosterone	남성호르몬제
Anexate inj	Flumazenil	해독제
Antiroid	Propylthiouracil	기타의 호르몬제
Aprotimbin inj	Aprotinin	기타의 순환계용약
Arduan inj	Pipecuronium Br	골격근이완제
Aredia inj	Pamidronate 2Na	대사성 의약품
Arelix cap	Piretanide	이뇨제
Artamin	D-Penicillamine	해독제
Artane, Trihexin	Trihexyphenidyl HCl	진경제
Artz inj	Hyaluronic Na	대사성 의약품
Ascorbic acid tab, pow	Ascorbic acid	비타민 C 및 P제
Aspirin	Aspirin	기타의 순환계용약
Aspirin, Rhonal	Aspirin	해열, 진통, 소염제
Asthcontin	Aminophylline	강심제
Astrix	Aspirin	기타의 순환계용약
Atenolol	Atenolol	기타의 순환계용약
Atgam inj	Antithymocyte globulin	생물학적 제제
Ativan tab, inj	Lorazepam	정신신경용제
Atock	Formoterol fumarate	진해거담제
Atropine oph. sol, oph. oint	Atropine sulfate	안과용제
Atropine sulfate inj	Atropine sulfate	진경제
Atrovent aerosol	Ipratropium bromide	진해거담제
Aurorix	Moclobemide	정신신경용제
Axid	Nizatidine	소화성궤양용제
Azathioprine	Azathioprine	자극요법제
Azeptin	Azelastine HCl	기타의 알레르기용약
Azintal forte		이담제
Azmacort inhaler	Triamcinolone acetonide	부신호르몬제
B.C.G percutaneous inj		백신류
B.C.G vaccine inj		백신류

약품명	성분명	의약품 분류
Bactroban oint	Mupirocin	기타의 외피용약
Banan tab, dry syr	Cefpodoxime proxetil	주로 그람양성, 음성균에 작용
Bearse		건위소화제
Beecom		혼합비타민제
Beecom hexa inj		혼합비타민제
Bellergal		자율신경제
Bendaline	Bendazac lysine	안과용제
Benzac AC lotion, AC 2.5%	Benzoyl Peroxide	피부연화제
Benztropine	Benztropine mesylate	진경제
Berotec	Fenoterl HBr	진해거담제
Besacolin	Bethanechl Cl	자율신경제
Betadine gargle	Povidone iodine	치과구강용약
Betadine sol, scrup, oint, gargle	Povidone iodine	외피용 살균소독제
Betaferon inj	Interferon	기타의 생물학적 제제
Betagan oph.sol	Levobunolol HCl	안과용제
Betoptic-s oph.susp 0.25%	Betaxolol HCl	안과용제
BiCNU inj	Carmustine(BCNU)	항악성종양제
Bilenor		이담제
Biltricide	Praziquantel	구충제
Bithree		정장제
Blutal inj	Iron chodroitin sulfate colloid	무기질제제
Bonaling-A	Dimenhydrinate	진훈제
Bosmin sol	Epinephrine	부신호르몬제
Botropase inj	Hemocoagulase	지혈제
Brevibloc inj	Esmolol HCl	부정맥용제
Brexin	Piroxicam β-cyclodextrin	해열, 진통, 소염제
Bricanyl syr	Terbutaline sulfate	진해거담제
Bromidine	Bromocriptine mesylate	대사성 의약품
Brosporin	Cefotiam hexitil	주로 그람양성, 음성균에 작용
Bunol inj	Butorphanol tartrate	해열, 진통, 소염제
Bupinephrine inj	Bupivacaine, Epinephrine	국소마취제
Buscopan tab, inj	Scopolamine butylbromide	진경제
Ca gluconate inj	Ca gluconate	칼슘제
CaC12 inj	Cal. chloride	칼슘제
Cadef elixir	Digoxin	강심제
Cafergot		해열, 진통, 소염제
Cal. carbonate	Cal. carbonate	칼슘제
Calamine lot	Calamine + ZnO	진통, 진양, 수렴, 소염제

약품명	성분명	의약품 분류
Calcio cap, Bonky inj	Calcitriol	비타민 A 및 D제
Calcort	Deflazacort	부신호르몬제
Canesten powder	Clotrimazole	기생성 피부질환용제
Canesten vag. tab	Clotrimazole	비뇨생식기관용제
Cantan inj	Ascorbic acid	비타민 C 및 P제
Capril	Captopril	혈압강화제
Cardopamin	Denopamine	강심제
Carmazepine CR	Carbamazepine	항전간제
Carmine CR	Carbamazepine	항전간제
Carverject inj	Alprostadil(PGE1)	기타의 순환계용약
Cefaclor cap syr	Cefaclor	주로 그람양성, 음성균에 작용
Cefatrex inj	Cephapirin Na	주로 그람양성, 음성균에 작용
Cefazolin inj	Cefazolin Na	주로 그람양성, 음성균에 작용
Cefmetazone inj	Cefmetazole Na	주로 그람양성, 음성균에 작용
Cefpiran inj	Cefpiramide Na	주로 그람양성, 음성균에 작용
Ceftriaxone inj	Ceftriaxone Na	주로 그람양성, 음성균에 작용
Celance	Pergolide mesylate	기타의 중추신경용약
Celoslin inj	Ceftezole Na	주로 그람양성, 음성균에 작용
Ceradolan inj	Cefotiam 2HCl	주로 그람양성, 음성균에 작용
Chloramphenicl oph. sol	Chloramphenicol	안과용제
Chlorpromazine	Chlorpromazine HCl	정신신경용제
Chymodiactin inj	Chymopapain	효소제제
Cibacen	Benazepril	혈압강화제
Cigelton		기타의 순환계용약
Cisplan inj	Cisplatin	항악성종양제
Claforan inj	Cefotaxime Na	주로 그람양성, 음성균에 작용
Clarityne	Loratadine	항히스타민제
Cleboril-S		기타의 소화기관용약
Cleocin inj		기타의 항생물질제제
Cleocin-T lot	Clindamycin	기타의 항생물질제제
Climara patch	Estradiol	난포호르몬 및 황체호르몬제
Clomifen	Clomiphene citrate	난포호르몬 및 황체호르몬제
Clozaril	Clozapine	정신신경용제
Codeine	Codeine phosphate	아편알카로이드계 제제
Cofrel	Benproperine phosphate	진해거담제
Colchin	Colchicine	통풍치료제
Colimycin F otic. sol		이비후과용제
Comthyroid		갑상선, 부갑상선호르몬제

약품명	성분명	의약품 분류
Conray 60		X선 조영제
Copan tab, syr	Clenbuterol HCl	진해거담제
Copolang	Polysaccharide K	항악성종양제
Cordarone tab, inj	Amiodarone HCl	부정맥용제
Cormelian	Dilazep HCl	혈관확장제
Coumadin	Warfarin Na	혈액응고저지제
Cozaar	Losartan K	혈압강화제
Cravit	Levofloxacin	기타의 화학요법제
Curelen oph. sol		안과용제
Cycin inj	Ciprofloxacin HCl	기타의 화학요법제
Cyclogyl oph. sol	Cyclopentolate	안과용제
Cycrin	Medroxyprogesterone acetate	난포호르몬 및 황체호르몬제
Cytarabin		항악성종양제
Cytotec	Misoprostol	소화성궤양용제
D.D.S	Dapsone	치나제
D/S 5%	Dextrose-Normal saline 5%	혈액대용제
D/W 5%, 10%, 20% 50% inj	Dextrose 5%, 10%, 20%, 50%	혈액대용제
Daivonex oint	Calcipotriol	기타의 외피용약
Danazol	Danazol	기타의 호르몬제
Daonil	Glibenclamide	당뇨병용제
Daunoblastina inj	Daunorubicin	항악성종양제
Daunoblastina inj	Daunorubicin HCI	주로 악성종양에 작용
Denol	Tripotassium dicitrato bismuthtate	소화성궤양용제
Depakine inj	Valproate Na	항전간제
Depo-Medrol inj	Methylprednisolone acetate	부신호르몬제
Deponit-5 patch	Nitroglycerin	혈관확장제
Depovirin inj	Testosterone cypionate	남성호르몬제
Dermatop oint	Prednicarbate	기타의 외피용약
Dermovate sol	Clobetasol propionate	기타의 외피용약
Dexamethasone inj	Dexamethasone	부신호르몬제
Dextrose inj 5%,10%, 20%, 50%	Dextrose	당류제
DHC	Dihydrocodeine	아편알카로이드계 제제
Diamicron	Gliclazide	당뇨병용제
Diamox	Acetazolamide	이뇨제
Diazepam tab, inj	Diazepam	정신신경용제
Dicetel	Pinaverium Br	기타의 소화기관용약
Dichlozid tab	Hydrochlorothiazide	이뇨제
Dicknol inj	Diclofenac dimethylaminoethalol	해열, 진통, 소염제

약품명	성분명	의약품 분류
Diflucan cap, inj, pos dry syr	Fluconazole	기타의 화학요법제
Digoxin inj, Digosin	Digoxin	강심제
Dilatrend	Carvedilol	혈압강화제
Dinol	Etidronate 2Na	대사성 의약품
Disgren	Triflusal	기타의 순환계용약
Ditropan	Oxybutynin Cl	자율신경계
		난포호르몬 및 황체호르몬제
D-Mannitol 205 inj	D-Mannitol	당류제
Domenan	Ozagrel HCl	기타의 호흡기관용약
Donpel	Domperidone	기타의 소화기관용약
Dopram inj	Doxapram HCl	호흡촉진제
Dormicum inj	Midazolam	최면진정제
Doxium	Dobesilate Ca	기타의 순환계용약
DPT vaccine inj	Diphteria, pertussis, tetanus	독소류 및 톡소이드류
Droperidol inj	Droperidol	정신신경용제
DS insulin inj	Insulin	당뇨병용제
Dulcolax supp. Dulcolax S	Bisacodyl	하제, 완장제
Dulcolax supp, Dulcolax S	Castor oil	하제, 완장제
Dulcolax supp, Dulcolax S	Gas enema	하제, 완장제
Dulcolax supp, Dulcolax S	Mineral oil	하제, 완장제
Dulcolax supp, Dulcolax S	Olive oil	하제, 완장제
Duphalac	Lactulose	대사성 의약품
Duratears oph. oint		안과용제
Duricef cap, syr	Cefadroxil	주로 그람양성, 음성균에 작용
Durogesic TTS patch	Fentanyl citrate	합성마약
E.P.S inj, Lastet cap	Etoposide	항악성종양제
Ebastel	Ebastine	항히스타민제
Ebiose		건위소화제
Ecolicin oph. oint		안과용제
Eglandin inj	Alprostadil(PGEI)	기타의 순환계용약
Elcitonin inj	Elcatonin	대사성 의약품
Elen	Indeloxazine HCI	기타의 중추신경용약
Emazon	Emorfazone	해열, 진통, 소염제
Emcaine inj	Mepivacaine HCI	국소마취제
Empynase-s	Pronase B	효소제제
Enafon	Amitriptyline HCl	정신신경용제
Energen		단백 아미노산제제
Ensure liquid		단백 아미노산제제

약품명	성분명	의약품 분류
Entobar inj	Pentobarbital Na	최면진정제
Epinephrine inj	Epinephrine	부신호르몬제
Epocelin inj	Ceftizoxime Na	주로 그람양성, 음성균에 작용
Epogam solft cap (ped)	r-Linolenic acid	알레르기용약
Eprex inj	Erythropoietin α	기타의 호르몬제
Erdergine	Ergoloid mesylate	기타의 순환계용약
Erdos	Erdosteine	진해거담제
Eryc	Erythromycin	그람양성균, 리케치아, 비루스에 작용
Erythro-P syr	Erythromycin estolate	그람양성균, 리케치아, 비루스에 작용
Esperson oint, lot, gel	Desoxymethasone	기타의 외피용약
Essential forte		간장질환용제
Eulexin	Flutamide	기타의 호르몬제
Eumovate cream, oint	Clobetasone butyrate	기타의 외피용약
Excegran	Zonisamide	항전간제
Famvir	Famciclovir	기타의 화학요법제
Farlutal	Medroxyprogesterone acetate	항악성종양제
Fenatussin	Guaifenesin	진해거담제
Fenopron	Fenoprofen Ca	해열, 진통, 소염제
Fentanyl inj	Fentanyl citrate	합성마약
Fexadine	Fenoverine HCI	진경제
Flagyl inj	Metronidazole	항원충제
Flanin	Pranoprofen	해열, 진통, 소염제
Flasinyl tab	Metronidazole	항원충제
Fleet phosphosoda sol		X선 조영제
Flixotide	Fluticasone propionate	진해거담제
Flospan	Phloroglucinol	진경제
Fludarene	Chromocarb diethylamine	혈관보강제
Flumarin inj	Flomoxef Na	주로 그람양성, 음성균에 작용
Fluorometholone oph. sol	Fluorometholone	안과용제
Foipan	Camostat mesylate	대사성 의약품
Forane sol	Isoflurane	전신마취제
Fortimicin inj	Astromicin sulfate	주로 그람양성, 음성균에 작용
Foy inj	Gabexate mesylate	대사성 의약품
Fragmin inj	Dalteparin	혈액응고저지제
Freamine		단백 아미노산제제
Fucidin tab, syr, oint	Fusidic acid	주로 그람양성균에 작용
Fungizone inj	Amphotericin B	주로 곰팡이, 원충에 작용
Furtman inj		기타의 혈액 및 체액용약

약품명	성분명	의약품 분류
Furtulon	Doxifluridine	항악성종양제
Galantase pow	Galactosidase	정장제
Gamma globulin inj	Immunoglobulin r	혈액제제류
Gaster tab, inj	Famotidine	소화성궤양용제
Gastrografin		X선 조영제
Gelma susp		제산제
Gelofusin inj	Gelatin MFG	혈액대용제
Gentacin cream	Gentamicin sulfate	화농성 질환용제
Gentamicin inj	Gentamicin sulfate	주로 항산성균에 작용
Gerolan sol	Ethylether	전신마취제
Gisonine	Isoniazid(INAH)	항결핵제
Glucobay	Acarbose	당뇨병용제
Glucophage	Metformin	당뇨병용제
Glycerosteril inj		대사성 의약품
Glycopyrrolate inj	Glycopyrrolate	골격근이완제
Glyressin inj	Terlipressin acetate	뇌하수체호르몬제
Green eight inj	Antihemophilic CoagulationFactor VIII	혈액제제류
Gromin	Clomipramine HCI	정신신경용제
Gyno-Betadine sol	Povidone iodine	기타의 비뇨생식기 및 항문용약
Gyno-Betadine vag. supp	Povidone iodine	비뇨생식기관용제
H2 tab. inj	Cimetidine	소화성궤양용제
Haes-steril 6% inj	Pentastarch	기타의 혈액 및 체액용약
Halcion	Triazolam	최면진정제
Half saline inj	H/D	기타의 혈액 및 체액용약
Halothane sol	Halothane	전신마취제
Haloxin	Hydroxychloroquine sulfate	항원충제
Hartman sol inj		기타의 혈액 및 체액용약
Havrix inj	Hepatitis A virus vaccine	백신류
Helocetin	Chloramphenicol	주로 그람양성, 음성균에 작용
Hemocontin		무기질제제
Hemo-Q syr, susp	Iron proteinsuccinylate	무기질제제
Hemotrate B1, B2, F sol		인공신장관류용제
Hepabig inj	Human Antihepatitis B Ig	혈액제제류
Hepaccine-B inj	Hepatitis B virus vaccine	백신류
Heparin inj	Heparin Na	혈액응고저지제
Hepatamine		단백 아미노산제제
Hepavax-gene inj	Hepatitis B virus vaccine	백신류
Herben	Diltiazem HCl	혈관확장제

약품명	성분명	의약품 분류
Hexabrix		X선 조영제
Hexavitamin		혼합비타민제
Hibitan sol, Hibisol sol	Chlorhexidine gluconate	외피용살균소독제
Hibitier inj	H. Inflenza vaccine	백신류
Holoxan inj	Ifosfamide	항악성종양제
Homatropine oph.sol	Homatropine HBr	안과용제
Hydralazin tab, inj	Hydralazine HCl	혈압강화제
Hydrea	Hydroxyurea	항악성종양제
Hydrocortisone oint.lot(원)	Hydrocortisone	기타의 외피용약
Hypaque		X선 조영제
Hypertet inj	Antitetanus lg	혈액제제류
Hytrast		X선 조영제
Hytrin	Terazosin	혈압강화제
Imipramine	Imipramine HCl	정신신경용제
Immucyst inj	BCG strain connaught	기타의 종양 치료제
Imovane	Zopiclone	최면진정제
Implanta, Cipol-N	Cyclosporine A	자극요법제
Inderal inj	Propranolol HCl	부정맥용제
Indigo carmine 0.8% inj		기능검사용 시약
Infectoflam oh.sol, oph.oint	Flurometholone+Gentamicin	안과용제
Inflexin HA inj	Influenza virus vaccine	백신류
Inhibace	Cilazapril	혈압강화제
Insulatard inj	Insulin	당뇨병용제
Inteban spansule	Indomethacin	해열, 진통, 소염제
Intrafusin 10%(Amino acid 10%)		단백 아미노산제제
Intralipid 10%, 20% inj		기타의 자양강장변질제
Intron inj	Interferon α 2b	항악성종양제
Iodipine oph.oint	Apraclonidine HCl	안과용제
Irritren	Lonazolac Ca	해열, 진통, 소염제
Ismo	Isosorbide-5-mononitrate	혈관확장제
Isoket retard cap, spray, inj	Isosorbide dinitrate	혈관확장제
Isoprophyl alcohol		방역용 살균소독제
Isoptin SR tab, inj	Verapamil HCl	혈관확장제
Isovist 300		X선 조영제
Isuprel inj	Isoproterenol HCl	진해거담제
IVF-C inj	Human Chorionic Gonadotropin(H.C.G)	기타의 호르몬제
IVF-M inj	Menotropin	난포호르몬 및 황체호르몬제
Jetepar inj		간장질환용제

약품명	성분명	의약품 분류
Jumax	Selegiline HCl	기타의 중추신경용약
K-40 inj, K-contin	KCl	무기질제제
Kallimate	Polystyrene sulfonate Ca	기타의 순환계용약
Kanamycin inj	Kanamycin sulfate	주로 항산성균에 작용
Kedanone	Idebenone	기타의 중추신경용약
Kerlone	Betaxolol HCl	혈압강화제
Ketalar inj	Ketamine HCl	전신마취제
Ketotop plaster, Kenofen gel	Ketoprofen	진통, 진양, 수렴, 소염제
Klaricid	Clarithromycin	기타의 항생물질제제
Klenzo sol	Normalsaline irriga.	기타의 인공관류용제
Kymoxin cap. syr	Amoxicillin	주로 그람양성, 음성균에 작용
Kytril tab. inj	Granisetron	최토제, 진토제
Lacteol granule		정장제
Lacticare HC lot, tube	NaPCA Lactic acid	기타의 외피용약
Lacure oph. sol	Hyaluronate Na	안과용제
Lamicil cr 1%	Terbinafine HCl	기생성 피부질환용제
Lamicital	Lamotrigine	항전간제
Lamina G sol 5%	Alginate Na 5%	지혈제
Lanston	Lansoprazole	소화성궤양용제
Lanvis	6-Thioguanine	항악성종양제
Lasix tab, inj	Furosemide	이뇨제
Ledercort Tamceton inj	Triamcinolone	부신호르몬제
Legalon comp		간장질환용제
Lentinan inj	Lentinan, mannitol, Dextran	항악성종양제
Leunase inj	L-Asparaginase	항악성종양제
Levamisole	Levamisole	기타의 종양 치료제
Levophed inj	Norepinephrine bitartrate	부신호르몬제
Levopride	Levosulpiride	기타의 소화기관용약
Liberty	Chlordiazepoxide	정신신경용제
Librax		정신신경용제
Lidocaine inj	Lidocaine HCl	국소마취제
Lioresal	Baclofen	골격근이완제
Lipanthyl	Fenofibrate	동맥경화용제
Lipiodol		X선 조영제
Lithium carbonate	Lithium carbonate	정신신경용제
Livial	Tibolone	난포호르몬 및 황체호르몬제
Livital	Biphenyl dimethyl Deca	간장질환용제
Livostin nasal spray	Levocarvastine HCl	기타의 알레르기용약

약품명	성분명	의약품 분류
Livostin oph. sol	Levocabastine	안과용제
Lodine	Etodolac	해열, 진통, 소염제
Logina cream	Budesonide	기타의 외피용약
Loperin	Loperamide HCl	정장제
Lopid	Gemfibrozil	동맥경화용제
Loprox Nail Lacquer	Ciclopirox	기생성 피부질환용제
Lorabid cap, syr	Loracarbef	주로 그람양성, 음성균에 작용
Losec	Omeprazole	소화성궤양용제
Loxonin	Loxoprofen Na	해열, 진통, 소염제
Luminal inj	Phenobarbital	최면진정제
M.T.X inj	Methotrexate	항악성종양제
M.V.H inj		혼합비타민제
Macperan inj	Metoclopramide HCl	기타의 소화기관용약
Magcorol		X선 조영제
Magnesin inj	Mag. sulfate	진경제
Magnevist		X선 조영제
Maltose inj 10%	Maltose 10%	당류제
Marobiven		치질용제
Maxidex oph.sol		안과용제
Maxitrol oph.oint		안과용제
Medilac-S		정장제
Mefoxin inj	Cefoxitin Na	주로 그람양성, 음성균에 작용
Meiact	Cefditoren pivoxil	주로 그람양성, 음성균에 작용
Meicelin inj	Cefminox Na	주로 그람양성, 음성균에 작용
Melleril	Thioridazine HCl	정신신경용제
Melpros inj		기타의 순환계용약
Menoferil	Cyclofenil	기타의 호르몬제
Menozol vag.supp	Stilbestrol	비뇨생식기관용제
Mephirol syr		진해거담제
Meptin	Procaterol HCl	진해거담제
Mesexin	Methylol cephalexin lysinate	주로 그람양성, 음성균에 작용
Mestinon	Pyridostigmine Br	자율신경제
Methazolamide		안과용제
Methergin tab, inj	Methylergometrine maleate	자궁수축제
Methimazole	Methimazole	갑상선, 부갑상선호르몬제
Methocarbamol tab, inj	Methocarbamol	골격근이완제
Methoxsalen cap	Methoxsalen	기생성 피부질환용제
Mevacor	Lovastatin	혈관보강제

약품명	성분명	의약품 분류
Mevacor	Lovastatin	동맥경화용제
Mevalotin	Pravastatin Na	동맥경화용제
Mexitil	Mexiletine HCl	부정맥용제
Mexitil	Procainamide	부정맥용제
Miacalcic nasal spray	Salcatonin	갑상선, 부갑상선호르몬제
Micronomicin inj	Micronomicin sulfate	주로 항산성균에 작용
Midron	Midodrine HCl	기타의 순환계용약
Mikelan	Carteolol HCl	부정맥용제
Mikelan oph.sol	Carteolol HCl	안과용제
Milisrol inj	Nitroglycerin	혈관확장제
Minipress	Prazosin HCl	혈압강화제
Minirin	Desmopressin	뇌하수체호르몬제
Minocin	Minocycline HCl	그람양성, 음성균, 리케치아, 비루스에 작용
Mitomycin-C inj	Mitomycin	항악성종양제
Mivacron inj	Mivacurium	골격근이완제
MMR II inj	Measles, Mumps, Rubella vaccine	백신류
Modivid inj	Cefodizime	주로 그람양성, 음성균에 작용
Molsiton	Molsidomine	혈관확장제
Morphine inj	Morphine HCl	아편알카로이드계 제제
MS-contin	Morphine sulfate	아편알카로이드계 제제
Mucomyst	Acetylcysteine	진해거담제
Mucopect inj, tab	Ambroxol HCl	진해거담제
Mucoril	Thiocolchicoside	골격근이완제
Mucosta	Rebamipide	소화성궤양용제
Mutacil pow	Psyllium Husk	하제, 완장제
Myalone	Afloqualone	골격근이완제
Myambutol	Ethambutol HCl	항결핵제
Mycin inj	Benzathine penicillin G	주로 그람양성균에 작용
Mycospor cream, sol	Bifonazole	기생성 피부질환용제
Mycostatin oint	Nystatin	기생성 피부질환용제
Mycostatin tab, syr	Nystatin	주로 곰팡이, 원충에 작용
Mydocalm inj	Tolperisone HCl	골격근이완제
Mydrin	Miribolan	해열, 진통, 소염제
Mydrin-P oph. sol		안과용제
Myprodol cap	Codeine+paracetamol+lbuprofen	아편알카로이드계 제제
Myranta 400		제산제
Na-40 inj 0.45% NaCl inj	NaCl	무기질제제
Nalador inj	Sulprostone(PGE2)	기타의 호르몬제

약품명	성분명	의약품 분류
Naloxone inj	Naloxone HCl	해독제
Nasacort nasal inhaler	Triamcinolone acetonide	이비인후과용제
Navelbin inj	Vinorelbin	항악성종양제
Navelbine inj	Vinorelbine ditartrate	주로 악성종양에 작용
Navoban tab, inj	Tropisetron	최토제, 진토제
Naxen-F	Naproxen Na	해열, 진통, 소염제
Neoplatin inj	Carboplatin	항악성종양제
Neotigason	Acitretin	비타민 A 및 D제
Nephrovite	Vitamin B, C complex	혼합비타민제
Neponide	Nemonapride	정신신경용제
Nerisona oint	Diflucortolone valerate	기타의 외피용약
Netromycin inj	Netilmycin sulfate	주로 그람양성, 음성균에 작용
Neuer	Cetraxate HCl	소화성궤양용제
Neusillin A gran.	Alum. Mag. Silicate	제산제
Neutrogin inj	Lenograstim	기타의 혈액 및 체액용약
Newfactan	Surfectant(Bivon)	기타의 호흡기관용약
Niceten		치과구강용약
Nicetile	Acetyl-L-Carnitine	기타의 순환계용약
Nicostop 10/20/30 patch	Nicotine	치료를 주목적으로 하지 않는 의약품
Nimotop inj, tab	Nimodipine	혈관확장제
Nisolone	Prednisolone	부신호르몬제
Nitroglycerin	Nitroglycerin	혈관확장제
Nitropress inj	Nitroprusside Na	혈압강화제
Nizoral cream, sol	Ketoconazole	기생성 피부질환용제
Nolvadex	Tamoxifen	항악성종양제
Normal saline inj	NaCl 0.9%	혈액대용제
Norumo A tab		제산제
Novalgin inj	Sulpyrine	해열, 진통, 소염제
Novasc	Amlodipine	기타의 순환계용약
Novolet 30/70 inj	Insulin	당뇨병용제
Novolet N inj	Insulin	당뇨병용제
Nubain inj	Nalbuphine HCl	해열, 진통, 소염제
Ofloxacin oph.sol,oph.oint	Ofloxacin	안과용제
Olbetam	Acipimox	동맥경화용제
Omnipaque		X선 조영제
Oncovin inj	Vincristine sulfate	항악성종양제
One alpha	Alfacalcidol	비타민 A 및 D제
Opalmon	Limaprost alfadex	기타의 순환계용약

약품명	성분명	의약품 분류
Optagent oph.sol	Povidone	안과용제
Optanac oph.sol	Diclofenac sodium 0.1%	안과용제
Optiray 320		X선 조영제
Orfil retard, syr	Valproate Na	항전간제
Ornidazole inj	Ornidazole	항원충제
Oscal	Calcium	칼슘제
Oxytocin inj	Oxytocin	자궁수축제
Ozex	Tosufloxacin tosylate	기타의 화학요법제
P.P.Z	Perphenazine	정신신경용제
PAM-A inj	Pralidoxime chloride	해독제
Panslan inj	Pancuronium Br	골격근이완제
Papaverine	Papaverine HCl	진경제
PAS Ca granule	p-Aminosalicylic acid	항결핵제
Pazeron inj	Cefazedone Na	주로 그람양성, 음성균에 작용
Peflacin tab, inj	Pefloxacin	기타의 화학요법제
Penbrex inj	Ampicillin	주로 그람양성, 음성균에 작용
Penicillin G K inj	Penicillin G K	주로 그람양성균에 작용
Penid	Methylphenidate HCl	각성제, 흥분제
Peniramin tab, inj	Chlorpheniramine maleate	항히스타민제
Pentaspan inj	Pentastarch	기타의 혈액 및 체액용약
Pentazocine inj	Pentazocine HCl	해열, 진통, 소염제
Pentocainsteril inj	Tetracaine HCl	국소마취제
Pentothal inj	Thiopental Na	전신마취제
Perdipine	Nicardipine	기타의 순환계용약
Perdipine LA	Nicardipine HCl	혈압강하제
Peridol tab. inj	Haloperidol	정신신경용제
Peritosol 150, 250, 425		기타의 인공관류용제
Perivar		치질용제
Persantin tab, inj	Dipyridamole	혈관확장제
Pethidine inj	Pethidine HCl	합성마약
Pharmorubicin inj	Epirubicin	항악성종양제
Pharmorubicin inj	Epirubicin HCl	주로 악성종양에 작용
Phazyme 95		건위소화제
Phenobarbital	Phenobarbital	최면진정제
Phenylephrine inj	Phenylephrine HCl	혈관수축제
Phenylephrine oph.sol		안과용제
Phenytoin, Peniton inj	Diphenylhydantoin Na	항전간제
Phosgel G susp		제산제

약품명	성분명	의약품 분류
Phosphota inj	Pot. phosphate	기타의 혈액 및 체액용약
Pilocarpine oph.sol 1%, 2%, 4%	Pilocarpine	안과용제
PK-Merz	Amantadine Sulfate	기타의 중추신경용약
Plasma-a sol inj		혈액대용제
Plecton	Cicloxillic acid	간장질환용제
Pletaal	Cilostazol	기타의 혈액 및 체액용약
Pnu-lmune 23 inj	Pneumococcal vaccine	백신류
Pocral syr	Chloral hydrate	최면진정제
Pofol inj	Propofol	전신마취제
Polioral syrup	Polio vaccine	백신류
Polybutin	Trimebutine maleate	기타의 소화기관용약
Pontal	Mefenamic acid	해열, 진통, 소염제
Pranol	Propranolol HCl	부정맥용제
Premarin	Conjugated estrogen	난포호르몬 및 황체호르몬제
Prepulsid tab, syr	Cisapride	기타의 소화기관용약
Primidone	Primidone	항전간제
Prinosine	Inosiplex	기타의 화학요법제
Proamine		단백 아미노산제제
Proctosedyl oint, supp		치질용제
Profenid inj	Ketoprofen	해열, 진통, 소염제
Progest inj.	Progesterone	난포호르몬 및 황체호르몬제
Pronil	Propranolol HCl	부정맥용제
Prostandin inj.	Alprostadil(PGE1)	기타의 순환계용약
Prostarmon. F inj	Dinoprost(PGE2)	자궁수축제
Prostin E2 vag. tab	Dinoprostone(PGE2)	기타의 호르몬제
Prozac	Fluoxetin HCl	정신신경용제
Pseudafed	Pseudoephedrine HCl	진해거담제
Pucaine inj	Bupivacaine HCl	국소마취제
Pulmicort nasal aqua	Budesonide	이비인후과용제
Pulmicort turbuhaler, respule	Budesonide	진해거담제
Purinethol	Mercaptopurine	항악성종양제
Pyrazinamide	Pyrazinamide	항결핵제
Pyridostigmine inj	Pyridostigmine Br	자율신경제
Pyridoxine	Pyridoxine HCl	비타민 B제
Quinidine sulfate	Quinidine sulfate	부정맥용제
Racicrol inj		기타의 혈액 및 체액용약
Radacef inj	Ceforanide	주로 그람양성, 음성균에 작용
Remicut SR cap	Emedastine difumarate	항히스타민제

약품명	성분명	의약품 분류
Renitec	Enalapril maleate	혈압강하제
Rentibloc	Sotalol	부정맥용제
Rescough syr	Zipeprol HCl	진해거담제
Rheodex-D inj		혈액대용제
Rhinathiol cap	S-Carboxymethylcysteine	진해거담제
Ricriden syr 0.8%	Nifurzide	정장제
Rifodex	Rifampicin	주로 항산성균에 작용
Rilutex	Riluzole	기타의 중추신경용약
Rimso-50 sol	Dimethyl sulfoxide	기타의 비뇨생식기 및 항문용약
Risperidal	Risperidone	정신신경용제
Rivotril	Clonazepam	항전간제
Rize	Clotiazepam	정신신경용제
Roaccutane	Isotretinoin	비타민 A 및 D 제
Robin inj, tab	Leucovorin Ca	해독제
Romantase		건위소화제
Ronaben	Flurbiprofen	해열, 진통, 소염제
Roxan cap	Roxatidine acetate HCL	소화성궤양용제
Rozex gel	Metronidazole	기타의 외피용약
Rubella virus vaccine		백신류
Rulid	Roxithromycin	주로 그람양성, 음성균에 작용
Rytmonorm	Propafenone HCl	부정맥용제
S/D 1:2, 1:4, 1:6		기타의 혈액 및 체액용약
Sabril	Vigabatrin	항전간제
Salofalk tab, supp	Mesalazine	기타의 소화기관용약
Sandostatin inj	Octreotide	기타의 호르몬제
Sepamin inj	Chlorpromazine HCl	정신신경용제
Septrim syr. tab	Co-Trimaxazole	설파제
Serenace	Haloperidol	정신신경용제
Serevent inhaler	Salmeterol xinafoate	진해거담제
Seroxat	Paroxetine	정신신경용제
Shincef inj	Cefuroxime Na	주로 그람양성, 음성균에 작용
Sibelium	Flunarizine 2HCl	혈관확장제
Sigmart	Nicorandil	혈관확장제
Sinemet, CR		기타의 중추신경용약
Sirdalud	Tizanidine	진경제
Smecta susp	Dioctahedral smectite	정장제
Sodium bicarbonate inj	$NaHCO_3$(Bivon)	해독제
Sodium bicarbonate pow	Sodium bicarbonate	제산제

약품명	성분명	의약품 분류
Solcorin oph. sol	Solcoseryl	안과용제
Solotop		X선 조영제
Solu-Cortef inj	Hydrocortisone Na succinate	부신호르몬제
Spagerin	Flavoxate HCl	기타의 비뇨생식기 및 항문용약
Spamon comp.		진경제
Spamon inj	Caroverine HCl	진경제
Spara	Sparfloxacin	기타의 화학요법제
Spectinomycin inj	Spectinomycin HCl	기타의 항생물질제제
Spectravan Ultra 28 lot		기타의 외피용약
Splendil ER	Felodipine	혈압강화제
Sporanox cap	Itraconazole	기타의 화학요법제
Stieva-A cream	Tretinoin	기생성 피부질환용제
Stigmine inj	Neostigmine methylsulfate	자율신경제
Stilnox	Zolpidem tartrate	최면진정제
Streptomycin inj	Streptomycin	주로 항산성균에 작용
Succicholine inj	Suxamethonium	골격근이완제
Suduvaccine inj	Varicella vaccine	백신류
Sulperazone inj		기타의 항생물질제제
Suprax cap, granule	Cefixime	주로 그람양성, 음성균에 작용
Surgam tab, inj	Tiaprofenic acid	해열, 진통, 소염제
Synthyroid	Levothyroxine Na	갑상선, 부갑상선호르몬제
T.F.T oph. sol	Trifluridine	안과용제
Tambocor	Flecainide acetate	부정맥용제
Tanakan	Ginko biloba ext.	기타의 순환계용약
Tantum gargle	Benzydamine HCl	치과구강용약
Tarasyn tab, inj	Ketorolac tromethamine	해열, 진통, 소염제
Tarexin	Tolperisone HCl	골격근이완제
Targocid inj	Teicoplanin	주로 그람양성균에 작용
Tarigen	Talniflumate	해열, 진통, 소염제
Tarivid otic sol	Ofloxacin	이비인후과용제
Taxol inj	Paclitaxel	항악성종양제
Tazime inj	Ceftazidime	주로 그람양성, 음성균에 작용
Tazocin inj	Piperacilline+Tazobactam	주로 그람양성, 음성균에 작용
Tears Natural Free oph. sol		안과용제
Tears Naturale II oph. sol		안과용제
Telebrix 30		X선 조영제
Tenstaten	Cicletanine HCl	혈압강화제
Teracyclin	Tetracycline HCl	그람양성, 음성균, 리케치아, 비루스에 작용

약품명	성분명	의약품 분류
Testo	Testosterone propionate	남성호르몬제
Tetabulin inj	Antitetanus Ig	혈액제제류
Theolan cap	Theophylline	진해거담제
Thiamine		비타민 B1제
Thiaton	Tiquizium Br	진경제
Thromboject	Sod. Tetradecyl sulfate	기타의 혈액 및 체액용약
Thrombokinase	Thromboplastin	지혈제
Thymico		이비과용제
Tienam inj		주로 그람양성, 음성균에 작용
Tilcotil	Tenoxicam	해열, 진통, 소염제
Timentin inj		주로 그람양성, 음성균에 작용
Timoptic oph.oint	Timolol maleate	안과용제
Tinset	Oxatomide	항히스타민제
Tiropa	Tiropramide HCl	진경제
Tiroxin	Cefroxadine	주로 그람양성, 음성균에 작용
Tobra inj	Tobramycin	주로 항산성균에 작용
Tobra oph.sol	Tobramycin	안과용제
Toburex inj	Dobutamine HCl	강심제
Tomiporan inj	Cefbuperazone Na	주로 그람양성, 음성균에 작용
Tomiron	Cefteram pivoxil	주로 그람양성, 음성균에 작용
Trandate inj	Labetalol	혈압강화제
Transamine-S cap, inj	Tranexamic acid	지혈제
Trast patch	Piroxicam	진통, 진양, 수렴, 소염제
Traumasteril		단백 아미노산제제
Travogen cream	Isoconazole nitrate	기생성 피부질환용제
Trental	Pentoxifylline	기타의 순환계용약
Trestan		기타의 자양강장변질계
Tridol cap, inj	Tramadol HCl	해열, 진통, 소염제
Triquilar	Ethinyl estradiol	피임제
Triquilar	Levonorgestrel	피임제
Tritace	Ramipril	혈압강화제
Trittico	Trazodone HCl	정신신경용제
Tropin inj	Dopamine HCl	기타의 순환계용약
Tylenol ER, chewable(ped), syr	Acetaminophen	해열, 진통, 소염제
U.F.T		항악성종양제
Ucerax tab, inj	Hydroxyzine HCl	정신신경용제
Ulcerlmin susp	Sucralfate	소화성궤양용제
Ultravist 300		X선 조영제
Ultravist 370		X선 조영제
Unasyn inj, tab	Ampicillin+sulbactam	주로 그람양성, 음성균에 작용

약품명	성분명	의약품 분류
Uracin oint	Crotamiton	진통, 진양, 수렴, 소염제
Urokinase inj	Urokinase	기타의 순환계용약
Uromitexan inj	Mesna	해독제
Urota inj	Protamine sulfate	기타의 혈액 및 체액용약
Ursa	Ursodesoxycholic acid	간장질환용제
Utrogestan cap	Progesterone	난포호르몬 및 황체호르몬제
Van base	Hydrophillic base	연고기제
Vancocin inj	Vancomycin HCl	주로 그람양성균에 작용
Varidase		효소제제
Vaseline	White petrolatum	연고기제
Vasopressin inj	Vasopressin	뇌하수체호르몬제
Vastinan	Trimetazidine HCl	혈관확장제
Vecaron inj	Vecuronium Br	골격근이완제
Velosulin inj	Insulin	당뇨병용제
Venitol	Diosmine+Hesperidin	혈관보강제
Veno Gamma inj	Immunoglobulin r	혈액제제류
Ventolin sol	Salbutamol sulfate	진해거담제
Verrumal		피부연화제
Vessel Due	Sulodexide	동맥경화용제
Vibramycin inj	Doxycycline hyclate	그람양성, 음성균, 리케치아, 비루스에 적용
Vistimon	Mesterolone	남성호르몬제
Vitamedin		비타민 B제
Vitamin K1 inj	Phytonadione	비타민 E 및 K제
Winstal		이담제
Xanax	Alprazolam	정신신경용제
XL-l gel	Fluocionide	기타의 외피용약
Xylocaine pump spray	Lidocaine 10%	국소마취제
YAL sol		하제, 완장제
Yamatetan inj	Cefotetan 2Na	주로 그람양성, 음성균에 작용
Yumerol inj	Methylprednisolone Na succinate	부신호르몬제
Yutopar cap, inj	Ritodrine	기타의 비뇨생식기 및 항문용약
YuYu clid	Ticlopidine HCl	기타의 혈액 및 체액용약
Zaditen tab, syr	Ketotifen fumarate	진해거담제
Zantac tab, inj	Ranitidine HCl	소화성궤양용제
Zarontil	Ethosuximide	항전간제
Zenol ccol patch		진통, 진양, 수렴, 소염제
Zinnat	Cefuroxime Axetil	주로 그람양성, 음성균에 작용
Zithromax cap, syr	Azithromycin	주로 그람양성, 음성균에 작용

약품명	성분명	의약품 분류
Zocor	Simvastatin	동맥경화용제
Zofran tab, inj	Ondansetron	최토제, 진토제
Zoladex inj	Goserelin acetate	항악성종양제
Zoladin inj	Acetazolamide Na	이뇨제
Zoloft	Sertraline HCl	정신신경용제
Zostrix HP cr 0.07%, 0.025%	Capsaicin	진통, 진양, 수렴, 소염제
Zovirax cream	Acyclovir	기타의 외피용약
Zovirax oph.oint	Acyclovir	안과용제
Zovirax tab, inj	Acyclovir	기타의 화학요법제
Zyloric	Allopurinol	통풍치료제
Zyrtec tab, syr	Cetirizine 2HCl	항히스타민제

참고문헌

1. 김광애 외	의학용어	현문사, 2006
2. 이성란	병원통계	신광출판사, 2004
3. 오송자 외	의학약어	현문사, 1997
4. 이성란	질병분류	신광출판사, 2005
5. 박찬웅	약리학	신광출판사, 1996
6. 서울대학교 의과대학편	심장학	서울대학교 출판부, 1995
7. 이우주	의학사전	도서출판 아카데미서적, 1996
8. 이영숙 외	여성건강간호학	현문사, 2000
9. 이성란	암등록	도서출판 진우, 2007
10. 주황기 외	임상약리학 및 실습	수문사, 1996
11. 한국표준질병사인분류	대한의무기록협회	대한의무기록협회 출판부, 1995
12. 홍준현	질병분류	고문사, 1987
13. 이성란	의무기록관리학	신광출판사, 2005

14. American Hospital Discharge Date Set, Chicago, 1994
15. American Medical Record Association, Evaluating the Quality of Medical Record Services, 1994
16. Arthur C. Guyton, M.D. Textbook of Medical Terminology, sixth edition, W.B. Saunders Company, 1997
17. Davi-Ellen Chabner, The Language of Medicine, W.B. Saunders Company, 1996
18 Ednarn K. Huffman, Medical Record Management, Berwgn, Physician's Record Company, 1985
19. Feighner JP, Robins E, Guse SB, et al. Dianostic criteria for use in psychiatric research, arch Gen psychiatry 1992
20. Frances A. An Introduction to DSM-IV, Hosp community psychiatry, 1990
21. Human anatomy and physiology, Elaine N. Marieb, The Benjamin/Cummings Publishers, 1991
22. Huffman, Health information Management Tenth ed, physicians' Record Company, 1994
23. Leonard, Building a Medical Vocabulary, W.B. Saunders Company, 1996
24. Lester Breslow, A Guide for the Tumor Registry Secretary in Recording Stage, Califor-nia tumor Registry, 1995
25. Miriam G. Austrin, Young's Learning Medical Terminology, The C.V. Mosby Company, 1995
26. Robbins LN, et al. National institute of mental health diagnostic interview schedule, Arch Gen Psychiatry, 1994
27. Stereotactic surgery Neurosurgery, 1994
28. Understanding medical terminology(8th), agnes clare frenay, Wm C. Brown Pulishers, 1995

실전문제 정답

1장 내과계

전체 차트							요약 차트
유수호	오대승	이천운	윤달인	하만세	복덩이	장천수	장만복
1. ④	1. ④	1. ②	1. ③	1. ④	1. ③	1. ②	1. ④
2. ③	2. ③	2. ④	2. ②	2. ①	2. ②	2. ④	2. ③
3. ①	3. ②	3. ②	3. ①	3. ③	3. ③	3. ②	3. ②
4. ④	4. ③	4. ⑤	4. ②	4. ④	4. ④	4. ②	4. ①
5. ③	5. ④	5. ③	5. ③	5. ③	5. ③	5. ④	5. ③
6. ②	6. ①	6. ①	6. ②	6. ②	6. ②	6. ③	6. ④
7. ④	7. ②	7. ③	7. ④	7. ④	7. ①	7. ①	
8. ①	8. ①	8. ②	8. ③	8. ④	8. ④	8. ②	
9. ③	9. ②	9. ③	9. ①	9. ②	9. ②	9. ④	
10. ②	10. ③	10. ①	10. ④	10. ①	10. ④	10. ③	

2장 외과계

전체 차트							요약 차트
최은인	신나라	이대길	황금빛	오합격	유기적	금수저	진장수
1. ④	1. ②	1. ①	1. ②	1. ②	1. ④	1. ③	1. ④
2. ①	2. ④	2. ②	2. ④	2. ②	2. ①	2. ③	2. ⑤
3. ②	3. ④	3. ③	3. ③	3. ④	3. ④	3. ②	3. ③
4. ③	4. ⑤	4. ③	4. ③	4. ③	4. ②	4. ④	4. ②
5. ①	5. ①	5. ①	5. ②	5. ③	5. ②	5. ④	5. ⑤
6. ③	6. ②	6. ④	6. ①	6. ③	6. ④	6. ②	6. ①
7. ④	7. ⑤	7. ④	7. ④	7. ④	7. ①	7. ①	
8. ⑤	8. ①	8. ②	8. ①	8. ①	8. ③	8. ②	
9. ⑤	9. ③	9. ③	9. ①	9. ③	9. ②	9. ②	
10. ②	10. ①	10. ②	10. ④	10. ②	10. ③	10. ①	

3장 산부인과계

전체 차트						요약 차트
김말복	빛나리	이태양	전완승	한승리	상한가	신승자
1. ②	1. ③	1. ①	1. ③	1. ①	1. ④	1. ③
2. ②	2. ②	2. ③	2. ②	2. ③	2. ③	2. ⑤
3. ①	3. ①	3. ③	3. ②	3. ②	3. ②	3. ①
4. ②	4. ③	4. ②	4. ①	4. ②	4. ①	4. ②
5. ③	5. ①	5. ④	5. ④	5. ②	5. ②	5. ①
6. ①	6. ④	6. ①	6. ①	6. ①	6. ④	6. ④
7. ④	7. ①	7. ②	7. ①	7. ①	7. ③	
8. ③	8. ②	8. ④	8. ②	8. ④	8. ②	
9. ①	9. ②	9. ③	9. ③	9. ②	9. ①	
10. ④	10. ①	10. ④	10. ④	10. ①	10. ①	

4장 기타계

전체 차트				요약 차트
박신통 아기	이필승	정대승	신완판	장역전
1. ③	1. ①	1. ③	1. ④	1. ③
2. ①	2. ④	2. ④	2. ③	2. ⑤
3. ④	3. ①	3. ②	3. ②	3. ②
4. ③	4. ②	4. ①	4. ④	4. ④
5. ①	5. ③	5. ④	5. ②	5. ⑤
6. ④	6. ④	6. ④	6. ②	6. ①
7. ①	7. ④	7. ②	7. ①	
8. ④	8. ③	8. ③	8. ③	
9. ③	9. ③	9. ①	9. ①	
10. ②	10. ②	10. ②	10. ②	

저자소개

이성란 (공주대학교 교수)

조혜영 (신한대학교 교수)

최원창 (대전과학기술대학교 교수/원장)

신연순 (공주대학교 교수)

조은희 (원광보건대학교 교수)

이경미 (연성대학교 교수)

김광애 (전 경북전문대학교 교수)

이해하기 쉽게 풀이한

최신 의무기록실무

인　쇄 | 2018년 5월 14일

발　행 | 2018년 5월 18일

공　저 | 이성란 조혜영 최원창 신연순 조은희 이경미 김광애

발행인 | 유 해 영

발행처 | **현 문 사**

주　소 | 서울시 송파구 송파대로 201 테라타워 2차 A동 1401호 (문정동) 우) 05854

전　화 | 02－511－5394－5　Fax | 02－517－4462

출판등록 | 1989년 3월 10일 제2017－000062호

Homepage | http://www.hyunmoon.co.kr

E-mail | hyunmoon@hyunmoon.co.kr

정가 32,000원

ISBN 979-11-5989-795-5